Updates in the Management of Breast Cancer

Editors

ANNA S. SEYDEL
LEE G. WILKE

SURGICAL CLINICS
OF NORTH AMERICA

www.surgical.theclinics.com

Consulting Editor
RONALD F. MARTIN

February 2023 • Volume 103 • Number 1

ELSEVIER

1600 John F. Kennedy Boulevard • Suite 1800 • Philadelphia, Pennsylvania, 19103-2899

http://www.surgical.theclinics.com

SURGICAL CLINICS OF NORTH AMERICA Volume 103, Number 1
February 2023 ISSN 0039–6109, ISBN-13: 978-0-323-93957-7

Editor: John Vassallo, j.vassallo@elsevier.com
Developmental Editor: Arlene Campos

Surgical Clinics of North America (ISSN 0039–6109) is published bimonthly by Elsevier Inc., 360 Park Avenue South, New York, NY 10010-1710. Months of publication are February, April, June, August, October, and December. Business and Editorial Offices: 1600 John F. Kennedy Blvd., Suite 1800, Philadelphia, PA 19103-2899. Periodicals postage paid at New York, NY and additional mailing offices. Subscription prices are $479.00 per year for US individuals, $1045.00 per year for US institutions, $100.00 per year for US & Canadian students and residents, $575.00 per year for Canadian individuals, $1327.00 per year for Canadian institutions, $580.00 for international individuals, $1327.00 per year for international institutions and $250.00 per year for foreign students/residents. To receive student/resident rate, orders must be accompanied by name of affiliated institution, date of term, and the *signature* of program/residency coordinator on institution letterhead. Orders will be billed at individual rate until proof of status is received. Foreign air speed delivery is included in all *Clinics* subscription prices. All prices are subject to change without notice. POSTMASTER: Send address changes to *Surgical Clinics*, Elsevier Health Sciences Division, Subscription Customer Service, 3251 Riverport Lane, Maryland Heights, MO 63043. **Customer Service (orders, claims, online, change of address): Telephone: 1-800-654-2452 (U.S. and Canada); 314-447-8871 (outside U.S. and Canada). Fax: 314-447-8029. E-mail: journalscustomerservice-usa@elsevier.com (for print support); journalsonlinesupport-usa@elsevier.com (for online support).**

Reprints. For copies of 100 or more, of articles in this publication, please contact the Commercial Reprints Department, Elsevier Inc., 360 Park Avenue South, New York, New York 10010-1710. Tel. 212-633-3874, Fax: 212-633-3820, E-mail: reprints@elsevier.com.

Surgical Clinics of North America is also published in Spanish by McGraw-Hill Interamericana Editores S.A., P.O. Box 5-237 06500 Mexico D.F. Mexico; and in Portuguese by Interlivros Edicoes Ltda., Rua Comandante Coelho 1085, CEP 21250, Rio de Janeiro, Brazil; and in Greek by Paschalidis Medical Publications, Athens Greece.

Surgical Clinics of North America is covered in *MEDLINE/PubMed (Index Medicus)*, *EMBASE/Excerpta Medica*, *Current Contents/Clinical Medicine*, *Current Contents/Life Sciences*, *Science Citation Index*, and *ISI/BIOMED*.

Contributors

CONSULTING EDITOR

RONALD F. MARTIN, MD, FACS
Colonel (Retired), United States Army Reserve, Department of General Surgery, Pullman Regional Hospital and Clinic Network, Pullman, Washington

EDITORS

ANNA S. SEYDEL, MD, FACS
Director, Surgical Breast Services, Marshfield Medical Center, Marshfield, Wisconsin

LEE G. WILKE, MD, FACS
Senior Medical Director, Clinical Cancer Services, Hendricks Chair in Breast Cancer Surgery Research, Vice Chair of Research, Professor, Department of Surgery, University of Wisconsin-Madison School of Medicine and Public Health, University of Wisconsin Carbone Cancer Center, Madison, Wisconsin

AUTHORS

JAMES ABDO, MD
Marshfield Medical Center, Marshfield, Wisconsin

OMID BAKHTAR, MD, MS
Sharp Healthcare, Surgical Pathology and Laboratory Medicine, Pathologist and Outreach Laboratory Medical Director, San Diego, California

ANDERSON BAUER, MD
Radiation Oncology Department, Interim Medical Director, Marshfield Clinic Health System, Marshfield, Wisconsin

MICHELE CARPENTER, MD
Center for Cancer Prevention and Treatment, St. Joseph Hospital, Orange, California; Department of Surgery, David Geffen School of Medicine at UCLA, Los Angeles, California

NICHOLAS W. CLAVIN, MD
Assistant Professor, Department of Plastic Surgery, Atrium Health, Charlotte, North Carolina

CHANDLER S. CORTINA, MD, MS, FSSO
Assistant Professor, Department of Surgery, Division of Surgical Oncology, Medical College of Wisconsin, Milwaukee, Wisconsin

VIJAYAKRISHNA K. GADI, MD, PhD
Division of Hematology and Oncology, University of Illinois Chicago, Translational Oncology Program, University of Illinois Cancer Center, Chicago, Illinois

MENG S. GUO, MD
Department of Plastic Surgery, Medical College of Wisconsin, Milwaukee, Wisconsin

ABHIGNA KODALI, MD
Division of Hematology and Oncology, Maimonides Cancer Center, Brooklyn, New York

AMANDA L. KONG, MD, MS, FACS, FSSO
Professor, Department of Surgery, Division of Surgical Oncology, Medical College of Wisconsin, Milwaukee, Wisconsin

JULIE LE, MD
Department of Surgery, David Geffen School of Medicine at UCLA, Los Angeles, California

CLAYTON T. MARCINAK, MD
Department of Surgery, Center for Human Genomics and Precision Medicine, University of Wisconsin-Madison, Madison, Wisconsin

MAX O. MENEVEAU, MD, MS
Department of Surgery, Division of Surgical Oncology, Cancer Center, University of Virginia, Charlottesville, Virginia

KRISLYN N. MILLER, DO
Breast Surgical Oncology Fellow, Department of Surgery, Duke University Medical Center, Durham, North Carolina

MUHAMMED MURTAZA, MBBS, PhD
Department of Surgery, Center for Human Genomics and Precision Medicine, University of Wisconsin-Madison, Madison, Wisconsin

ANAND K. NARAYAN, MD, PhD
Vice Chair of Equity, Associate Professor, Department of Radiology, University of Wisconsin-Madison, Madison, Wisconsin

HEATHER B. NEUMAN, MD, MS
Associate Professor, Wisconsin Surgical Outcomes Research Program, Department of Surgery, University of Wisconsin Carbone Cancer Center, Madison, Wisconsin

SARAH NIELSEN, DO
Section Head–Breast Imaging, Department of Radiology, Marshfield Clinic Health System, Marshfield Clinic–Wausau Center, Wausau, Wisconsin

HOLLY ORTMAN, MD
Marshfield Medical Center, Marshfield, Wisconsin

ANNE WARREN PELED, MD
Co-Director, Sutter Health California Pacific Medical Center Breast Cancer Program, San Francisco, California

JENNIFER K. PLICHTA, MD, MS
Director of the Breast Risk Assessment Clinic, Associate Professor, Department of Surgery, Duke Cancer Institute, Department of Population Health Sciences, Duke University Medical Center, Durham, North Carolina

EMILY P. RABINOVICH, MS
University of Virginia School of Medicine, Charlottesville, Virginia

ELIZABETH O. RIORDAN, MD
Marshfield Medical Center, Marshfield, Wisconsin

NATALIA RODRIGUEZ, MD
Marshfield Medical Center, Marshfield, Wisconsin

MARGUERITE M. ROONEY, BS
Medical Student, Department of Surgery, Duke University Medical Center

JESSICA R. SCHUMACHER, PhD
Associate Professor, Wisconsin Surgical Outcomes Research Program, Department of Surgery, University of Wisconsin Carbone Cancer Center, Madison, Wisconsin

ANNA S. SEYDEL, MD, FACS
Director, Surgical Breast Services, Marshfield Medical Center, Marshfield, Wisconsin

SHAYNA L. SHOWALTER, MD
Department of Surgery, Division of Surgical Oncology, Cancer Center, University of Virginia, Charlottesville, Virginia

SARAH P. SHUBECK, MD, MS
Assistant Professor, Department of Surgery, University of Chicago, Chicago, Illinois

SARAH E. TEVIS, MD
Assistant Professor, Division of Surgical Oncology, Department of Surgery, University of Colorado Denver, Aurora, Colorado

SAM Z. THALJI, MD
Department of Surgery, Division of Surgical Oncology, Medical College of Wisconsin, Milwaukee, Wisconsin

RACHEL TILLMAN, MD
Marshfield Medical Center, Marshfield, Wisconsin

MARY A. VARSANIK, MD
House Officer, Department of Surgery, University of Chicago, Chicago, Illinois

RICK D. VAVOLIZZA, MD
Department of Surgery, Division of Surgical Oncology, Cancer Center, University of Virginia, Charlottesville, Virginia

SUDHEER R. VEMURU, MD
General Surgery Resident, Department of Surgery, University of Colorado Denver, Aurora, Colorado

LEE G. WILKE, MD, FACS
Senior Medical Director, Clinical Cancer Services, Hendricks Chair in Breast Cancer Surgery Research, Vice Chair of Research, Professor, Department of Surgery, University of Wisconsin-Madison School of Medicine and Public Health, University of Wisconsin Carbone Cancer Center, Madison, Wisconsin

Contents

> Although the normal anatomy of the breast is relatively simple, a myriad of hyperplastic, atypical, and frankly malignant processes exist. Though a histologic continuum exists, the natural progression of breast disease is not always on a continuum. Moreover, the distinction between hyperplastic, atypical, and frankly malignant processes rests on subtle qualitative and sometimes quantitative features. The treatment of breast-related lesions has always been, and continues to be, a multidisciplinary task. A general understanding of histopathologic features of breast disease will allow clinicians to identify scenarios that are potentially inconsistent with the working diagnosis.

> Randomized clinical trials have been essential in guiding the surgical and systemic treatment of breast cancer, with most focusing on de-escalation. Here, we discuss key clinical trials that have shaped the modern approach to the treatment of breast cancer, focusing on studies that are more recent.

> Genetic testing plays an important role in assessing breast cancer risk and often the risk of other types of cancers. Accurate risk assessment and stratification represents a critical element of identifying who is best served by increased surveillance and consideration of other prevention or treatment options while also limiting overtreatment and unnecessary testing. The indications for testing will likely continue to expand, and ideally, more women with a genetic predisposition to breast cancer will be identified before they are diagnosed with breast cancer and thus have the option to consider effective screening and prevention management strategies.

The cancer genome plays an increasingly large role in the care of patients with breast cancer. Commercially available gene-expression profiling assays are now a part of staging and treatment guidelines, and their use continues to be examined in large-scale studies. With the advent of next-generation sequencing, the cancer genome can now be examined more quickly, less invasively, and in much greater detail. These technologies have led to a more nuanced understanding of molecular pathways, allowing providers to better match patients to clinical trials. Furthermore, a new era of diagnostics based on liquid biopsies is expected to revolutionize disease detection and clinical care.

Among women, breast cancer remains the second leading cause of cancer death in the United States. Mammography remains the only validated screening tool to reduce breast cancer mortality. The American Society of Breast Surgeons recommends that average-risk women undergo breast cancer screening every year starting at age 40. This article reviews the fundamentals of mammography screening, current age-based mammography screening recommendations, supplemental breast cancer screening recommendations in high-risk women, and novel imaging technologies. This review summarizes recommendations from the American Society of Breast Surgeons and published guidelines from major societies to reflect a range of evidence-based perspectives regarding mammographic screening.

The potential value of de-escalation in breast cancer therapy cannot be overstated. From reducing complications and morbidity of surgical therapy to the avoidance of chemotherapy in certain populations, the benefits of eliminating low-value therapies are significant. Further, those interventions that have minimal to no benefit may also further low-risk care cascades resulting in additional treatments or interventions without associated value, with increased financial toxicity, and resulting excess health care expenditures.

Traditionally, surgical therapy for primary breast lesions in stage IV breast cancer has been reserved for palliation. Several retrospective studies have suggested a possible survival benefit with surgical resection of the primary tumor in patients with distant metastases. However, evidence from prospective, randomized controlled trials suggest that locoregional control provides no clear survival advantage for patients with stage IV breast cancer. Future areas of inquiry include identification of subsets of patients who may derive a survival benefit from locoregional control.

New innovations aid the breast surgeon with better ability to localize tumors using wireless techniques, reduce re-excision rates by intraoperative margin evaluation and perform aesthetically; pleasing, and safe surgeries. In addition to improving oncological outcomes, we can continue to improve the quality of life for our patients through evolving surgeries including nerve-sparing mastectomies, robotic mastectomies, and lymphovascular surgeries (LYMPHA). Our article reviews current and evolving techniques and technology that all breast surgeons should add to his or her armamentarium to provide optimal surgical care.

Although surgery of the breast and axilla is generally well-tolerated by patients, the breast surgeon recognizes that complications can occur even when operating with experience on the lowest risk patients. The operative repertoire ranges from breast conserving surgery, mastectomy (including skin-sparing and nipple-sparing types), to modified radical mastectomy, with each procedure carrying a different expected surgical morbidity. Patients and families who are fully informed of potential complications before their operation describe greater trust in their surgeon and are better able to co-manage complications with the surgical team, when they occur.

As breast oncologic surgical procedures and approaches have evolved in recent years, so have breast reconstruction techniques. Newer advances focus on expanding the options of reconstructive approaches and patient selection, optimizing quality of life, and helping improve postsurgical survivorship. These advances span from techniques to expand criteria for nipple-sparing mastectomies, optimizing and enhancing oncoplastic surgery, evolving autologous reconstruction options, and preserving and restoring sensation after mastectomy.

Breast surgeons are trained in diagnostic modalities, treatment effectiveness, patient safety, and operative techniques, with emphasis on "the right treatment at the right time for the right patient." But delivering quality breast cancer care means more than achieving good outcomes. Physicians have routinely measured disease-free survival and overall survival to determine success in treating breast cancer. Patients are demanding attention to "quality of life" outcomes as well. As clinicians caring for patients with breast cancer, our focus must shift from early detection to survivorship to re-evaluate our own definition of cure and address the important issues affecting the quality of life of all of our patients.

Survivorship focuses on individual's health and well-being. Assessing for cancer recurrence is a follow-up priority for survivors and providers. However, providers also emphasize the importance of assessing for adherence to ongoing treatment. Providers should also assess for sequelae of local-regional and systemic treatment. Assessing for mental health is important, as many cancer survivors experience anxiety or depression. Finally, survivors should be encouraged to have ongoing visits with their primary care to ensure screening for other health conditions. This article reviews the recommendations for survivorship and the level of evidence supporting each aspect of high-quality survivorship care.

Radiation treatment is a well-established component of breast cancer treatment, in both breast conservation and also for many patients who have had mastectomy as well as those with metastatic disease. The basis for this was established in multiple large meta-analyses, and multiple modern studies have further defined the role of radiation. The radiation must be delivered to the area at risk, which can include the partial breast, whole breast, chest wall, and/or regional lymph nodes. There are a number of acceptable radiation treatment techniques and dose-fractionation schedules that can be individualized to each patient. Radiation can also play an important role in patients with metastatic cancer.

The indications for preoperative/neoadjuvant systemic therapy in breast cancer have changed over the past few years. In this article, the authors review the current data for use of neoadjuvant therapy in inoperable and operable settings. The evolution of various neoadjuvant regimens used in triple-negative breast cancer, human epidermal growth factor receptor 2 (HER2) overexpressing/gene-amplified (HER2+) tumors, and hormone receptor positive breast cancer is discussed as well as the role of neoadjuvant chemotherapy in tailoring adjuvant treatment.

SURGICAL CLINICS
OF NORTH AMERICA

SURGICAL CLINICS
OF NORTH AMERICA

SERIES OF RELATED INTEREST

Advances in Surgery
http://www.advancessurgery.com/
Surgical Oncology Clinics
http://www.surgonc.theclinics.com/
Thoracic Surgery Clinics
http://www.thoracic.theclinics.com/

Foreword
Breast Cancer

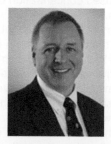

Ronald F. Martin, MD, FACS
Consulting Editor

Life is cyclical. The examples are endless: tides, planetary motion, seasons, birth and death, and so on. Lifelong learning is also cyclical—or at least it should be. Most learning models are predominantly linear in that we build a foundational base and then add on to it in some vertical manner. Perhaps at some point in development the foundation is expanded horizontally, or we join two existing structures. Some efforts lead to a coherent architecture, and sometimes we create bizarre patterns of foot traffic and hallways that lead to nowhere. As occasionally happens with buildings, people frequently forget to go back and look at the structures that underpin our further learning that we are building upon.

If one works in health care as someone who provides direct care to patients, there is rarely cause to think about the physical space one practices in unless something specific isn't working. If one works in health care at a system level (whether in a clinical capacity or not), one must be very concerned about the physical space—and its maintenance. If the assumed behind-the-scenes and taken-for-granted items malfunction, one will rapidly realize that a failing heater/chiller system, problematic air handlers, failing medical gas lines, unreliable water supplies, and so forth, can be far more detrimental to a health care platform than provider performance, personnel-related problems, or even pandemic-level patient stresses we face.

In medical education, and in particular continuing medical education, I am not so sure we fully grasp the idea and necessity of knowledge foundation maintenance at the system level. We are very interested in shiny objects and new and different (which is fine). We do not appear to share the same enthusiasm for keeping the base of knowledge secure and well maintained.

I have spent most of my medical career in some manner of formal medical education. A significant part of my job was to moderate the morbidity and mortality conference and our conferences on indications. During that time, more of the marginal clinical outcomes, or questionable decisions in general, I saw could be traced back to a

Surg Clin N Am 103 (2023) xiii–xiv
https://doi.org/10.1016/j.suc.2022.10.001
0039-6109/23/© 2022 Published by Elsevier Inc.

surgical.theclinics.com

suboptimal understanding of basic foundational knowledge or failure to apply that knowledge appropriately rather than lack of knowledge of the cutting-edge topics. We tend to assume all of us who reach a certain level of career development have that solid base of knowledge and it has been well maintained. The reality is, for some of us, time has made our foundation less stable, while for others, perhaps their foundation was a little wobbly at the outset. In either case, focused concentration on improving the knowledge base would be good for both groups.

At the *Surgical Clinics*, our fundamental model is to return to most topics on about a 5- to 7-year interval. We pick that timeframe because it about matches the length of training of most surgeons who start off in general surgery. We choose to come back to broad topics—often from a slightly altered perspective—because we feel that the foundations of our knowledge perpetually need examination and improvement; not just for some of but for all of us. Of course, we also try to combine this with updating our platforms on what is new (shiny or not) and what is on the cusp.

In the previous issue of the *Surgical Clinics*, we focused on the benign disorders of the breast. In this issue, we flip the coin to the malignant breast disorders. If ever there were a field of surgical thought that needed great attention to its foundational basis, breast surgery may well be the poster child. It does not take too close a look to realize the breast cancer models of the Halsted era bear little to no resemblance to our current understanding today, and today's model probably won't look much like those in the not-too-distant future.

Drs Seydel and Wilke, along with their collaborators, have compiled an excellent collection of articles that range from the absolutely fundamental to the edge of where we are heading. I am grateful to all of them for their efforts. The interested reader who devours these articles should be able to significantly improve or reinforce her/his understanding of this topic.

In an idealized world, all surgeons and other physicians would be allowed to, if not required to, take some time to go back to "medical school" on some regular interval with the intent of rebuilding the foundations of our knowledge as we did originally. I can hear the cries of incredulity as I type this. It's too expensive, it's too disruptive, it's logistically challenging, "we already do this by other means," "I don't need/want to," and so forth. All these claims are valid to some extent. Yet still we must find ways to not just add on knowledge but also truly reinvent and reinforce the base of our knowledge. I am not convinced we do that as well as we could.

In the meanwhile, we at the *Surgical Clinics* shall continue our efforts to examine the entire spectrum of surgical knowledge as best we can. We remain grateful to all those who have collaborated in making these issues possible. We remain even more grateful to those who use these materials as part of their toolset to improve the care of their patients and their communities.

Ronald F. Martin, MD, FACS
Colonel (retired), United States Army Reserve
Department of General Surgery
Pullman Surgical Associates
Pullman Regional Hospital and Clinic Network
825 Southeast Bishop Boulevard, Suite 130
Pullman, WA 99163, USA

E-mail address:
rfmcescna@gmail.com

Preface

Changing Landscape of Breast Cancer Management

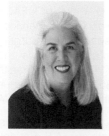
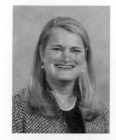

Anna S. Seydel, MD, FACS   Lee G. Wilke, MD, FACS
Editors

As surgeons who trained in general surgery before breast surgery became its own discipline, we as editors of this *Surgical Clinics* issue find the expanse of changes benefiting individuals with breast cancer to be remarkable. The surgical giants, Drs Seymour Schwartz, Folkert Belzer, and David Sabiston, could never have foreseen the advancements in specialty breast cancer care. It is hard to believe that we began our training before the routine use of core needle biopsy, sentinel lymph node biopsy, and full-panel genetic testing. Indeed, many of the debates of our training, is axillary node dissection diagnostic or therapeutic?, do you have to take the nipple areolar complex at the time of mastectomy?, can chemotherapy be given prior to surgery?, have now been clinically proven. The evolution of breast cancer surgery has followed the results of clinical trials, which have proven "less is more" in a much needed effort to improve cosmetic outcomes and quality of life for our patients.

This review is meant to be a resource for surgeons treating breast cancer patients today, recognizing clinical trials and innovation will change this landscape even further next year. Breast surgeons are expected to master current surgical techniques while also being mindful of the impact our treatments have on the quality of life of our patients. As such, this issue of *Surgical Clinics* incorporates articles on survivorship medicine, a burgeoning area of practice in the management of breast cancer. We have also included standard articles on updated pathology and current radiology, a discussion about practice changing clinical trials, and systemic medical management. We are excited about the discussion on new surgical techniques and novel approaches to breast reconstruction. Finally, the article on deescalation will have all of us continuing to reevaluate and examine our role as surgeons in the future care of individuals with breast cancer.

Surg Clin N Am 103 (2023) xv–xvi
https://doi.org/10.1016/j.suc.2022.08.012
0039-6109/23/© 2022 Published by Elsevier Inc.   **surgical.theclinics.com**

We hope you enjoy this review of breast cancer management as much as we have enjoyed working with our colleagues to put this together.

Anna S. Seydel, MD, FACS
Surgical Breast Services
Marshfield Medical Center
1000 North Oak Avenue
Marshfield, WI 54449, USA

Lee G. Wilke, MD, FACS
Clinical Cancer Services
UW Department of Surgery
University of Wisconsin School of Medicine and
Public Health
600 Highland Avenue
Madison, WI 53792, USA

E-mail addresses:
seydel.anna@marshfieldclinic.org (A.S. Seydel)
wilke@surgery.wisc.edu (L.G. Wilke)

Pathology of Breast Cancer
Subtypes, Receptors, Biologic Markers, and Staging

Omid Bakhtar, MD, MS

KEYWORDS

- Pathology • Breast • Subtype • Markers

KEY POINTS

- Some breast cancer subtypes have distinct clinical, prognostic, and predictive features.
- Management of many lesions requires histologic, radiographic, and clinical correlation.
- A variety of malignant papillary lesions exist and the management of many of these is akin to those of DCIS.

NORMAL HISTOLOGY

At the histologic level, the adult female breast is composed of a ductal-lobular system. Acinar structures in their clustered forms compose lobules. These lobules are then interconnected by a network of ductules and ducts. The point at which the ducts meet the lobules is referred to as a terminal duct and the terminal ductal lobular unit (TDLU) serves as an area of immense importance as it is the site at which most pathology occurs (**Fig. 1**A). In turn, ductules drain into ducts while ducts coalesce into collecting ducts that terminate at the nipple. Although this orderly description may lead one to believe that the breast is anatomically composed of distinct segments that originate from the collecting ducts of the nipple, the practical anatomy of the breast shows overlapping networks of ducts and ductules making separation of one segment from another largely impossible.

The acinar structures/lobules, ductules, ducts, and collecting ducts of the breast display a very characteristic 2-layer pattern composed of so-called luminal epithelial cells and an outer, almost mesh-like layer of myoepithelial cells (**Fig. 1**B). The luminal cells can undergo an array of hyperplastic, metaplastic, and neoplastic change. That being said, the vast majority of duct-based pathology arises from the TDLU, one notable exception being the solitary intraductal papilloma that arises from the larger

Sharp Healthcare, Surgical Pathology and Laboratory Medicine, 5651 Copley Drive, Suite B, San Diego, CA 92111, USA
E-mail address: Omid.Bakhtar@Sharp.com

Surg Clin N Am 103 (2023) 1–15
https://doi.org/10.1016/j.suc.2022.08.001
0039-6109/23/© 2022 Elsevier Inc. All rights reserved.

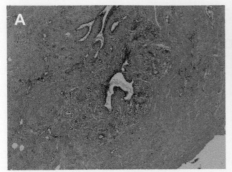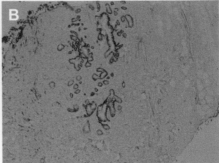

Fig. 1. Terminal ductal lobular unit. (A) The H&E image shows ducts terminating into a lobular unit. (B) The immunostain (calponin) highlights the myoepithelium surrounding this benign anatomical structure.

ducts of the breast. The myoepithelial layer of the breast is capable of contracting, a process that allows for the expulsion of milk from the lactating breast.

As will be discussed later in this article, the myoepithelial layer also serves as an important diagnostic feature as invasive carcinomas of the breast are devoid of a myoepithelial layer while the vast majority of benign and in situ lesions of the breast display a myoepithelial layer, albeit sometimes diminished.

The ductal and lobular structures of the breast are surrounded by stromal tissue. The lobules are surrounded by specialized, loose, and mildly cellular intralobular stroma that contrasts with the more collagenous and paucicellular interlobular stroma. This appearance makes the lobular units easy to identify, even at low-power magnifications.

INTRADUCTAL PROLIFERATIONS

The TDLU is responsible for a variety of metaplastic, hyperplastic, and frankly neoplastic processes. Hyperplastic processes arise when there is proliferation of epithelial cells leading to multilayering of the luminal cells (**Fig. 2**A). In its simplest form, ductal hyperplasia refers to proliferation of a few layers of epithelial cells, with minimal distention of the involved spaces and limited clinical significance. As this proliferation intensifies, the layering of the cells tends to distend the affected spaces with

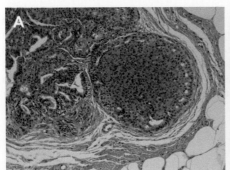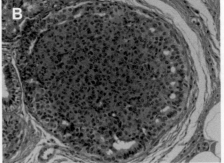

Fig. 2. Usual ductal hyperplasia. (A) Florid ductal hyperplasia of the usual type. Note the pronounced hyperplastic change with luminal cells replacing the entire caliber of the lumen. (B) Slitlike spaces are present at the edge of the expanded duct with swirling architectural pattern of the cells showing no significant rigidity of nuclear membranes.

microcyst formation, cyst rupture, and scarring/fibrosis of the surrounding stromal tissue. The clinical counterpart to this histologic change is "fibrocystic disease" or the more appropriately used terminology "fibrocystic change." Although it can be bothersome to the affected patient, it only carries a nominal increased risk (1.5–2.0x) of subsequent breast cancer. The intersection between histology, descriptive terms, and clinical scenario can cause confusion. In discussing the clinical and histologic scenarios, it is important to keep in mind that (usual) ductal hyperplasia can become florid and cause the clinical scenario of fibrocystic change. Therefore, the terms (usual) ductal hyperplasia and florid (usual) ductal hyperplasia are similar, though not as encompassing, as nonproliferative fibrocystic change and proliferative fibrocystic change.

Florid ductal hyperplasia (proliferative fibrocystic change) results in a proliferation of luminal cells that show variably sized cells distributed in solid, slitlike, or micropapillary architecture. These cells have a somewhat "swirling" appearance and tend to be distributed in a haphazard manner (**Fig. 2B**).

Although this haphazard and swirling distribution of cells seems more of artistic consequence, it serves as the diagnostic histopathologic change that determines a hyperplastic versus an atypical proliferation.

ATYPICAL INTRADUCTAL PROLIFERATIONS AND DUCTAL CARCINOMA IN SITU

Atypical intraductal proliferations cease to have the swirling and haphazard pattern seen in hyperplastic processes. Instead, atypical intraductal proliferations follow a more organized histologic hierarchy resulting in an element of secondary structuring. For instance, atypical intraductal proliferations tend to show increased "rigidity" of cells with more pronounced cell membranes, so-called cookie-cutter fenestrations, and secondary structures such as micropapillary proliferations. Depending on the extent and quantity of these atypical structures, a distinction is made between atypical ductal hyperplasia (ADH) and ductal carcinoma in situ (DCIS).

ADH consists of a proliferation of cells that share features with those of low-grade DCIS but also includes a population of cells that are more characteristic of usual ductal hyperplasia or "normal" luminal cells. So long as the atypical cells are histologically similar to those of low-grade ductal carcinoma, and some, but not all, features of DCIS are present, a diagnosis of ADH can be rendered. Therefore, the distinction between ADH and low-grade DCIS is largely based on the extent of atypia and the overall size of the focus of atypia, the size criteria being one that has been controversial and difficult to clearly define. When the quantitative features of low-grade DCIS are fulfilled, one finds a more expansive proliferation of atypical cells with low-grade histologic features that oftentimes create intraductal architectural structures (**Fig. 3**). These structures include proliferations that are solid, cribriform, papillary, and micropapillary. However, unlike the intermediate grade and high-grade counterparts, necrosis is generally absent, albeit not completely exclusionary.

When confronted with intermediate grade and high-grade histology, the quantitative rules applied in distinguishing ADH from low-grade DCIS are no longer of consequence. Any quantity of an atypical intraductal process that clearly shows intermediate-grade or high-grade features is sufficient to warrant a diagnosis of intermediate-grade/high-grade DCIS. The same architectural hierarchy that is seen in low-grade DCIS can be seen in high-grade DCIS. However, high-grade lesions are composed of more pleomorphic cells, increase mitotic activity and necrosis (**Figs. 4A, B**). This necrosis can be expansive and is often associated with microcalcifications. High-grade DCIS can also result in dense fibrosis/desmoplasia that can be so prominent it results in a palpable,

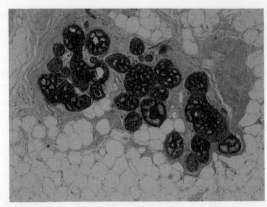

Fig. 3. Ductal carcinoma in situ. Secondary structures are present and many spaces are involved. The findings constitute low-grade DCIS.

mass-forming process. Therefore, unlike low-grade DCIS, a mass-forming lesion includes the differential diagnosis of high-grade DCIS.

LOBULAR LESIONS, NONINVASIVE

Atypical lobular hyperplasia (ALH) and lobular carcinoma in situ (LCIS) are breast lesions composed of identical cells and are differentiated solely by the extent of lobular unit involvement. These cells are characterized by their relatively small size, monotony, dyshesive nature, and occasional intracytoplasmic vacuoles. The dyshesive nature of the cells is owed to loss of cell membrane E-cadherin protein with E-cadherin immunostain showing loss of membrane staining. As such, e-cadherin is frequently used as an immunostain in distinguishing lobular lesions from ductal lesions. However, some cases of lobular neoplasia can express E-cadherin staining, so most pathologists continue to use histologic features as the defining characteristic of lobular lesions.

Given that the cells are often superimposed on acini within a lobule, the distinction between LCIS and ALH is based on the degree of lobular distention, albeit a subjective

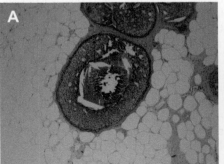
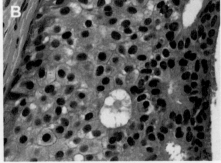

Fig. 4. Intermediate grade DCIS. (*A*) Central necrosis is present, a feature more commonly seen with higher grade DCIS. (*B*) Note the high-power view (40x) showing rigidity of cells as evidenced by clearly identifiable nuclear membranes. There is secondary structuring in the form of lumens, structures that recapitulate the duct-forming elements of the breast.

process. Most experts agree that if at least half of the acini in the lobule are distended by the aforementioned cells, the findings qualify as LCIS(**Fig. 5**). Lesser degrees of distension warrant a diagnosis of ALH.

It bears mentioning that the previous description relates to the "classic" variant of lobular carcinoma and that other variants exist (eg, pleomorphic and florid). Although the microscopic description of these variants is beyond the scope of this publication, the reader should be aware that these variants are of consequence as the management may differ significantly from that of classical lobular lesions.[1]

INVASIVE LESIONS

As mentioned previously, most invasive carcinomas arise from the terminal lobular unit. Therefore, the classification of invasive ductal versus invasive lobular carcinoma is based on histologic appearance and not the site of origin of the tumor. Many invasive lobular carcinomas are not thought to be derived from LCIS. Moreover, DCIS is not an obligate precursor of invasive ductal carcinoma.

Most invasive carcinomas of the breast are adenocarcinomas and as such the 2 largest histologic categories are that of invasive ductal carcinoma and invasive lobular carcinoma. In all invasive scenarios, these tumors are devoid of a myoepithelial layer (**Fig. 6D**). In fact, in cases where the invasive quality of tumor cells is not readily identifiable, immunophenotypic markers demonstrating the presence/absence of myoepithelial cells allow for classification of the tumor type (**Fig. 6A–D**).

Invasive Ductal Carcinoma

When invasive tumors show a histologic tendency toward those of "normal" breast epithelium, they are classified as invasive ductal carcinoma. Invasive ductal carcinoma represents a heterogeneous group of tumors that range from well-differentiated ("grade 1") tumors to more poorly differentiated ("grade 3") types. The grading of such tumors approximates the tendency of the tumor to form structures similar to those of the normal breast. Therefore, grade 1 tumors form ductal/acinar structures, whereas higher-grade tumors show less architecture (clusters, sheets, and single cells).

The grading of these tumors is based on 3 distinct features (tubule formation, nuclear pleomorphism, and mitotic activity). Each feature is scored and the overall score determines the grade of the tumor. In summary, grade 1 tumors tend to form ductal/acinar structures (**Fig 7**) while demonstrating little pleomorphism and low mitotic

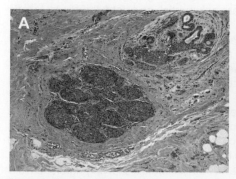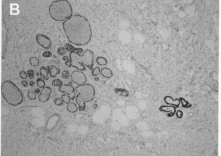

Fig. 5. Lobular carcinoma in situ. (*A*) Acinar structures significantly distended by lobular neoplasia. (*B*) Note the loss of e-cadherin (with retention of e-cadherin in a nearby duct).

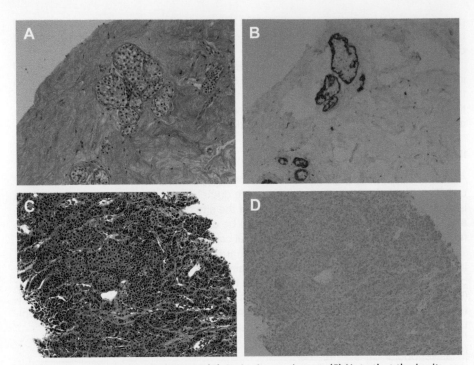

Fig. 6. In situ and invasive carcinomas. (*A*) An in situ carcinoma. (*B*) Note that the in situ carcinoma is enveloped by myoepithelial cells (brown immunostain). (*C*) An invasive carcinoma. (*D*) Note the absence of myoepithelium (absence of stain present in Fig. 6B).

activity, whereas grade 3 tumors show single cell/sheeting type morphology with increased pleomorphism and mitotic activity.

Some invasive ductal carcinomas display histologic (and clinical) features that allow them to be categorized into specialized subtypes. Approximately three-quarters of invasive ductal carcinomas fall into the "no special type" category while the remaining show histopathologic features that are adequate to place them into distinct subtypes. Care must be taken to strictly follow the rules established for classifying tumors into special subtypes as these subtypes often display distinct immunophenotypic and clinical properties. As such, it is not uncommon for pathologists to use the distinction "with features of" when histologic criteria are only partial, and not fully, characteristic of a tumor of special type.

This classification system is based largely on histologic characteristics and more current classification systems that are based on biomarkers and molecular features are now available. Although there is great overlap between histologic features and biomarker/molecular features, these systems are not always perfectly aligned.

The vast majority of low-grade/well-differentiated/grade 1 invasive ductal carcinomas express estrogen receptor and progesterone receptor in tumor cells. Although this expression diminishes in the high-grade/poorly differentiated/grade 3 invasive ductal carcinomas, many grade 3 tumors continue to express these hormone receptors. Overall, approximately 75% of invasive ductal carcinomas express estrogen receptor. The more poorly differentiated tumors (many of which carry the HER2 molecular phenotype) overexpress HER2 protein. These tumors represent approximately 15% of invasive

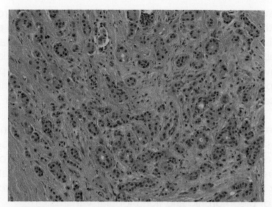

Fig. 7. Invasive ductal carcinoma. This well-differentiated/grade 1 invasive ductal carcinoma forms ductal structures. Note the presence of lumens which recapitulate breast ductal elements.

ductal carcinomas. The remaining 10% comprise the "triple-negative" category that is negative for hormone receptors and HER2.

Invasive Lobular Carcinoma

Invasive lobular carcinomas comprise approximately 10% of invasive lesions of the breast. As compared to invasive ductal carcinoma, these lesions are more commonly multifocal and are frequently poorly delimited. This characteristic is secondary to the asymmetric growth pattern and pattern of infiltration. In its classic form, invasive lobular carcinoma is composed of uniform, small, rounded cells with occasional intra-cytoplasmic droplets. The cells are distributed in linear arrays (**Fig 8**) and can encircle other breast structures in an "onion-skin" fashion.

As mentioned earlier, the growth pattern and dyshesive nature of invasive lobular carcinoma is due to the loss of membranous expression of e-cadherin. Although this finding can be demonstrated by immunohistochemical methods, the distinction between a diagnosis of invasive ductal carcinoma versus invasive lobular carcinoma

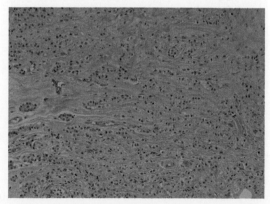

Fig. 8. Invasive lobular carcinoma. Note the linear arrays and dyshesive/single-cell characteristics.

is of less clinical importance to the surgeon than that of the overall growth pattern. For instance, stating that an invasive ductal carcinoma demonstrates a growth pattern similar to an invasive lobular carcinoma is more surgically relevant than whether it truly has ductal or lobular differentiation. Therefore, while some clinicians occasionally request that an invasive mammary carcinoma with lobular growth pattern be tested for e-cadherin to prove its lobular subtype, an invasive ductal carcinoma with lobular growth pattern can mimic many of the clinical features of an invasive lobular carcinoma.

In its classic form, invasive lobular carcinomas typically show strong and diffuse estrogen and progesterone receptor expression and are generally negative for HER2. Several variants of invasive lobular carcinoma exist and some of these variants demonstrate differences in histopathologic features and are associated with different hormone receptor phenotypes. The reader is referred to other sources with more in-depth discussion of pleomorphic and florid lobular variants.[1]

Invasive Mammary Carcinoma with Mixed Ductal and Lobular Features

Some invasive tumors fail to follow the pure histologic features defined for invasive ductal or invasive lobular carcinomas. In fact, it is not uncommon to see tumors that show mixed ductal and lobular features (**Fig 9**). These tumors are best classified as such. Again, it is important to stress to the clinician that the local growth features of a tumor are more defined by the microscopic growth features than the actual subtype. Therefore, it should come as no surprise that the biological characteristics of tumors that show mixed ductal and lobular features can mimic those of an invasive lobular carcinoma.[2]

Invasive Ductal Carcinomas of Special Type

Although invasive carcinomas showing ductal, lobular, or mixed ductal and lobular features comprise 90-95% of invasive tumors, there are invasive tumors that show distinct histopathologic (and clinical) features. To allow for a quick assessment of these features, invasive breast carcinomas of special type are listed below with only a brief synopsis of histopathology and a listing of relevant biomarkers and clinical pearls.

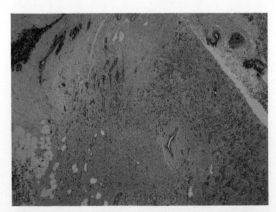

Fig. 9. Invasive mammary carcinoma with mixed ductal and lobular features. This invasive tumor shows mixed characteristics. The right side of the image shows ductal differentiation, whereas the central portion shows lobular characteristics.

Tubular carcinoma
Histology. Well-formed/low-grade tubular structures with apical snouts and haphazard distribution in a desmoplastic stroma.

Biomarkers. Almost always estrogen receptor-positive, progesterone receptor-positive, and HER2-negative. This phenotype is so consistent that divergent results should serve as a "red flag" in either the diagnosis or the quality of the biomarker testing.

Clinical pearls
- Question the diagnosis of tubular carcinoma if estrogen receptor is negative or if HER2 analysis is positive
- Benign entities in the differential diagnosis include sclerosing lesions and microglandular adenosis
- Microglandular adenosis is devoid of a myoepithelial layer (representing one of the few benign entities devoid of myoepithelium). As such, the use of myoepithelial markers is of no help in making the distinction between microglandular adenosis and tubular carcinoma. However, microglandular adenosis should be negative for estrogen receptor while tubular carcinoma almost always shows strong and diffuse estrogen reactivity
- The distinction between tubular carcinoma and grade 1 invasive ductal carcinoma of no special type is important as tubular carcinomas show less aggressive clinical course than grade 1 invasive ductal carcinoma of no special type. However, this distinction is best made on an excisional specimen and not on core biopsy samplings

Cribriform carcinoma
Histology. Strikingly similar histologic features to that of cribriform DCIS. Tumor nests tend to have a more angulated pattern than DCIS and additional patterns of invasive tumor and DCIS are not uncommonly present.

Biomarkers. These tumors are generally ER/PR positive and HER2 negative.

Clinical pearls
- Generally ER/PR-positive, HER2-negative tumors
- May be occult
- May be mistaken for cribriform variant of DCIS and may represent a subset of supposed DCIS cases that have lymph node metastases

Mucinous carcinoma
Histology. Characterized by low- to intermediate-grade ductal carcinomas embedded within pools of mucin. By definition, the vast majority (>90%) of the tumor should display the characteristic histologic features. Adherence to this criterion is important given that the clinical course of mucinous carcinoma is favorable. Benign lesions and intraductal carcinomas associated with mucin can make diagnosis challenging.

Biomarkers. These tumors are typically ER/PR positive and HER2 negative.

Clinical pearls
- Generally ER/PR positive
- Tendency to occur in older patients
- May be difficult to distinguish from benign mucinous proliferation (mucocele-like lesion) when tissue sampling is limited to needle core biopsy

Medullary carcinomas

Histology. Strict adherence to histologic criteria is necessary in diagnosing medullary carcinomas. By definition, these tumors should be high grade and must display the following features:

- Syncytial growth pattern
- Lymphoplasmacytic inflammation
- Well delimited borders
- No glandular/tubular differentiation

Biomarkers. The tumors are classically negative for ER/PR and HER2.

Clinical pearls
- Strict adherence to the histologic requirements is necessary in making this diagnosis
- BRCA germline mutations are associated with this tumor type
- "Triple-negative" phenotype is expected

Invasive micropapillary carcinoma

Histology. This tumor displays a very characteristic growth pattern of tumor clusters in clear spaces; a feature that histologically resembles lymphovascular invasion. When endothelial markers are used, these clear spaces often lack endothelium, suggesting against lymphovascular invasion. Nevertheless, the frequent association with lymph node metastases suggests that at least some of these spaces likely represent true lymphovascular invasion.

Biomarkers. Generally ER/PR positive with HER2 variability.

Clinical pearls
- Lymph node involvement at presentation is common
- Any component of micropapillary carcinoma ("with micropapillary features") is of importance as it increases the likelihood of nodal metastases

Metaplastic carcinoma

Histology. This entity represents more of a category of tumor types than a single histologic entity. Any malignant entity that shows an epithelial phenotype that has undergone transformation into either a nonglandular lineage or a mesenchymal lineage is included in this category. Therefore, a variety of malignant lesions inclusive of squamous cell carcinoma, adenosquamous carcinoma, metaplastic squamous cell carcinoma, and malignant spindle cell lesions with epithelial markers are included in this category.

Biomarkers. Generally negative for ER/PR and HER2.

Clinical pearls
- This category contains multiple tumor types and does not represent a single entity. However, sampling by needle biopsy may make it difficult to define the entities present.
- Mesenchymal component may be benign or malignant (sarcoma).
- Spread may follow that of carcinoma or sarcoma depending on the types of tumor present

Adenoid cystic carcinoma

Histology. Virtually identical to their salivary gland counterparts with solid, cribriform, and tubular epithelial components. Unlike their salivary gland counterparts, lymphovascular invasion is not a frequent finding.

Biomarkers. Generally negative for ER/PR and HER2.

Clinical pearls
- Despite the triple-negative phenotype, these tumors have an excellent prognosis with little propensity to spread. Care should be taken to not overtreat patients because of their triple-negative status.

Phyllodes Tumor

Phyllodes tumors are composed of epithelial and stromal components. Unlike fibroadenomas, these tumors display clinical characteristics that range from low-grade/benign behavior to overt malignancy. At the low-grade/benign end of the spectrum is an entity that shares many characteristics with fibroadenomas. In fact, the distinction between a low-grade/benign phyllodes tumor and fibroadenoma may be difficult, if not impossible based solely on a core biopsy.[3] There are excisional specimens that straddle the line between fibroadenomas and benign phyllodes tumors. Phyllodes tumors are defined by their tumor border, stromal cellularity, stromal atypia, stromal mitotic activity, and stromal overgrowth.

The reader is referred to the WHO criteria for further discussion around the features that define the spectrum of phyllodes tumors.[4]

It should be noted that not all criteria need be present for a diagnosis of phyllodes tumor and that the overall grade of the tumor is often dictated by the most aggressive feature present.

PAPILLARY LESIONS

There has been a significant change in the classification of, and the approach to, papillary lesions of the breast. These lesions also range from benign entities (intraductal papilloma) to atypical entities (atypical papilloma) and more aggressive lesions that act akin to carcinoma in situ or frankly invasive lesions.

Intraductal Papilloma (with and Without Atypia/Ductal Carcinoma in Situ)

Intraductal papillomas consist of ductal spaces involved by proliferating epithelial cells overlying fibrovascular cores. As with (most) other benign lesions, these lesions are enveloped in myoepithelium. The papillary proliferation is usually confined to a ductal space, but in the case of peripheral papillomatosis, it may involve many peripheral spaces. Intraductal papillomas may involve central or peripheral ducts. More centrally located lesions can result in nipple discharge. As with other proliferative lesions of the breast, intraductal papillomas can harbor atypical features ("atypical papilloma") prompting management similar to that seen in cases of ADH. Unlike other breast entities, the absence of myoepithelial cells (within papillae) in papillary lesions only denotes atypia and is insufficient, in and of itself, to define an invasive process. At the far end of the spectrum is papilloma with DCIS. The exact distinction between atypical papilloma and papilloma with DCIS is controversial. A size threshold of 3 mm has been set for the distinction between ADH versus DCIS within a papilloma.[5]

Papillary Ductal Carcinoma in Situ

Papillary DCIS is an entity that is best clustered with the architectural variants of DCIS and its inclusion in this section is meant solely to draw attention to this fact. This is a distinctly different lesion than intraductal papilloma with DCIS as there is no underlying papilloma. Instead, the papillary component represents a secondary structure of the DCIS (DCIS recapitulating a secondary structure of the breast). Papillary DCIS should be treated as other cases of DCIS.

Papillary Carcinomas (Encapsulated Papillary Carcinoma and Solid Papillary Carcinoma)

Encapsulated papillary carcinomas were previously designated intracystic/encysted papillary carcinomas. By definition, these papillary lesions are well-delimited and are surrounded by a capsule. Most cases of encapsulated papillary carcinoma should be treated as in situ carcinomas as the risk for metastatic disease is low. Distinction should be drawn between well-delimited cases of solid papillary carcinoma and cases that harbor foci of frankly invasive carcinoma. In such cases, a focus of "conventional" type invasion is seen near the capsule. These cases are best categorized as invasive carcinoma with the measurement of the invasive component being that of the conventional invasion.[6]

Solid papillary carcinomas are often multinodular and do not display the papillary secondary structures seen in other papillary lesions. Instead, the epithelial component tends to be more compact and fibrovascular cores are evident between the compact epithelial proliferation. Unlike encapsulated carcinomas, solid papillary carcinoma frequently grows as multiple nests with circumscribed/contoured margins. When there is loss of the classic, well-rounded and delimited contour resulting in a so-called "jagged" pattern, a diagnosis of invasive carcinoma should be rendered. These cases should be treated as invasive carcinomas with the measurement of the "jagged" invasive component used for staging purposes.[4]

Receptors and prognostic/predictive panels

The terms prognostic and predictive are often misunderstood. Prognostic factors predict the course that a disease will take in the absence of therapy, especially in terms of recurrence and mortality. Predictive factors forecast the likelihood that a patient will benefit from a given therapy.[7] Prognostic and predictive factors are not mutually exclusive, and many factors can be both prognostic and predictive.

Prognostic factors often include clinical factors (age, comorbidities) or tumor-related features outlined within pathology synoptic reports (tumor size, histologic grade, nodal burden). In addition, molecular tests that provide risk of recurrence also provide prognostic data.

Predictive factors assess the likelihood of benefit from therapeutics (hormonal, chemotherapeutic, targeted). These are generally assessed by immunohistochemical methods (estrogen/progesterone/HER2) or molecular methods (Her2, PDL1, etc.). It should be noted that these same predictive factors can also provide a level of prognostic data.

A variety of multigene assays exist with some noteworthy differences in their predictive and prognostic value. However, the distinction between these assays is beyond the scope of this discussion.

Anatomic staging remains an increasingly important determinant of survival and is based on the AJCC stage as defined by T/N/M categories. Prognostic staging uses anatomic staging coupled with tumor grade and biomarker (ER/PR/HER2) status.

The reader is referred to AJCC Cancer Staging Manual (8th edition) tables to stage their individual patients, especially when prognostic staging is being performed.[8]

Estrogen, progesterone, and HER2 analysis can all be performed using immunohistochemical methods. Both estrogen receptor and progesterone receptor immunostains are based on nuclear reactivity and are scored from 0% to 100%.[9] It is essential to note internal controls on cases that are hormone receptor negative (<1%) as normal breast elements should show low-level reactivity (~10%–40% of benign breast epithelial elements should stains with ER/PR). ER/PR immunostains also show varying degrees of intensity that are generally scored as weak/

intermediate/strong (**Fig 10**). A pitfall of significant importance are cases that are mistakenly diagnosed as negative when weak/blush intensity is present. For instance, a case can show very faint nuclear reactivity in 80% of tumor cells, but if this faint reactivity is missed, the case can be diagnosed as negative (0%).

HER 2 analysis by immunohistochemical methods is based on the scoring of membranous reactivity. Cases with circumferential and complete membranous reactivity in >10% of tumor cells are deemed HER2 positive (3+, **Fig 11**), whereas those with no staining or incomplete staining in <10% of cells and those with incomplete membrane staining that is faint in >10% of tumor cells are deemed negative (0+ versus 1+). Equivocal type cases that show weak to moderate staining in >10% of tumor cells are generally reflexed to in situ methodology for additional testing.[10]

In situ methodology is generally performed using fluorescent methods, though chromogenic methods are also available. Most in situ approaches use dual probe technology to enumerate Her2 gene copies and chromosome copies (generally by CEP 17 probe). A ratio between HER2 and chromosome enumeration probes places the tumor in 1 of 5 groups defined by the American Society of Clinical Oncology/College of American Pathologists Clinical Practice Guideline Focused Update. Although groups 1 (positive) and 5 (negative) constitute endpoints of HER2 testing, groups 2, 3, and 4 require additional workup.[10]

MOLECULAR CLASSIFICATION

Over the last two decades, novel laboratory techniques have allowed for reclassification of breast cancers based on molecular footprints. mRNA analysis has allowed for molecular classification which closely approximates predictive and prognostic groups identified by earlier technologies. The associated genes tend to cluster based on estrogen receptors, keratin expression, and HER2 protein, all of which used to serve as more classic phenotypic markers for classifying breast cancers. In fact, the molecular categories have immunohistochemical counterparts (see below). Breast cancers expressing luminal keratins comprise the largest groups. The 4 main categories include luminal A, luminal B, HER2, and basal-like.[11]

Luminal A and luminal B subgroups share luminal keratin expression (cytokeratins 8 and 18) and estrogen expression. Luminal B subtype tumors differ in that they are driven by proliferation-related proteins not seen in the luminal A type. Moreover, a subset of luminal B tumors express HER2 (so-called "triple-positive" cancers).

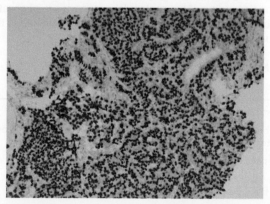

Fig. 10. Estrogen receptor. Strong nuclear immunoreactivity of estrogen receptor in virtually all tumor cells.

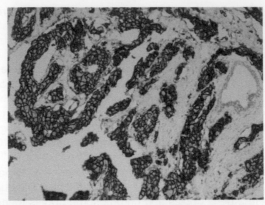

Fig. 11. HER2 immunostain. This HER2 case was scored 3+ because of the circumferential and complete membranous reactivity in virtually all tumor cells.

As the name implies, the Her2 molecular group tumors (generally) overexpress HER2. These tumors are high grade and demonstrate high proliferation rates.

Basal-like tumors also display high-grade histology, but unlike luminal B subgroup tumors, these tumors express basal-like keratins (cytokeratins 5, 14, and 17). These tumors generally lack estrogen and progesterone receptor expression and are thus dubbed "triple-negative" tumors. However, not all triple-negative tumors belong to the basal-like category.

Although immunohistochemical methods can be used as surrogates for the molecular counterparts, this correlation is far from perfect. Immunohistochemical methods reveal phenotypic characteristics and there are many reasons why genotypic and phenotypic characteristics do not always match. Nevertheless, the following immunohistochemical counterparts exist:

Luminal A: ER+, HER2-, low ki67. Luminal B: ER+, HER2-, high ki67 or ER+, HER2+, high ki67. HER2: ER-, HER2+, high ki67. Basal-like: ER- HER2-, high ki67.

The molecular classification of breast tumors serves to emphasize that breast carcinomas include a myriad of distinct categories. Each category has distinctive molecular footprints resulting in unique diagnostic, prognostic, predictive, and clinical attributes. Although surgical pathology reports do not generally categorize tumors in this manner, an understanding of the molecular categories is of great research importance and can be of benefit in guiding treatment, especially in cases that do not have a clear histologic counterpart.

CLINICS CARE POINTS

- Low-grade breast cancers are generally estrogen receptor positive
- The distinction between ADH and DCIS can be difficult and can rest on qualitative and quantitative factors
- In situ lobular lesions generally require a different approach than in situ ductal lesions
- Care should be taken to ensure that the findings in the prognostic breast panel are congruent with the type of cancer
- The distinction between a fibroadenoma and a benign/low-grade phyllodes tumor is not always possible on core biopsy

- Papillary lesions of the breast have many subtypes and some of the malignant forms are best treated in a manner akin to DCIS

DISCLOSURE

The author has nothing to disclose.

REFERENCES

1. Schnitt SJ, Brogi E, Chen YY, et al. American registry of pathology expert opinions: the spectrum of lobular carcinoma in situ: diagnostic features and clinical implications. Ann Diagn Pathol 2020;45:151481.
2. Arps DP, Jorns JM, Zhao L, et al. Re-excision rates of invasive ductal carcinoma with lobular features compared with invasive ductal carcinomas and invasive lobular carcinomas of the breast. Ann Surg Oncol 2014;21(13):4152–8.
3. Krings G, Bean GR, Chen YY. Fibroepithelial lesions; The WHO spectrum. Semin Diagn Pathol 2017;34(5):438–52.
4. WHO Classification of Tumors Editorial Board. WHO classification of tumors. 5th edition. Lyon: International Agency for Research on Cancer; 2019. Breast tumors.
5. Page DL, Salhany KE, Jensen RA, et al. Subsequent breast carcinoma risk after biopsy with atypia in a breast papilloma. Cancer 1996;78(2):258–66.
6. Li X, Xu Y, Ye H, et al. Encapsulated papillary carcinoma of the breast: A clinico-pathological study of 49 cases. Curr Probl Cancer 2018;42(3):291–301.
7. Oldenhuis CN, Oosting SF, Gietema JA, et al. Prognostic versus predictive value of biomarkers in oncology. Eur J Cancer 2008;44(7):946–53.
8. Amin MB, Edge SB, Greene FL, et al, editors. AJCC cancer staging manual. 8th edition. New York: Springer; 2017.
9. Allison KH, Hammond MEH, Dowsett M, et al. Estrogen and progesterone receptor testing in breast cancer: american society of clinical oncology/college of american pathologists guideline update. Arch Pathol Lab Med 2020;144(5):545–63.
10. Wolff AC, Hammond MEH, Allison KH, et al. Human epidermal growth factor receptor 2 testing in breast cancer: american society of clinical oncology/college of american pathologists clinical practice guideline focused update. Arch Pathol Lab Med 2018;142(11):1364–82.
11. Peppercorn J, Perou CM, Carey LA. Molecular subtypes in breast cancer evaluation and management: divide and conquer. Cancer Invest 2008;26(1):1–10.

Clinical Trials in Breast Cancer

Practice Changing, Landmark with a Focus on More Current Trials

Rick D. Vavolizza, MD[a], Emily P. Rabinovich, MS[b,1],
Max O. Meneveau, MD, MS[a], Shayna L. Showalter, MD[a,*]

KEYWORDS

- Landmark clinical trials • Current management of breast cancer
- Breast conserving surgery • Radiation therapy • Sentinel node biopsy
- Local-regional recurrence • Axillary lymph node dissection

KEY POINTS

- Surgery of the breast: In patients who are eligible for and desire breast conserving therapy (breast conserving surgery [BCS] + radiation therapy [RT]), BCS plus RT provides equivalent disease-free survival (DFS), overall survival (OS), and risk of local-regional recurrence (LRR) when compared with mastectomy. Ongoing trials are evaluating minimally invasive procedures (eg, cryoablation, radiofrequency ablation [RFA]) for small, early-stage invasive breast cancer and nonoperative management for low-risk ductal carcinoma in situ.
- Surgery of the axilla: In patients with clinically node-negative disease found to have 1 to 2 positive lymph nodes on sentinel node biopsy (SLNB), axillary lymph node dissection (ALND) does not provide an advantage with respect to locoregional control or OS compared with SLNB. Ongoing trials aim to clarify the role of ALND and regional nodal RT for patients with confirmed positive axillary disease who receive neoadjuvant chemotherapy and have subsequent complete pathologic response in the axilla versus residual disease.
- Radiation therapy: RT reduces the rate of LRR after BCS or mastectomy. Recent and ongoing trials focus on hypofractionation and partial breast radiation.

Continued

---

[a] Department of Surgery, Division of Surgical Oncology, Cancer Center, University of Virginia, PO Box 80709, Charlottesville, VA 22908, USA; [b] University of Virginia School of Medicine, Charlottesville, VA, USA
[1] Present address: 725 Walker Square Apartment 2A, Charlottesville, VA 22903.
* Corresponding author. Department of Surgery, Breast and Melanoma Surgery Division, University of Virginia, PO Box 800709, Charlottesville, VA 22908.
E-mail address: SNL2T@virginia.edu

Surg Clin N Am 103 (2023) 17–33
https://doi.org/10.1016/j.suc.2022.08.002
0039-6109/23/© 2022 Elsevier Inc. All rights reserved.

surgical.theclinics.com

Continued

- Chemotherapy: In patients with locally advanced breast cancer, chemotherapy significantly improves DFS and OS and can downstage disease in the breast and axilla in the neoadjuvant setting. Recent and ongoing trials have focused on limiting the use of chemotherapy to high-risk patients and immunotherapy.
- Endocrine therapy: In patients with hormone-receptor positive invasive breast cancer, endocrine therapy provides a 50% reduction in the risk of recurrence and has been shown to significantly improve DFS and OS.

INTRODUCTION

The multidisciplinary management of breast cancer has been in constant evolution since Halsted first described the radical mastectomy.[1,2] There continues to be a trend toward de-escalation of both surgical and systemic treatments in order to mitigate morbidities while preserving oncologic and cosmetic outcomes.

The objectives of this review are to address the landmark trials used to guide the current management of (1) surgery of the breast, (2) surgery of the axilla, (3) radiation therapy (RT), and (4) systemic therapies (endocrine and chemotherapy) while also discussing the future directions for each.

SURGERY OF THE BREAST—FROM RADICAL MASTECTOMY TO BREAST CONSERVING THERAPY

Until the late 1960s, Halsted's radical mastectomy (removal of the breast, overlying skin, pectoralis major and minor muscles, and levels I–III axillary lymph nodes) was considered the standard of care for the treatment of breast cancer, regardless of the stage of disease.[1,2] This was an exceptionally morbid procedure and mortality remained high. In the late 1960s, advances in the understanding of breast cancer biology and clinical outcomes challenged the notion that breast cancer spreads by a contiguous process from the breast to regional lymph nodes via lymphatic vessels and eventually to distant sites. An alternative hypothesis proposed that breast cancer is a systemic disease from its earliest stages and can metastasize without always involving regional lymph nodes.[3–6] This change, coupled with the desire to reduce morbidity and improve oncologic outcomes, led to the development of randomized control trials (RCT), which have formed the current standard of care for the surgical and systemic treatment of breast cancer.

The first significant shift away from radical mastectomy began in 1971, with the initiation of the National Surgical Adjuvant Breast and Bowel Project (NSABP) B-04 Trial.[7–9] Participants with clinically node-negative disease were randomized to undergo radical mastectomy, mastectomy plus postmastectomy RT (PMRT), or mastectomy alone. Participants with clinically node-positive disease were randomized to either radical mastectomy or total mastectomy plus PMRT. The aim was to determine whether patients who received local-regional treatment other than radical mastectomy had similar outcomes to those undergoing radical mastectomy. After 25 years of follow-up, there was no difference in disease-free survival (DFS), distant-disease-free survival (DDFS), or overall survival (OS) for participants undergoing radical mastectomy compared with total mastectomy, regardless of nodal status.[9] Furthermore, the results suggested that routine axillary lymph node dissection (ALND) for patients with clinically node-negative disease was unnecessary and could be performed only if clinically evident disease developed in the axilla without impacting OS.[9] In fact, 40% of the clinically node-negative patients who underwent radical mastectomy had pathologically positive axillary nodes. However, only 19% of those randomized to total mastectomy alone (who presumably also had a 40% positive node rate) developed a local-regional recurrence (LRR) in the axilla. This suggests that leaving behind occult positive nodes does not always result in axillary recurrence or significantly decrease OS. Finally, NSABP B-04 demonstrated that PMRT provided no survival benefit for patients with clinically node-negative disease. However, clinically node-negative patients who underwent mastectomy plus PMRT had a lower rate of LRR (5%) compared with those who underwent radical mastectomy (9%) or mastectomy alone (13%; $P = .002$).

After the B-04 trial demonstrated that less radical surgery was effective, some argued that breast conserving surgery (BCS) was a feasible option that may provide adequate oncologic results. The shift from routine total mastectomy to breast conserving therapy (BCS plus RT; BCT) came to fruition with the NSABP B-06[10] and NSABP B-17[11] trials for invasive breast cancer and ductal carcinoma in situ (DCIS), respectively. In the NSABP B-06 trial, participants with tumors 4 cm or greater were randomized to undergo BCS and ALND (with or without RT) or mastectomy and ALND. Participants with positive axillary nodes received adjuvant systemic therapy with fluorouracil and melphalan. After 20 years of follow-up, the NSABP B-06 trial demonstrated no difference in DFS, DDFS, or OS after BCS and ALND with or without RT compared with mastectomy and ALND.[10] However, the addition of RT after BCS significantly decreased the rate of LRR (39% vs 14%; $P < .0001$).[10] After the results of these trials were published, the NCCN guidelines were updated to state that BCT is the preferred treatment option when feasible.[12] Subsequent studies have replicated these results.[13–16] Similar to the NSABP B-06 trial for invasive cancer, the NSABP B-17 trial reported that RT significantly reduced the rate of recurrence for patients with DCIS compared with BCS alone.[11]

LRR is a risk factor for distant metastasis and death.[17] It has been estimated that for every 4 LRRs, 1 patient will die of breast cancer.[18] The importance of RT after BCT was underscored in a meta-analysis performed by the Early Breast Cancer Trialists' Collaborative Group (EBCTCG). The EBCTCG reported that RT after BCT significantly reduced the rate of any recurrence (local-regional or distant) from 35% to 19% with an absolute risk reduction (ARR) of 15.7% ($P < .00001$) as well as moderately reducing the risk of death from breast cancer (15-year ARR 3.8%; $P = .00005$).[18] More recent studies have reported lower LRR rates of 2% to 6% at 10-year follow-up[19,20] because of more effective and longer durations of systemic treatment. The above trials have provided the foundation for the modern approach to the surgical treatment of breast cancer by demonstrating that BCT offers acceptable oncologic and cosmetic outcomes.

DCIS is a nonobligate precursor to invasive breast cancer and represents 20% to 25% of all new breast cancer diagnoses,[21] with 14% to 53% of DCIS progressing to invasive cancer over a period of 10 or more years.[22] During the past decade, there has been ongoing debate regarding the possible overdiagnosis and, thus, overtreatment of DCIS. Consequently, there is increasing interest in de-escalating the management of DCIS, including possible nonoperative management for low-grade and intermediate-grade DCIS (low-risk DCIS). Four RCTs assessing nonoperative treatment of low-risk DCIS are underway in the United States (Comparison of Operative versus Monitoring and Endocrine Therapy, COMET),[23] United Kingdom (LORIS),[24] Europe (LORD),[25] and Japan (LORETTA).[26] The COMET trial is a phase III RCT for low-risk DCIS in which participants either undergo surgery (lumpectomy or mastectomy) plus RT when appropriate or active surveillance alone.[23] Both groups are eligible for adjuvant endocrine therapy (AET), as appropriate. The COMET trial is projected to complete accrual by July 2023.

SURGERY OF THE AXILLA—FROM ROUTINE AXILLARY LYMPH NODE DISSECTION TO SELECTIVE AXILLARY LYMPH NODE DISSECTION AND SENTINEL NODE BIOPSY

Axillary surgery in patients with breast cancer serves both diagnostic and therapeutic purposes. The involvement of axillary lymph nodes is a crucial prognostic factor for LRR and OS. Historically, ALND was routinely performed to assess axillary status for staging purposes, to aid in decision-making for adjuvant treatment recommendations, and to provide regional control of disease. ALND is associated with high morbidity including lymphedema, shoulder dysfunction, pain, and paresthesias.[27,28]

The NSABP B-32 trial was designed to determine whether sentinel lymph node biopsy (SLNB) provided the same oncologic benefits to that of ALND but with fewer side effects in patients with clinically node-negative disease.[29] In this phase III trial, 5611 participants were randomized to undergo either SLNB plus immediate ALND or SLNB followed by ALND only in the setting of a positive sentinel node. There was no statistically significant difference in OS, DFS, and regional recurrence between the 2 groups.[29] The NSABP B-32 trial demonstrated that SLNB was a safe and effective approach for clinically node-negative patients, and that the addition of ALND in patients with a negative SLNB did not improve outcomes but did increase morbidity.

After the results from NSABP B-32 were published in 2010, SLNB became the standard of care for patients with clinically node-negative disease. As the next step in de-escalation of local therapy, the ACOSOG Z0011 trial sought to determine whether clinically node-negative patients with a positive SLNB could be spared completion ALND.[30] ACOSOG Z0011 was a multicenter noninferiority trial, which enrolled 891 participants with T1–T2 ($\leq$5 cm), N0, and M0 invasive breast cancer undergoing BCT. All participants received BCS followed by whole breast radiation (WBI), and recommendations for adjuvant systemic therapy were made at the discretion of the treating provider. Participants with 1 to 2 positive SLNs were randomized to undergo ALND or no further axillary surgery. The initial[30,31] and long-term follow-up data[32] published in 2010 and 2016, respectively, demonstrated that among participants with 1 to 2 positive SLNs, ALND does not provide an advantage with respect to LRR or OS compared with SLNB alone. As such, it is currently the standard of care that SLNB alone is adequate treatment after BCS in clinically node-negative patients with up to 3 positive nodes who will receive WBI.[33,34] Several studies have reported the impact of ACOSOG Z0011 in clinical practice. MD Anderson Cancer Center reported their rate of ALNDs in SLNB-positive patients to be 85% 1 year before Z0011, 24% 1 year after Z0011 results were released, and 8% as of 2016.[35] Furthermore, among 27,635 patients identified from the National Cancer Database who met Z0011 criteria, ALND nonadherence to Z0011 has decreased from 34.0% in 2012% to 22.7% in 2015.[36]

In 2002, the European Organization for Research and Treatment of Cancer initiated the AMAROS trial, which was designed to assess the safety of RT versus ALND among patients with a positive SLN.[34] The AMAROS trial was a multicenter, open-label, phase III noninferiority trial, which randomized 4806 patients with T1–T2, clinically node-negative invasive breast cancer to undergo either ALND or axillary RT. Of the total cohort, 1425 participants were found to have 1 to 2 positive nodes after SLNB and were analyzed for the study. At 5 years, axillary recurrence was 0.43% (95% CI 0.00–0.92) after ALND and 1.19% (95% CI 0.31–2.08) after axillary RT.[34] However, lymphedema was 28% versus 14% after ALND compared with axillary RT, respectively. The results of this trial demonstrated that axillary RT provides equivalent regional control with less morbidity compared with ALND in patients with a positive SLN. Unlike the ACOSOG Z0011 trial, the AMAROS trial enrolled both participants who underwent BCS (n = 1166; 609 in ALND group and 557 in RT group) and mastectomy (n = 248; 127 in ALND group and 121 in RT group). This has provided data to support omission of ALND in patients who undergo a mastectomy, contingent on the receipt of PMRT.

The shift toward less axillary surgery continued when in 2016, the Society of Surgical Oncology and the Choosing Wisely campaign published guidelines recommending against the routine use of SLNB in clinically node-negative patients aged 70 years or older with early-stage, hormone receptor (HR)-positive, HER2-negative invasive breast cancer treated with BCS and AET.[37] This recommendation was supported by data from the CALGB 9343 trial,[38] which demonstrated no survival benefit among participants who underwent ALND versus no axillary surgery. Although the primary goal of CALGB 9343 was to establish whether RT was beneficial in this patient population, the trial showed only a marginally higher axillary recurrence rate among women who did not undergo axillary evaluation. In contrast, participants with tumors with high-risk features (ie, larger tumors, HER2-positive, triple negative) can still be considered for SLNB to help guide decisions regarding adjuvant chemotherapy as mortality in these patients remains high.[39]

Because the use of neoadjuvant chemotherapy (NAC) increased, the utility of SLNB in the postneoadjuvant setting was called into question. The ACOSOG Z1071 trial sought to determine the false-negative rate (FNR) of SLNB after NAC in women who were initially pathologically node-positive.[40] From 2009 to 2011, 687 patients underwent SLNB followed by ALND. Among patients with disease confined to the SLNs, the FNR was 12.6% (39/310). The FNR decreased with the use of dual tracers (radiocolloid and blue dye; 10.8% in combination versus 20.3% with single agent) and when 3 or more SLNs were removed (9.1% for 3 or more SLNs vs 21.1% for 2 SLNs).[40] A similar trial, SENTINA, demonstrated that if the dual tracer technique was used, the FNR was 8.6%, and the FNR decreased as the number of SLNs removed increased.[41] As a result of these trials, for patients with pathologically node-positive disease at diagnosis who undergo NAC, SLNB is considered acceptable for nodal staging using the following criteria[42]: (1) use of clinical axillary examination and axillary ultrasound to guide patient selection for SLNB, (2) placement of a clip in the biopsy-proven positive node at diagnosis and resecting the clipped node at the time of the SLNB, (3) dual tracer lymphatic mapping, and (4) ensuring 2 or more SLNs are removed.

Several trials are currently evaluating further de-escalation of axillary surgery. These include Alliance A011202[43] and NSABP B-51/RTOG 1304,[44] both of which are now closed to accrual. Alliance A011202 is a phase III RCT that aims to clarify the role of ALND for patients with biopsy-proven node-positive disease (T1–T3, N1, M0) who, despite converting to clinically node-negative after NAC, have a positive SLN at surgery. Participants were randomized to either (1) completion ALND plus regional nodal irradiation (RNI) or (2) axillary RT plus RNI. The primary endpoint is determining invasive breast cancer recurrence-free interval. NSABP B-51/RTOG 1304 is a phase III RCT evaluating if PMRT + RNI or the additional of RNI to WBI after BCS reduces invasive breast cancer recurrence-free interval in participants with pathologically positive nodes who convert to pathologically nega-tive nodes after NAC. For participants undergoing mastectomy, random assign-ment is to no chest wall RT + RNI or to chest wall RT + RNI. For participants undergoing BCS, random assignment is to WBI or WBI + RNI. Data from both studies are forthcoming and may change the management of the axilla in node-positive patients treated with NAC.

RADIATION THERAPY

In the late 1990s, several studies examined the effect of RT on LRR after mastectomy when combined with chemotherapy.[45] The Danish Breast Cancer Cooperative Group (DBCG) 82B trial demonstrated a significant reduction in LRR and distant metastases among premenopausal participants who received RT and adjuvant chemotherapy following mastectomy for pathologic stage II/III disease compared with chemotherapy alone (9% vs 32%; $P < .001$). The trial also demonstrated a significant improvement in DFS irrespective of tumor size, histopathological grade, or number of positive nodes among these participants.[46] Although the efficacy of RT for premenopausal women with breast cancer had been studied, there was a paucity of data regarding its efficacy among postmenopausal women.

To evaluate the association between PMRT and rates of LRR and OS among post-menopausal women who had undergone mastectomy, the DBCG 82C trial enrolled 1375 postmenopausal women with stage II/III breast cancer between 1982 and 1990. Participants were randomized to receive tamoxifen plus RT versus tamoxifen alone. There was a substantial reduction in LRR among participants who received RT plus tamoxifen compared with tamoxifen alone (8% vs 35%; $P < .001$), as well as a significant improvement in DFS and OS at 10-year follow-up.[47] As previously described in detail, the NSABP B-04 and B-06 trials were instrumental in driving the paradigm shift and de-escalation of surgical management from radical mastectomy to total mastectomy, and ultimately, BCT, due to the role RT played in reducing LRR following more conservative surgical management.

The CALGB 9343 and PRIME II studies built on findings from NSABP B-04 and B-06 by focusing on older women with early-stage breast cancer to determine the benefit of adjuvant RT in women treated with BCS and AET. The CALGB 9343 trial enrolled 636 women aged 70 years or older with ER-positive/HER2-negative, clinically node-negative breast cancer with tumors 2 cm or greater to receive or not receive RT after BCS. All women were treated with adjuvant tamoxifen.[48] At 5-year and 10-year follow-ups, there was small but significant decrease in LRR among participants who received tamoxifen plus RT when compared with the cohort who received tamoxifen alone.[38,48] There were no significant differences in time to mastectomy, overall breast preserva-tion, time to distant metastasis, or OS.[38] The PRIME II trial was performed in parallel in Europe with a similar study design and assessed whether RT versus no RT following BCT would influence ipsilateral breast tumor recurrence (IBTR) among women aged 65 years or older with ER-positive, clinically node-negative breast cancer with tumors 3 cm or greater. Similar to the CALGBB 9343 results, at 5-year follow-up, there was a small decrease in IBTR among participants who received RT compared with those treated with AET alone (1.3% vs 4.1%; $P = .0002$). Again, there were no significant dif-ferences in OS, LRR, distant metastases, contralateral breast cancers, or new breast cancers.[49] The authors of both of these studies concluded that RT omission is reason-able in women aged 70 years or older with early-stage, ER-positive tumors, and the NCCN guidelines were subsequently updated to include consideration of RT omission in this population.[50]

In the 1980s, despite known advantages of BCT and standard fractionated RT (SF-WBI), less than half of eligible patients were reported to receive the full treatment regimen due to the 6 to 7-week course of traditional WBI.[51,52] The challenges posed by traditional WBI with regards to patient convenience and cost led to the introduction of several trials examining the efficacy of hypofractionated WBI (HF-WBI) during approximately 4 weeks. One such study randomized 1234 participants with early-stage breast cancer to receive SF-WBI or HF-WBI. At 10-year follow-up, the study reported that the risk of LRR with HF-WBI was comparable to that following SF-RT (6.7% vs 6.2%),[53] which corroborated findings from earlier trials in the United Kingdom.[54,55]

Given that many LRRs and IBTRs occur close to the primary tumor site, accelerated partial breast irradiation (APBI) has been explored as an alternative to WBI. Several forms of APBI have been developed to meet patient demand for convenience and to spare normal tissues (heart, skin, chest wall). Several trials published during the past decade have demonstrated comparable local control rates, shortened treatment timelines, diminished toxicities to surrounding tissues, and positive cosmetic outcomes associated with APBI administered via brachytherapy, intraoperative radiotherapy (IORT), and external beam RT.[56] The NSABP B-39 trial was a randomized, phase III trial to investigate whether APBI was equivalent to WBI in preventing IBTR after BCS for patients with DCIS or stage I or II breast cancer.[57] At a median follow-up of 10.2 years, 90 (4%) of 2089 women eligible for the primary outcome in the APBI cohort and 71 (3%) of 2036 women in the WBI cohort had an IBTR (HR 1.22, 90% CI 0.94–1.58). Although APBI did not meet their criteria for equivalence to WBI in controlling IBTR, the absolute difference in the 10-year cumulative incidence of IBTR was less than 1%. Furthermore, the trial reported that distant disease-free interval, OS, and DFS were not different for APBI versus WBI.

IORT represents the most condensed form of APBI, providing only one dose of radiation given at the time of BCS. The single dose targeted IORT during lumpectomy TARGIT-IORT trial evaluated women aged 45 years or older diagnosed with invasive ductal carcinoma and eligible for BCT to determine whether IORT delivered during BCS could effectively replace daily fractionated whole breast external beam radiotherapy (EBRT) for early-stage breast cancer. A total of 2298 women were randomized. With long-term follow-up, IORT was found to be noninferior to EBRT with no difference in RFS, DFS, OS, and breast cancer specific mortality. Rates of LRR were comparable among participants in the IORT and EBRT cohorts (2.11% vs 0.95%, $P = .28$).[58] Concurrently, the ELIOT phase III trial randomized 1305 women to either APBI with IORT or WBI and included women aged 48 to 75 years with unicentric breast cancers less than 25 mm, clinically negative nodes, and suitable for BCT. This trial revealed an increased rate of IBTR among participants treated with IORT when compared with WBI; however, IORT was comparable among women at very low risk of recurrence (less than 1.3% risk at 10 years) with small (<1 cm), well-differentiated, luminal A tumors with a low proliferative index.[59]

SYSTEMIC THERAPIES
Chemotherapy

The widespread use of adjuvant chemotherapy began in the 1970s with the introduction of cyclophosphamide plus methotrexate and fluorouracil. In the 1990s, adverse effects and poor tolerance resulted in a shift toward the use of anthracycline-based and taxane-based regimens, and it was recommended that most women with breast cancer be offered adjuvant chemotherapy.[60] More recent advancements in gene expression assays such as Mammaprint and Oncotype DX and recurrence score risk stratification models have provided a foundation for personalized systemic therapy and de-escalation of chemotherapy regimens.[61]

Until the early 2000s, most women with invasive breast cancer were treated with adjuvant chemotherapy. Around this time, gene-expression assays were developed with the intention of more deliberate decisions regarding systemic therapy. The Oncotype DX, a 21-gene assay was of particular interest given its accuracy and had been shown in retrospective studies to predict chemotherapy benefit among women with HR-positive disease and high recurrence scores.[61,62] In 2006, a randomized prospective trial (Trial Assigning Individualized Options for Treatment; TAILORx) was initiated to determine the benefit of chemotherapy among women with midrange recurrence scores on the Oncotype DX panel.[63] In this study, 6,711 participants with ER-positive, HER-2 negative, node-negative breast cancer and a midrange recurrence score of 11 to 25 were randomized to receive either chemoendocrine therapy or endocrine therapy alone. At long-term follow-up of 9 years, the 2 treatment groups had comparable rates of invasive DFS, DDFS, LRR, and OS. In this population, absolute benefit of chemotherapy was amplified with increasing recurrence score.[63]

Although Oncotype DX was shown to be beneficial in making adjuvant chemotherapy decisions for women with HR-positive node-negative disease, another gene assay, MammaPrint (70-genes), was investigated among women with up to 3 positive nodes and stratified participants according to risk group, HR status, nodal involvement, HER2 status, and age. As such, the MINDACT phase III trial[64] was designed to identify the utility of MammaPrint combined with clinical features in selecting women for adjuvant chemotherapy. The trial enrolled 6,693 participants between 2007 and 2011. This trial used MammaPrint to reduce the proportion of participants identified as "high-risk" based on clinical parameters, with comparable OS and DDFS; however, DFS was higher among participants who were identified as "high-risk" clinically and received chemotherapy, regardless of genomic risk.[64]

The trials described above laid the foundation for current trials such as RxPONDER, a randomized phase III trial, which aims to determine the optimal recurrence score cutoffs for predicting chemotherapy benefit with these prognostic assays.[65] Gene expression panels such as Oncotype DX and MammaPrint have demonstrated promising metric performances in the prediction of prognosis and determining more personalized treatment regimens, with multiple recent trials corroborating these results.[66]

Human epidermal growth factor receptor 2 (HER2)-positive cancers, which involve amplification of the HER2 gene, are associated with a higher propensity for disease recurrence.[67] Trastuzumab is a humanized monoclonal antibody that binds the extracellular domain of HER2 and has been reported to significantly increase OS and DFS compared with chemotherapy alone.[61,68] The North Central Cancer Treatment Group N9831 Alliance trial published in 2015 enrolled 1615 participants with operable node-positive or high-risk node-negative HER2-positive breast cancer. Participants were randomized to receive chemotherapy alone with doxorubicin and cyclophosphamide, followed by paclitaxel, or the same regimen followed by trastuzumab. Concurrently, the NSABP B-31 trial included 1736 participants with a similar study design. Joint analysis of data from these 2 trials demonstrated a significant improvement in DFS with trastuzumab plus chemotherapy, with a 39% reduction in death rate with the addition of trastuzumab ($P < .001$).[69]

Current trials investigating the management of locally advanced unresectable or metastatic breast cancer involve the phase III DESTINY-Breast04 trial, which has been among the first studies to yield clinically significant improvements in PFS and

OS following administration of trastuzumab deruxtecan, regardless of HR status, in patients previously treated with up to 2 lines of chemotherapy.[70] The KATHERINE trial is a phase III open-label trial, which randomized 1486 participants with HER2-positive, early-stage breast cancer who were found to have residual invasive disease after NAC to receive trastuzumab emtansine or trastuzumab alone in the adjuvant setting. Interim analysis, published in 2019, showed a significant increase in DFS among patients who received the trastuzumab emtansine derivative.[56]

Neoadjuvant Chemotherapy

By the 1980s, the benefits of adjuvant chemotherapy had been established and results from the NSABP B-07 trial supported the use of BCT. In an effort to increase the number of women eligible for BCT, the NSABP B-18 trial sought to evaluate the benefit of NAC with the use of doxorubicin (also known as adriamycin) and cyclophosphamide (AC).[71] Between 1988 and 1993, 1523 participants with early-stage breast cancer were enrolled and randomized to receive either preoperative or postoperative AC. LRR, DFS, and OS were comparable between the 2 groups. A larger proportion of participants treated with NAC underwent BCT (68% and 60%; $P = .001$), particularly among those with tumors 5 cm or greater at diagnosis.[71,72] Participants who received NAC were more likely to have negative nodes at the time of surgery compared with those who received adjuvant chemotherapy. Furthermore, those who achieved a pathologic complete response (pCR) experienced a significantly longer DFS and OS.[72] Subsequent trials have validated these findings, revealing a significant benefit of NAC in downstaging breast and axillary disease to facilitate BCT, and decreasing morbidity associated with axillary surgery by allowing for SLNB rather than ALND in select patients.[73]

Triple-negative breast cancers (TNBC) comprise approximately 12% to 20% of all breast cancers diagnosed each year worldwide,[74] and patients often present with locally advanced disease. NAC regimens among patients with TNBC have demonstrated relatively high rates of pCR.[74] Compared with HER-2-positive and HR-positive disease, TNBCs lack treatable molecular targets. The lack of target receptors coupled with diminished disease-free intervals in the adjuvant and neoadjuvant settings make surgery and chemotherapy 2 of the only available treatment modalities. Traditional chemotherapy regimens for TNBC include platinum compounds, taxanes, and anthracyclines. Several studies have demonstrated additional benefit of adjuvant capecitabine, a chemotherapeutic agent, which works synergistically with taxanes, in patients with residual disease after NAC.[61] The CREATE-X trial, which included women with stage I-IIIB breast cancer who underwent NAC and did not have a pCR, demonstrated significant improvement in 5-year DFS (74.1% vs 67.6%; HR 0.70; $P = .01$) and OS (89.2% vs 83.3%; HR = 0.59; $P = .01$) among participants who received adjuvant capecitabine.[75]

Recently, immunotherapy has revolutionized the treatment of many cancers, especially in the neoadjuvant setting. The KEYNOTE-522 trial is an ongoing, phase III randomized, double-blind study, which aims to assess the use of immunotherapy in participants with TNBC. Preliminary reports revealed improved outcomes and pCR rates among participants with TNBC who received neoadjuvant or adjuvant immunotherapy plus NAC compared with NAC alone.[76]

Endocrine Therapy

Approximately 65% of all breast cancers are HR-positive. Early-stage, HR-positive disease is generally associated with an excellent prognosis.[77] Hormone therapies with selective estrogen receptor (ER) modulators (SERM) and aromatase inhibitors

(AI) are now the gold-standard for treatment in patients with ER-positive breast cancer.[78]

In 1983, the Nolvadex Adjuvant Trial Organization enrolled 1285 women with stage I/II breast cancer who were treated by mastectomy with either axillary node clearance or axillary node sampling and then randomized to receive either tamoxifen for 2 years or no further treatment. This trial demonstrated that treatment failure (recurrent disease or death) at 21 months was significantly reduced in participants receiving tamoxifen compared with controls (14.2% vs 20.5%; $P = .01$).[79,80] Further trials by the EBCTCG revealed a 47% reduction in LRR with 5 years of tamoxifen treatment.[80,81] Although tamoxifen has been demonstrated to have significant efficacy in improving DFS and OS in patients with ER-positive tumors, it has adverse partial estrogenic effects in the uterus and vascular system, increasing the risk of endometrial hyperplasia and cancer as well as venous thromboembolism and hot flashes.[82]

Given the unfavorable side effect profile associated with long-term tamoxifen therapy and partial antiestrogenic effects, the utility of AIs rather than SERMs has been studied. The use of AIs was initially reported in the early 1970s.[83] AIs have demonstrated comparable or increased DFS and OS compared with tamoxifen therapy alone with a more manageable side-effect profile.[80] The Arimidex, Tamoxifen Alone or in Combination (ATAC) trial revealed significantly improved DFS at 3-year follow-up among participants treated with adjuvant anastrozole versus tamoxifen alone (89.4% vs 87.4%; $P = .013$). Anastrozole use was associated with a significantly reduced incidence of hot flashes, endometrial cancer, vaginal bleeding and discharge, venous thromboembolic events, and cerebrovascular events.[84] These therapies have become standard of care for postmenopausal women with HR-positive breast cancer, given that a primary source of estrogen production in this population is via peripheral conversion of androgens to estrogens by the enzyme aromatase.[83]

Given the encouraging outcomes in NAC trials, administration of neoadjuvant endocrine therapy (NET) has also been explored among patients with HR-positive breast cancer because they generally do not derive significant benefit from NAC. Several landmark trials have demonstrated the efficacy of NET in decreasing HR-positive breast cancers and facilitating BCT.[85] In 2001, the P024 trial reported the efficacy of 4 months of neoadjuvant letrozole versus tamoxifen among 337 postmenopausal women with HR-positive breast cancers who were not considered eligible for BCT. In this trial, neoadjuvant letrozole was shown to reduce tumor volume more effectively than neoadjuvant tamoxifen. Participants who underwent treatment with neoadjuvant letrozole were more likely to undergo BCT than their counterparts who underwent treatment with tamoxifen (45% vs 35%; $P = .022$).[86]

The Immediate Preoperative Anastrozole, Tamoxifen, or Combined with Tamoxifen multicenter trial assessed the role of neoadjuvant tamoxifen, anastrozole, or the combination of both in the improvement of objective response rate, as well as the identification of potential endpoints that would adequately predict clinical outcomes in the adjuvant setting.[87] In concordance with prior studies, women who were randomized to receive neoadjuvant anastrozole were more likely to undergo BCT than those who received neoadjuvant tamoxifen (46% vs 22%; $P = .022$). Further biomarker studies revealed that participants who received anastrozole had more significant suppression of Ki67 following treatment, an objective measure of response, which was associated with recurrence free survival (log rank $P = .008$).[72]

Studies currently in progress such as ALTERNATE[88] and NBRST[89] are seeking to determine the effects of NET among postmenopausal women, and whether molecular subtyping can predict response to NET and chemotherapy.

SUMMARY

The modern approach to the treatment of breast cancer has been guided by numerous clinical trials that have largely sought to de-escalate therapy while improving oncologic outcomes. Here, we have reviewed several modern trials, which inform the current standard of care for patients with breast cancer. Future trials are seeking to further de-escalate therapy and will continue to push toward personalized, patient-specific treatments.

CLINICS CARE POINTS

- When an eligible patient is deciding between breast conserving surgery (BCS) and mastectomy, it is crucial to discuss that breast conserving therapy (BCS + radiation therapy (RT); BCT) provides equivalent disease-free survival (DFS), overall survival (OS), and risk of local-regional recurrence (LRR) when compared to mastectomy.

- The current standard of care for patients with ductal carcinoma in situ (DCIS) is BCT or mastectomy. The ongoing COMET trial, a phase III randomized control trial, is enrolling patients with low-risk DCIS and randomizing participants to either undergo surgery (BCS+RT or mastectomy) or active surveillance.

- For patients with pathologically node-positive disease at diagnosis who undergo neoadjuvant chemotherapy (NAC), sentinel lymph node biopsy (SLNB) is considered acceptable for nodal staging using the following criteria: (1) use of clinical axillary exam and axillary ultrasound to guide patient selection for SLNB, (2) placement of a clip in the biopsy-proven positive node at diagnosis and resecting the clipped node at the time of the SLNB, (3) dual tracer lymphatic mapping, and (4) ensuring ≥ 2 SLNs are removed.

- Patients who are clinically node-positive at diagnosis benefit from NAC to down stage the axilla and to avoid axillary lymph node dissection (ALND) if they have a complete pathologic response (pCR). Results from two cooperative group trials aimed at clarifying the role of ALND and regional nodal RT for patients with confirmed positive axillary disease who receive NAC but still have a positive SLNB at the time of surgery (Alliance A011202) or are found to have achieved a pCR in the axilla (NSABP B-51/RTOG 1304) are forthcoming.

- Patient-centered discussions regarding various types of RT (i.e. hypofractionated whole breast radiation, accelerated partial breast irradiation, and intraoperative radiotherapy) may improve patient convenience and spare normal tissues (heart, skin, chest wall) from radiation while preserving oncologic and cosmetic outcomes.6. Patients with hormone-receptor positive breast cancer benefit from endocrine therapy as it provides a 50% reduction in risk of recurrence and has been shown to significantly improve DFS and OS.

DISCLOSURE

The authors have nothing to disclose.

REFERENCES

1. Halsted WSI. The Results of Operations for the Cure of Cancer of the Breast Performed at the Johns Hopkins Hospital from June, 1889, to January, 1894. Ann Surg 1894;20(5):497–555.
2. Lewis D, Rienhoff WF. Results of Operations at the Johns Hopkins Hospital for Cancer of the Breast: Performed at the Johns Hopkins Hospital from 1889 to 1931. Ann Surg 1932;95(3):336–400.

3. Fisher B, Redmond C, Fisher ER. The contribution of recent NSABP clinical trials of primary breast cancer therapy to an understanding of tumor biology–an overview of findings. Cancer 1980;46(4 Suppl):1009–25.

4. Fisher B, Fisher ER. Transmigration of lymph nodes by tumor cells. Science 1966; 152(3727):1397–8.

5. Fisher B, Fisher ER. Experimental evidence in support of the dormant tumor cell. Science 1959;130(3380):918–9.

6. Fisher B, Fisher ER. The interrelationship of hematogenous and lymphatic tumor cell dissemination. Surg Gynecol Obstet 1966;122(4):791–8.

7. Fisher B, Montague E, Redmond C, et al. Comparison of radical mastectomy with alternative treatments for primary breast cancer. A first report of results from a prospective randomized clinical trial. Cancer 1977;39(6 Suppl):2827–39.

8. Fisher B, Redmond C, Fisher ER, et al. Ten-year results of a randomized clinical trial comparing radical mastectomy and total mastectomy with or without radiation. N Engl J Med 1985;312(11):674–81.

9. Fisher B, Jeong JH, Anderson S, et al. Twenty-five-year follow-up of a randomized trial comparing radical mastectomy, total mastectomy, and total mastectomy followed by irradiation. N Engl J Med 2002;347(8):567–75.

10. Fisher B, Anderson S, Bryant J, et al. Twenty-year follow-up of a randomized trial comparing total mastectomy, lumpectomy, and lumpectomy plus irradiation for the treatment of invasive breast cancer. N Engl J Med 2002;347(16):1233–41.

11. Fisher B, Costantino J, Redmond C, et al. Lumpectomy compared with lumpectomy and radiation therapy for the treatment of intraductal breast cancer. N Engl J Med 1993;328(22):1581–6.

12. National Comprehensive Cancer Network. Clinical Practice Guidelines in Oncology: Breast Cancer (version 4.2022). https://www.nccn.org/professionals/physician_gls/pdf/breast.pdf.

13. Litière S, Werutsky G, Fentiman IS, et al. Breast conserving therapy versus mastectomy for stage I-II breast cancer: 20 year follow-up of the EORTC 10801 phase 3 randomised trial. Lancet Oncol 2012;13(4):412–9.

14. van Maaren MC, de Munck L, de Bock GH, et al. 10 year survival after breast-conserving surgery plus radiotherapy compared with mastectomy in early breast cancer in the Netherlands: a population-based study. Lancet Oncol 2016;17(8):1158–70.

15. Hartmann-Johnsen OJ, Kåresen R, Schlichting E, et al. Survival is Better After Breast Conserving Therapy than Mastectomy for Early Stage Breast Cancer: A Registry-Based Follow-up Study of Norwegian Women Primary Operated Between 1998 and 2008. Ann Surg Oncol 2015;22(12):3836–45.

16. Veronesi U, Cascinelli N, Mariani L, et al. Twenty-year follow-up of a randomized study comparing breast-conserving surgery with radical mastectomy for early breast cancer. N Engl J Med 2002;347(16):1227–32.

17. Fortin A, Larochelle M, Laverdière J, et al. Local failure is responsible for the decrease in survival for patients with breast cancer treated with conservative surgery and postoperative radiotherapy. J Clin Oncol 1999;17(1):101–9.

18. Darby S, McGale P, Correa C, et al. Effect of radiotherapy after breast-conserving surgery on 10-year recurrence and 15-year breast cancer death: meta-analysis of individual patient data for 10,801 women in 17 randomised trials. Lancet 2011; 378(9804):1707–16.

19. Poortmans PMP, Arenas M, Livi L. Over-irradiation. Breast 2017;31:295–302.

20. Mittendorf EA, Buchholz TA, Tucker SL, et al. Impact of chemotherapy sequencing on local-regional failure risk in breast cancer patients undergoing breast-conserving therapy. Ann Surg 2013;257(2):173–9.

21. McCormick B, Winter K, Hudis C, et al. RTOG 9804: a prospective randomized trial for good-risk ductal carcinoma in situ comparing radiotherapy with observation. *J Clin Oncol* Mar 2015;33(7):709–15.

22. Erbas B, Provenzano E, Armes J, et al. The natural history of ductal carcinoma in situ of the breast: a review. Breast Cancer Res Treat 2006;97(2):135–44.

23. Hwang ES, Hyslop T, Lynch T, et al. The COMET (Comparison of Operative versus Monitoring and Endocrine Therapy) trial: a phase III randomised controlled clinical trial for low-risk ductal carcinoma in situ (DCIS). BMJ Open 2019;9(3): e026797.

24. Francis A, Thomas J, Fallowfield L, et al. Addressing overtreatment of screen detected DCIS; the LORIS trial. Eur J Cancer 2015;51(16):2296–303.

25. Elshof LE, Tryfonidis K, Slaets L, et al. Feasibility of a prospective, randomised, open-label, international multicentre, phase III, non-inferiority trial to assess the safety of active surveillance for low risk ductal carcinoma in situ - The LORD study. Eur J Cancer 2015;51(12):1497–510.

26. Kanbayashi C, Thompson AM, Hwang E-SS, et al. The international collaboration of active surveillance trials for low-risk DCIS (LORIS, LORD, COMET, LORETTA). J Clin Oncol 2019;37(15_suppl):TPS603.

27. Fleissig A, Fallowfield LJ, Langridge CI, et al. Post-operative arm morbidity and quality of life. Results of the ALMANAC randomised trial comparing sentinel node biopsy with standard axillary treatment in the management of patients with early breast cancer. Breast Cancer Res Treat 2006;95(3):279–93.

28. Lucci A, McCall LM, Beitsch PD, et al. Surgical complications associated with sentinel lymph node dissection (SLND) plus axillary lymph node dissection compared with SLND alone in the American College of Surgeons Oncology Group Trial Z0011. J Clin Oncol 2007;25(24):3657–63.

29. Krag DN, Anderson SJ, Julian TB, et al. Sentinel-lymph-node resection compared with conventional axillary-lymph-node dissection in clinically node-negative patients with breast cancer: overall survival findings from the NSABP B-32 randomised phase 3 trial. Lancet Oncol 2010;11(10):927–33.

30. Giuliano AE, McCall L, Beitsch P, et al. Locoregional recurrence after sentinel lymph node dissection with or without axillary dissection in patients with sentinel lymph node metastases: the American College of Surgeons Oncology Group Z0011 randomized trial. *Ann Surg* Sep 2010;252(3):426–32 ; discussion 432-3.

31. Giuliano AE, Hunt KK, Ballman KV, et al. Axillary dissection vs no axillary dissection in women with invasive breast cancer and sentinel node metastasis: a randomized clinical trial. Jama 2011;305(6):569–75.

32. Giuliano AE, Ballman K, McCall L, et al. Locoregional Recurrence After Sentinel Lymph Node Dissection With or Without Axillary Dissection in Patients With Sentinel Lymph Node Metastases: Long-term Follow-up From the American College of Surgeons Oncology Group (Alliance) ACOSOG Z0011 Randomized Trial. *Ann Surg* Sep 2016;264(3):413–20.

33. Galimberti V, Cole BF, Zurrida S, et al. Axillary dissection versus no axillary dissection in patients with sentinel-node micrometastases (IBCSG 23-01): a phase 3 randomised controlled trial. Lancet Oncol 2013;14(4):297–305.

34. Donker M, van Tienhoven G, Straver ME, et al. Radiotherapy or surgery of the axilla after a positive sentinel node in breast cancer (EORTC 10981-22023

AMAROS): a randomised, multicentre, open-label, phase 3 non-inferiority trial. Lancet Oncol 2014;15(12):1303–10.

35. Weiss A, Mittendorf EA, DeSnyder SM, et al. Expanding Implementation of ACO-SOG Z0011 in Surgeon Practice. Clin Breast Cancer 2018;18(4):276–81.

36. Tseng J, Alban RF, Siegel E, et al. Changes in utilization of axillary dissection in women with invasive breast cancer and sentinel node metastasis after the ACO-SOG Z0011 trial. Breast J 2021;27(3):216–21.

37. Five Things Physicians and Patients Should Question 2016. https://www.choosingwisely.org/wp-content/uploads/2016/07/SSO-5things-List_2021-Updates.pdf. [Accessed 18 May 2022].

38. Hughes KS, Schnaper LA, Bellon JR, et al. Lumpectomy plus tamoxifen with or without irradiation in women age 70 years or older with early breast cancer: long-term follow-up of CALGB 9343. J Clin Oncol 2013;31(19):2382–7.

39. Blair SL, Tsai C, Tafra L. ASBRS Great Debate: Sentinel Node Biopsy in Patients Over 70 Years of Age. Ann Surg Oncol 2018;25(10):2813–7.

40. Boughey JC, Suman VJ, Mittendorf EA, et al. Sentinel lymph node surgery after neoadjuvant chemotherapy in patients with node-positive breast cancer: the ACOSOG Z1071 (Alliance) clinical trial. Jama 2013;310(14):1455–61.

41. Kuehn T, Bauerfeind I, Fehm T, et al. Sentinel-lymph-node biopsy in patients with breast cancer before and after neoadjuvant chemotherapy (SENTINA): a prospective, multicentre cohort study. Lancet Oncol 2013;14(7):609–18.

42. Fisher CS, Margenthaler JA, Hunt KK, et al. The Landmark Series: Axillary Management in Breast Cancer. *Ann Surg Oncol* Mar 2020;27(3):724–9.

43. NCT01901094: Comparison of axillary lymph node dissection with axillary radiation for patients with node-positive breast cancer treated with chemotherapy. Available at: https://clinicaltrials.gov/ct2/show/NCT01901094. Accessed April 5, 2022.

44. NCT01872975: Standard or comprehensive radiation therapy in treating patients with early-stage breast cancer previously treated with chemotherapy and surgery. https://clinicaltrials.gov/ct2/show/NCT01872975. [Accessed 18 May 2022].

45. Joshi SC, Khan FA, Pant I, et al. Role of radiotherapy in early breast cancer: an overview. Int J Health Sci (Qassim) 2007;1(2):259–64.

46. Overgaard M, Hansen PS, Overgaard J, et al. Postoperative radiotherapy in high-risk premenopausal women with breast cancer who receive adjuvant chemotherapy. Danish Breast Cancer Cooperative Group 82b Trial. N Engl J Med 1997;337(14):949–55.

47. Overgaard M, Jensen MB, Overgaard J, et al. Postoperative radiotherapy in high-risk postmenopausal breast-cancer patients given adjuvant tamoxifen: Danish Breast Cancer Cooperative Group DBCG 82c randomised trial. Lancet 1999; 353(9165):1641–8.

48. Hughes KS, Schnaper LA, Berry D, et al. Lumpectomy plus Tamoxifen with or without Irradiation in Women 70 Years of Age or Older with Early Breast Cancer. N Engl J Med 2004;351(10):971–7.

49. Kunkler IH, Williams LJ, Jack WJ, et al. Breast-conserving surgery with or without irradiation in women aged 65 years or older with early breast cancer (PRIME II): a randomised controlled trial. *Lancet Oncol* Mar 2015;16(3):266–73.

50. Gradishar WJ, Moran MS, Abraham J, et al. NCCN Guidelines® Insights: Breast Cancer, Version 4.2021: Featured Updates to the NCCN Guidelines. J Natl Compr Cancer Netw 2021;19(5):484–93.

51. Njeh CF, Saunders MW, Langton CM. Accelerated Partial Breast Irradiation (APBI): A review of available techniques. Radiat Oncol 2010;5(1):90.

52. Legorreta AP, Liu X, Parker RG. Examining the use of breast-conserving treatment for women with breast cancer in a managed care environment. Am J Clin Oncol 2000;23(5):438–41.

53. Whelan TJ, Pignol J-P, Levine MN, et al. Long-Term Results of Hypofractionated Radiation Therapy for Breast Cancer. N Engl J Med 2010;362(6):513–20.

54. Bentzen SM, Agrawal RK, Aird EG, et al. The UK Standardisation of Breast Radiotherapy (START) Trial B of radiotherapy hypofractionation for treatment of early breast cancer: a randomised trial. *Lancet* Mar 2008;371(9618):1098–107.

55. Bentzen SM, Agrawal RK, Aird EG, et al. The UK Standardisation of Breast Radiotherapy (START) Trial A of radiotherapy hypofractionation for treatment of early breast cancer: a randomised trial. Lancet Oncol 2008;9(4):331–41.

56. Tann AW, Hatch SS, Joyner MM, et al. Accelerated partial breast irradiation: Past, present, and future. World J Clin Oncol 2016;7(5):370–9.

57. Vicini FA, Cecchini RS, White JR, et al. Long-term primary results of accelerated partial breast irradiation after breast-conserving surgery for early-stage breast cancer: a randomised, phase 3, equivalence trial. Lancet 2019;394(10215): 2155–64.

58. Vaidya JS, Bulsara M, Baum M, et al. Long term survival and local control outcomes from single dose targeted intraoperative radiotherapy during lumpectomy (TARGIT-IORT) for early breast cancer: TARGIT-A randomised clinical trial. BMJ 2020;370:m2836.

59. Orecchia R, Veronesi U, Maisonneuve P, et al. Intraoperative irradiation for early breast cancer (ELIOT): long-term recurrence and survival outcomes from a single-centre, randomised, phase 3 equivalence trial. Lancet Oncol 2021;22(5): 597–608.

60. Verrill M. Chemotherapy for early-stage breast cancer: a brief history. *Br J Cancer* Sep 2009;101(Suppl 1):S2–5.

61. Hensing W, Santa-Maria CA, Peterson LL, et al. Landmark trials in the medical oncology management of early stage breast cancer. Semin Oncol 2020;47(5): 278–92.

62. Paik S, Tang G, Shak S, et al. Gene Expression and Benefit of Chemotherapy in Women With Node-Negative, Estrogen Receptor–Positive Breast Cancer. J Clin Oncol 2006;24(23):3726–34.

63. Sparano JA, Gray RJ, Makower DF, et al. Adjuvant Chemotherapy Guided by a 21-Gene Expression Assay in Breast Cancer. N Engl J Med 2018;379(2):111–21.

64. Cardoso F, van't Veer LJ, Bogaerts J, et al. 70-Gene Signature as an Aid to Treatment Decisions in Early-Stage Breast Cancer. N Engl J Med 2016;375(8):717–29.

65. Kalinsky K, Barlow WE, Gralow JR, et al. 21-Gene Assay to Inform Chemotherapy Benefit in Node-Positive Breast Cancer. N Engl J Med 2021;385(25):2336–47.

66. Xin L, Liu YH, Martin TA, et al. The Era of Multigene Panels Comes? The Clinical Utility of Oncotype DX and MammaPrint. World J Oncol 2017;8(2):34–40.

67. Bradley R, Braybrooke J, Gray R, et al. Trastuzumab for early-stage, HER2-positive breast cancer: a meta-analysis of 13 864 women in seven randomised trials. Lancet Oncol 2021;22(8):1139–50.

68. Krop I, Ismaila N, Andre F, et al. Use of Biomarkers to Guide Decisions on Adjuvant Systemic Therapy for Women With Early-Stage Invasive Breast Cancer: American Society of Clinical Oncology Clinical Practice Guideline Focused Update. J Clin Oncol 2017;35(24):2838–47.

69. Perez EA, Romond EH, Suman VJ, et al. Four-year follow-up of trastuzumab plus adjuvant chemotherapy for operable human epidermal growth factor receptor 2-

positive breast cancer: joint analysis of data from NCCTG N9831 and NSABP B-31. J Clin Oncol 2011;29(25):3366–73.

70. Modi S, Ohtani S, Lee C, et al. Abstract OT1-07-02: A phase 3, multicenter, randomized, open-label trial of [fam-] trastuzumab deruxtecan (T-DXd; DS-8201a) vs investigator's choice in HER2-low breast cancer (DESTINY-Breast04). Cancer Res 2020;80(4_Supplement):OT1-07-02.

71. Fisher B, Brown A, Mamounas E, et al. Effect of preoperative chemotherapy on local-regional disease in women with operable breast cancer: findings from National Surgical Adjuvant Breast and Bowel Project B-18. J Clin Oncol 1997;15(7): 2483–93.

72. Haddad TC, Goetz MP. Landscape of neoadjuvant therapy for breast cancer. Ann Surg Oncol 2015;22(5):1408–15.

73. JAvd Hage, Velde CJHvd, Julien J-P, et al. Preoperative Chemotherapy in Primary Operable Breast Cancer: Results From the European Organization for Research and Treatment of Cancer Trial 10902. J Clin Oncol 2001;19(22):4224–37.

74. Wahba HA, El-Hadaad HA. Current approaches in treatment of triple-negative breast cancer. Cancer Biol Med 2015;12(2):106–16.

75. Masuda N, Lee S-J, Ohtani S, et al. Adjuvant capecitabine for breast cancer after preoperative chemotherapy. N Engl J Med 2017;376(22):2147–59.

76. Schmid P, Cortes J, Pusztai L, et al. Pembrolizumab for early triple-negative breast cancer. N Engl J Med 2020;382(9):810–21.

77. McAndrew NP, Finn RS. Clinical review on the management of hormone receptor–positive metastatic breast cancer. JCO Oncol Pract 2021;21:00384.

78. Chang Y-C, Cheung CHA, Kuo Y-L. Tamoxifen Rechallenge Decreases Metastatic Potential but Increases Cell Viability and Clonogenicity in a Tamoxifen-Mediated Cytotoxicity-Resistant Subline of Human Breast MCF7 Cancer Cells. Original Research. Frontiers in cell and developmental biology 2020;8. https://doi.org/10.3389/fcell.2020.00485.

79. Organisation NAT. Controlled trial of tamoxifen as adjuvant agent in management of early breast cancer: interim analysis at four years by nolvadex adjuvant trial organisation. Lancet 1983;321(8319):257–61.

80. Gradishar W. Landmark trials in endocrine adjuvant therapy for breast carcinoma. Cancer 2006;106(5):975–81.

81. Group EBCTC. Tamoxifen for early breast cancer: an overview of the randomised trials. Early Breast Cancer Trialists' Collaborative Group. Lancet 1998;351(9114): 1451–67.

82. Lorizio W, Wu AH, Beattie MS, et al. Clinical and biomarker predictors of side effects from tamoxifen. Breast Cancer Res Treat 2012;132(3):1107–18.

83. Chumsri S, Howes T, Bao T, et al. Aromatase, aromatase inhibitors, and breast cancer. J Steroid Biochem Mol Biol 2011;125(1–2):13–22.

84. Baum M, Budzar AU, Cuzick J, et al. Anastrozole alone or in combination with tamoxifen versus tamoxifen alone for adjuvant treatment of postmenopausal women with early breast cancer: first results of the ATAC randomised trial. Lancet 2002;359(9324):2131–9.

85. Sella T, Weiss A, Mittendorf EA, et al. Neoadjuvant Endocrine Therapy in Clinical Practice: A Review. JAMA Oncol 2021;7(11):1700–8.

86. Eiermann W, Paepke S, Appfelstaedt J, et al. Preoperative treatment of postmenopausal breast cancer patients with letrozole: A randomized double-blind multicenter study. Ann Oncol 2001;12(11):1527–32.

87. Barchiesi G, Mazzotta M, Krasniqi E, et al. Neoadjuvant Endocrine Therapy in Breast Cancer: Current Knowledge and Future Perspectives. Int J Mol Sci 2020;16(10):21.
88. ClinicalTrials.gov. Fulvestrant and/or Anastrozole in Treating Postmenopausal Patients With Stage II-III Breast Cancer Undergoing Surgery. https://www.clinicaltrials.gov/ct2/show/NCT01953588. [Accessed 18 May 2022].
89. Whitworth P, Beitsch P, Mislowsky A, et al. Chemosensitivity and Endocrine Sensitivity in Clinical Luminal Breast Cancer Patients in the Prospective Neoadjuvant Breast Registry Symphony Trial (NBRST) Predicted by Molecular Subtyping. Ann Surg Oncol 2017;24(3):669–75.

Genetics of Breast Cancer
Risk Models, Who to Test, and Management Options

Marguerite M. Rooney, BS[a], Krislyn N. Miller, DO[a],
Jennifer K. Plichta, MD, MS[a,b,c],*

KEYWORDS

- Breast cancer risk • Breast cancer genetics • Genetic testing
- Breast cancer prevention • Breast cancer screening

KEY POINTS

- Women age ≥25 years old should undergo breast cancer risk assessment, particularly those with a family history of cancer.
- Multiple risk models exist to help evaluate a patient's risk of developing breast cancer, and they differ based on the risk factors included and the types of risk calculations provided.
- Not all risk models are appropriate for assessing breast cancer risk for every patient.
- Depending on risk level or known genetic mutation, increased imaging surveillance may be recommended.
- Depending on risk level or known genetic mutation, bilateral risk-reducing mastectomy may be considered.

INTRODUCTION

Breast cancer is the most common noncutaneous cancer in women, with more than 285,000 estimated cases to be diagnosed in 2022 in the United States.[1] Efforts to improve breast cancer treatment and increase survival focus not only on treatment development and early detection but also on the identification of patients at a higher risk of developing breast cancer. Breast cancer risk factors can include hormonal and lifestyle factors, family history, and/or known germline mutations in a breast-cancer-related gene.[2] Current research has identified several germline mutations that contribute to a patient's risk of developing breast cancer.[3,4] In addition to known genetic mutations, patients can also be considered high risk based on family history alone.[5]

[a] Department of Surgery, Duke University Medical Center, Durham, NC 22710, USA; [b] Duke Cancer Institute, Duke University Medical Center, Durham, NC 22710, USA; [c] Department of Population Health Sciences, Duke University Medical Center, Durham, NC 27710, USA
* Corresponding author. Department of Surgery, Duke University Medical Center, DUMC 3513, Durham, NC 22710.
E-mail address: jennifer.plichta@duke.edu

Surg Clin N Am 103 (2023) 35–47
https://doi.org/10.1016/j.suc.2022.08.016
0039-6109/23/© 2022 Elsevier Inc. All rights reserved.

In all, approximately 5% to 10% of breast cancers are from identifiable germline genetic causes.[6] As such, many breast cancer risk models have been developed to combine risk factors to estimate an individual's risk of developing breast cancer, risk of carrying a BRCA1 or BRCA2 mutation, or the risk of both. These tools can assist clinicians when selecting which patients to refer for genetic counseling and when patients may qualify for genetic testing, increased imaging surveillance, and/or consideration of other medical or surgical interventions, thus helping to guide testing, treatment, and screening recommendations for these patients. Several organizations, including the National Comprehensive Cancer Network (NCCN), recommend genetic risk evaluation for selected patients. The American Society for Breast Surgeons (ASBrS) recommends that all women aged 25 years or more undergo formal risk assessment for breast cancer with updates based on changes in family or personal medical history.[7] The United States Preventive Services Task Force, meanwhile, recommends risk assessment only for patients with a personal or family history of breast, ovarian, tubal, or peritoneal cancers, or for those with ancestry associated with mutations, such as Ashkenazi Jews.[8,9]

At present, the NCCN does not recommend universal germline genetic testing for all patients with breast cancer, although the ASBrS does recommend offering genetic testing to all patients with breast cancer, recognizing insurance coverage may not consistently support this universal approach. The NCCN guidelines describe criteria for genetic testing based on a family history of several different cancers with associated ages at diagnosis for the affected family members. If patients do not meet the criteria set forth by the NCCN but do have a greater than 5% probability of a BRCA1/2 mutation based on risk models, testing may still be indicated, and it may even be considered for those patients with a 2.5% to 5% probability of a BRCA1/2 mutation based on these models.[10] Although there are many models, this article describes several of the most relevant and validated (**Table 1**).

MODELS: BREAST CANCER AND GENETIC RISK
Family History Assessment Tool

The Family History Assessment Tool (FHAT) is a validated scoring tool initially developed to help clinicians identify which patients would most benefit from a referral to genetic counseling based on family cancer history.[11] As expected with a first-pass screening tool, FHAT has high sensitivity (94%; specificity 51%), and as such does typically identify several false-positives.[12] Unlike the other models discussed later, this tool does not provide a percent likelihood of developing breast cancer but rather has a scoring threshold after which genetic counseling is recommended.

Breast Cancer Risk Assessment Tool

One of the earliest breast cancer risk models, Breast Cancer Risk Assessment Tool (BCRAT), based on the Gail Model, estimates the risk of developing invasive breast cancer in the next 5 years and through age 90 years (lifetime risk) for women older than 35 years using personal reproductive history and family history of first-degree relatives.[13] This model uses hormonal risk factors (age at menarche, age at first live birth) and pathologic (personal history of breast disease and breast biopsy). This model was initially developed on 280,000 white women aged 35 to 74 years in the Breast Cancer Detection Demonstration Project and Surveillance, Epidemiology, and End Results Program as a joint National Cancer Institute and American Society of Breast Cancer screening study.[14] Later, it was extended via smaller studies (ranging from 1563–3244 patients) to include risk assessment for black, Asian, Pacific Islander, and Hispanic women.[15–17] However, it is thought to underestimate risk for black women.[18]

Table 1

Selected breast cancer risk assessment models: model outputs, included personal and family risk factors, excluded populations

Model	FHAT[11]	BCRAT[13]	Claus Model[20,23]	BRCAPRO[66]	BOADICEA[27,67,68]	Tyrer-Cuzick[69]
Risk evaluation						
Evaluates risk of developing breast cancer	✓	✓	✓	✓	✓	✓
Evaluates risk of having BRCA1 or BRCA2				✓	✓	✓
Personal risk factor inclusion						
Age		✓	✓	✓	✓	✓
Race/ethnicity		✓		✓		✓
BMI						✓
Age at menarche		✓				✓
Age at first live birth		✓				✓
Age at menopause						✓
Hormone replacement therapy use						✓
Breast density						✓
History of prior breast biopsy		✓				✓
History of atypical ductal hyperplasia		✓				✓[a]
History of lobular carcinoma in situ						✓[a]
Family history inclusion						
First-degree relatives	✓	✓	✓	✓	✓	✓
Second-degree relatives	✓		✓	✓	✓	✓
Third-degree relatives	✓				✓	

(continued on next page)

Table 1
(continued)

Model	FHAT[11]	BCRAT[13]	Claus Model[20,23]	BRCAPRO[66]	BOADICEA[27,67,68]	Tyrer-Cuzick[69]
Age at onset of breast cancer	✓		✓	✓	✓	✓
Bilateral breast cancer	✓			✓	✓	✓
Ovarian cancer	✓			✓	✓	✓
Male breast cancer				✓	✓	
Excluded populations		• Personal history of breast cancer, DCIS, LCIS • Known BRCA1/2 mutation • Past chest radiation	• Patients without a family history of breast cancer			

Abbreviations: BCRAT, Breast Cancer Risk Assessment Tool; BMI, body mass index; BOADICEA, Breast and Ovarian Analysis of Disease Incidence and Carrier Estimation Algorithm; DCIS, ductal carcinoma in situ; FHAT, Family History Assessment Tool; LCIS, lobular carcinoma in situ.
[a] May overestimate risk in this population and therefore not be appropriate for use.

This model has also been demonstrated to underestimate the risk for women with atypical hyperplasia.[19]

Claus model
The Claus model was developed using a population-based, case-control study (Cancer and Steroid Hormone Study [CASH]), conducted by the Centers for Disease Control and Prevention.[20,21] This model does not include nonhereditary risk factors in determining lifetime risk of breast cancer and should be used only for women with at least 1 female first- or second-degree relative with breast cancer, based on the assumption that breast cancer is transmitted in an autosomal dominant manner.[12,22] There are 2 versions of the Claus model: risk tables ("Claus tables"), which are based on the model, and the model itself.[23]

MODELS: BREAST CANCER AND GENETIC RISK
BRCAPRO

BRCAPRO predicts a patient's probability of carrying a *BRCA1* or *BRCA2* mutation, the probability of developing invasive breast cancer or ovarian cancer (if not diagnosed with breast cancer), and the probability of developing a contralateral breast cancer (if breast cancer is present).[24,25] The model relies on family history (including relation, age at diagnosis, pathologic markers, race, ethnicity, and treatment), as well as prevalence and penetrance of *BRCA1* and *BRCA2* and baseline breast cancer rates in the population. The model then applies Bayes theorem.

Breast and Ovarian Analysis of Disease Incidence and Carrier Estimation Algorithm

Breast and Ovarian Analysis of Disease Incidence and Carrier Estimation Algorithm (BOADICEA) is intended for women with a family history that may suggest an increased risk of breast or ovarian cancer, to predict the probability of a *BRCA1* or *BRCA2* mutation and risk of developing breast cancer.[26,27] BOADICEA uses family history of breast and ovarian cancer to calculate risk.

Tyrer-Cuzick Model (International Breast Cancer Study)

The Tyrer-Cuzick model estimates a patient's risk of a *BRCA1* or *BRCA2* mutation and risk of developing an invasive or in situ cancer over time by using genetic and hormonal risk factors. Tyrer-Cuzick is particularly useful in populations that are at high risk based on family history where models such as the BCRAT are not as effective.[13] In addition, it predicts the risk of both invasive and in situ cancers rather than just invasive cancers. Importantly, this model has been demonstrated to overestimate invasive cancer risk in women with lobular carcinoma in situ and atypical hyperplasia, and other models may be more accurate for these patient populations.[28,29]

GERMLINE GENETIC TESTING

Genetic testing for breast cancer has grown considerably in recent history. When genetic testing for breast cancer was first available, only limited gene panels, typically evaluating only *BRCA1* and *BRCA2*, were available. However, only up to 30% of *genetically linked* breast cancers are driven by germline *BRCA1/2* mutations.[6] Now, multigene assays evaluating for high-, moderate-, and low-penetrance genes beyond just *BRCA1/2* are available. Therefore, there is a potential group of patients who received limited or single-gene genetic testing before 2014 who may benefit from repeat/expanded testing.[30]

Although expanding the criteria for germline genetic testing is gaining popularity and the NCCN guidelines become more inclusive every year, there remain several obstacles to testing. One of the main concerns is who will perform the genetic counseling and testing. Although there were an estimated 4700 genetic counselors in the United States in 2019, 17 states had 20 or fewer genetic counselors in the entire state, and 4 states had 5 or less.[31] Furthermore, many genetic counselors are not involved in direct patient care, opting instead to work for companies in industry or pharma; and of those seeing patients, many work in noncancer areas, such as prenatal genetics. To combat this problem, some have advocated for physicians to perform their own counseling and testing,[32] which is supported by several organizations in official statements and by providing education.[7,9,32] Beyond those limitations, cost also remains a concern. After identifying the association of *BRCA1* and *BRCA2* with breast cancer in the 1990s,[33,34] 1 company was performing all *BRCA1/2* testing. However, in 2013, the supreme court invalidated the gene patents for that company,[35] thus opening the door for new companies to offer genetic testing related to cancer; this ultimately led to the rapid decline in the cost of genetic testing from more than $4000 for *BRCA1/2* testing alone to now offering multigene panels for $250.[36] Although still not free or feasible for some patients, it is certainly much more attainable for many. It is also worth noting that direct-to-consumer testing is available, but it has not been validated for clinical use, and any "positive" results from these tests should be confirmed in a clinically approved laboratory certified by the Clinical Laboratory Improvement Amendments.[10]

Of the numerous clinically approved testing companies currently offering germline genetic testing, options include both limited and expanded panels. Some favor a more limited approach, testing for only those genes that are most likely to be related to the history presented. However, others prefer to test all genes that may have implications for the patient, even if the risk of harboring such a mutation is low, particularly given the decreasing cost and minimal difference in risk to the patient. Once a test is selected, patient samples can now be provided via multiple methods, such as blood draws and buccal swabs, or even saliva samples, although blood samples tend to be the most reliable (ie, adequate for testing).

When the results from a test return, 5 possible outcomes may be reported for any given variant identified: benign, likely benign, pathogenic, likely pathogenic, or variant of uncertain significance (VUS). As the names imply, benign and likely benign variants are considered "negative," and no further recommendations are typically required. In contrast, pathogenic and likely pathogenic variants are considered "positive" test results, and providers can refer to national guidelines, such as those published by the NCCN, for management recommendations.[10] For VUS findings, it is important to remember that these are actually considered "negative" as well, meaning that no intervention or management decision should be altered based on this finding. Although VUS rates for *BRCA1* and *BRCA2* have steadily declined as more patients have been tested, the expansion of testing to many other genes has yielded a notable increase in overall VUS rates.[37] However, this should similarly decline as again more patients, and particularly more diverse patient populations, are tested.

In addition, racial and ethnic disparities exist in access to and uptake of genetic testing for all cancers and in breast cancer in particular, with previous work demonstrating racial and ethnic disparities in genetic testing for solid tumor malignancies.[38,39] In breast cancer, previous work has shown how contributing factors such as decreased provider referrals, access, and awareness has led to lower rates of genetic testing for black women compared with their white counterparts.[40–44] As genetic testing becomes more and more common, it will be critical to make sure that all patients from diverse ethnic backgrounds have equal access to testing and to ensure the risk models and testing reflect the diversity of potential outcomes and risks based on racial and ethnic origins.

Genetic testing and risk modeling demonstrate the need for interdisciplinary care for the patient at high risk for the development of breast cancer. Although access to a genetic counselor allows for increased genetic testing and timely counseling, not all centers and patients have access.[45,46] In this setting, surgeons can play a critical role in conducting initial risk assessment, identifying patients who may benefit from genetic counseling, and often recommending and ordering genetic testing.[32]

IMAGE-BASED SCREENING FOR BREAST CANCER IN HIGH-RISK POPULATIONS

In addition to the general population screening guidelines, the NCCN has screening guidelines for patients with high- or moderate-risk gene mutations related to breast cancer. According to the 2022 NCCN guidelines, patients with high-risk gene mutations (ie, ≥50% absolute lifetime risk of breast cancer [BRCA1, BRCA2, CDH1, PALB2, PTEN, and TP53]) should follow specific screening guidelines. The NCCN recommends that for BRCA1 and BRCA2 mutation carriers, breast awareness should start at age 18 years, with clinical breast examinations every 6 to 12 months starting at age 25 years. Furthermore, breast cancer imaging/screening for women aged 25 to 29 years should include an annual breast MRI with contrast, or if MRI is unavailable, annual mammogram, with consideration of tomosynthesis. Women aged 30 to 75 years should receive an annual mammogram with consideration of tomosynthesis and a breast MRI with contrast; beyond age 75 years, management should be conducted on an individual basis. Notably, these same screening guidelines apply to women with BRCA1/2 mutations even after a breast cancer diagnosis, if they have residual breast tissue (underwent lumpectomy or only a unilateral mastectomy). Patients with a high-risk TP53 mutation have similar recommendations as those patients who are BRCA1/2 mutation carriers except for clinical breast examinations beginning at an even earlier age (ie, age 20 years or at the age of the earliest diagnosed breast cancer in the family if younger than 20 years). The recommendations for those women with CDH1, PALB2, and PTEN mutations consist of an annual mammogram with consideration of tomosynthesis and breast MRI with contrast starting at age 30 years.[47]

The NCCN recommends that those patients with moderate-risk mutations (20% to 50% absolute lifetime risk of developing breast cancer, ie, ATM, BARD1, CDH1, CHEK2, and NF1) undergo annual screening mammography with consideration of tomosynthesis and breast MRI with contrast. The age of starting this screening depends on the gene mutation. For instance, those with CDH1 and NF1 are recommended to begin screening mammography and MRI at age 30 years, whereas women with ATM, CHEK2, and BARD1 mutations are recommended to begin at age 40 years.[47]

Because women with high-risk genes tend to develop breast cancer at a younger age when breast tissue is dense, the sensitivity of mammography alone is lower. In high-risk women, the sensitivity of MRI detecting a breast abnormality ranges from 77% to 100% with a specificity of 81% to 98.9%; this compares to mammography, which has a sensitivity of 12.5% to 40% and specificity of 93% to 100%. Therefore, mammography in association with MRI is the standard screening recommendation in these moderate- to high-risk women.[48] There are certain criteria required for the administration of a high-quality MRI screening, including regional availability, a radiologist with breast MRI imaging experience, the ability to perform biopsy under MRI guidance, and dedicated breast coils specific for breast imaging.[47] In addition to unavailability, reasons for declining MRIs for screening purposes include patient claustrophobia, patient time constraints, financial concerns, referral issues, body habitus, body implants, and frailty.[49]

Screening with whole breast ultrasonography (WBUS) is another imaging tool used for women who cannot or do not wish to undergo MRIs. Overall, this modality is well tolerated, widely available, relatively inexpensive, and does not require intravenous contrast or ionizing radiation. WBUS has been shown to detect cancers not seen on mammography with a greater sensitivity in dense breast. Concerns include the need for a highly experienced technologist and the inability to detect calcifications.[50]

Contrast-enhanced mammography (CEM), which uses modified digital mammography with the addition of an intravenous contrast agent, is another imaging modality that is not standard for breast cancer screening, yet shows promise for the future.[51] In a retrospective study by Sung and colleagues,[51] 904 patients received baseline CEM screenings with 1-year follow-up. Results showed a breast cancer detection rate of 15.5 of 1000, sensitivity increased from 50% with the standard mammography to 87.5% with CEM (p = 0.03), and specificity was 93.7% (95% confidence interval, 91.9%–95.3%).[51] Other imaging modalities, such as thermography, which detects localized skin temperature gradients and produces a heat map of the breast (thermogram), have been theorized to identify developing tumors; yet, there is insufficient evidence to support its use in breast cancer screening.[52]

ROLE OF RISK-REDUCING BREAST SURGERY

According to the NCCN guidelines, bilateral risk-reducing mastectomy (BRRM) may be considered and discussed with all women with a high-risk pathogenic/likely pathogenic germline genetic mutation, which includes *BRCA1, BRCA2, CDH1, PALB2, PTEN,* and *TP53.* Discussions should include the degree of protection, reconstruction options, and residual breast cancer risk with age and life expectancy.[47] Surgical risk-reducing mastectomies include simple, total, skin-sparing, or nipple-sparing mastectomies, all of which have been shown to be safe and feasible options for women choosing a risk-reducing surgery. Regardless of the type of mastectomy, the goal is to remove as much of the breast tissue as possible for the obvious reason of reducing the risk of developing breast cancer.[48] In a review of 201 BRCA1/2 carriers, Yao and colleagues demonstrated that nipple-sparing mastectomies have a low rate of complications and locoregional recurrence. Loss of the nipple areolar complex occurred in 1.8% of the patients, flap necrosis in 2.5%, and there were 4 recurrences (none at the nipple areolar complex and 3 in patients with cancer) over a mean follow-up time of 32.6 months.[53] Reconstruction options using implant-based (silicone or saline) prepectoral or postpectoral versus autogenous flap grafts should be part of the discussion with the patient when they are opting for BRRM.[48]

BRRM reduces the risk of developing breast cancer by more than 90%[54]; however, the survival benefit is unclear. According to Heemskerk-Gerritsen and colleagues,[55] who reviewed 2857 BRCA1/2 mutation carriers in the Netherlands, 42% of the *BRCA1* and 35% of the *BRCA2* mutation carriers received BRRMs. During a mean follow-up of 10 years, breast cancer-specific survival of women at age 65 years with *BRCA1* mutations was 93% for patients receiving surveillance versus 99.7% for those who had BRRM, in contrast to patients with a *BRCA2* mutation, for which rates were 98% and 100%, respectively. Overall, they concluded that BRRM for *BRCA1* mutation carriers was associated with lower mortality, but not necessarily for *BRCA2* mutation carriers.[55]

Consideration around unwanted secondary effects such as chronic pain, decreased body image, and decreased sexual satisfaction also needs to be part of the BRRM discussion. A 2018 Cochrane review looked at these psychosocial effects, reporting that generally, patients were satisfied with their decision for BRRM, but their psychological well-being was impacted.[54] In particular, Gahm and colleagues[56] demonstrated in their review of 59 women post-BRRM that 69% reported chronic pain, 71% reported discomfort in their breasts, and 85% had reduced sexual sensations, which all negatively impacted their enjoyment of sex. However, their quality of life and feelings of regret were not a factor.[56] An additional Cochrane review specifically focused on the psychosocial interventions and the effect these had on the quality of life and emotional well-being in female BRCA mutation carriers who underwent BRRM. Unfortunately, only 2 studies with small sample sizes fit the review criteria and no conclusions could be drawn from the data. These findings (or lack thereof) further emphasize the importance of supporting women when they choose this type of elective risk-reducing surgery and the need for further research in this area of long-term outcomes for risk-reducing surgery.[57]

TREATMENT OF BREAST CANCER IN HIGH-RISK PATIENTS

For women with a genetic predisposition to breast cancer who develop breast cancer, survival outcomes may vary. However, a systematic review and meta-analysis of 66 studies of patients with breast cancer and BRCA1/2 mutations noted that the evidence was inconclusive, because some studies suggested worse outcomes, whereas others demonstrated relatively more favorable survival outcomes.[58] Given no clear difference in survival outcomes, patients with BRCA1/2 mutations and breast cancer may still be eligible for breast-conserving therapy (lumpectomy and radiation), similar to those patients with breast cancer and no BRCA1/2 mutation.[59] However, patients with BRCA1/2 mutations do have an increased risk of developing a contralateral (or second primary) breast cancer, potentially as high as greater than 30%, depending on the age at diagnosis of the first breast cancer.[60] As such, many women with BRCA1/2 mutations and breast cancer may opt for bilateral mastectomies (1 therapeutic and 1 prophylactic) to reduce that risk of a second breast cancer.[61]

Beyond surgery, there are now systemic therapy options that are specific to women with a genetic predisposition to breast cancer. For example, the recently published OlympiA trial demonstrated that women with BRCA1/2 mutations and early breast cancer may benefit from 1 year of an adjuvant poly(adenosine diphosphate-ribose) polymerase inhibitor (PARPi).[62] Similar benefits were previously demonstrated for women with BRCA1/2 mutations and metastatic/advanced breast cancer as well.[63,64] In addition to its impact on systemic therapy options, the results of genetic testing may also impact radiation therapy recommendations, because women with TP53 mutations or homozygous ATM mutations are generally advised to avoid therapeutic radiation.[65] As more women with a genetic predisposition to (breast) cancer are identified, more research will undoubtedly reveal additional areas where we can personalize treatment recommendations for our patients.

SUMMARY

Genetic testing plays an important role in assessing breast cancer risk and often the risk of other types of cancers. Accurate risk assessment and stratification represents a critical element of identifying who is best served by increased surveillance and consideration of other prevention or treatment options while also limiting overtreatment and unnecessary testing. Given the implications of these types of genetic test results, the indications for testing will likely continue to expand, and ideally, more women with a genetic predisposition to breast cancer will be identified before they are diagnosed with breast cancer and thus have the option to consider effective screening and prevention management strategies.

CLINICS CARE POINTS

- Women aged 25 years or older should undergo breast cancer risk assessment, particularly those with a family history of cancer.
- Multiple risk models exist to help evaluate a patient's risk of developing breast cancer, and they differ based on the risk factors included and the types of risk calculations provided.
- Not all risk models are appropriate for assessing breast cancer risk for every patient.
- The indications for germline genetic testing are continually expanding.
- Depending on the risk level or known genetic mutation, increased imaging surveillance may be recommended.
- Depending on the risk level or known genetic mutation, BRRM may be considered.

DISCLOSURE

- The authors report no proprietary or commercial interest in any product mentioned or concept.
- Dr J.K. Plichta is a recipient of research funding by the Color Foundation (PI: J.K. Plichta). She serves on the National Comprehensive Cancer Network (NCCN) Breast Cancer Screening Committee.

REFERENCES

1. Breast cancer facts & figures, Am Cancer Soc, 2021, Available at: https://www.cancer.org/content/dam/cancer-org/research/cancer-facts-and-statistics/annual-cancer-facts-and-figures/2020/cancer-facts-and-figures-2020.pdf.   Accessed August 4, 2021.
2. Rojas K, Stuckey A. Breast cancer epidemiology and risk factors. Clin Obstet Gynecol 2016;59:651–72.
3. Shiovitz S, Korde LA. Genetics of breast cancer: a topic in evolution. Ann Oncol 2015;26:1291–9.
4. Valencia OM, Samuel SE, Viscusi RK, et al. The role of genetic testing in patients with breast cancer: a review. JAMA Surg 2017;152:589–94.
5. Keeney MG, Couch FJ, Visscher DW, et al. Non-BRCA familial breast cancer: review of reported pathology and molecular findings. Pathology 2017;49:363–70.
6. Economopoulou P, Dimitriadis G, Psyrri A. Beyond BRCA: new hereditary breast cancer susceptibility genes. Cancer Treat Rev 2015;41:1–8.
7. Consensus Guideline on Hereditary Genetic Testing for Patients With and Without Breast Cancer. Available at: https://www.breastsurgeons.org/about/statements/PDF_Statements/BRCA_Testing.pdf. Accessed August/13/2018.
8. Owens DK, Davidson KW, Krist AH, et al. Risk assessment, genetic counseling, and genetic testing for BRCA-related cancer. JAMA 2019;322:652.
9. Rajagopal PS, Nielsen S, Olopade OI. USPSTF recommendations for BRCA1 and BRCA2 testing in the context of a transformative national cancer control plan. JAMA Netw Open 2019;2:e1910142.
10. Daly MB, Pal T, Berry MP, et al. Genetic/familial high-risk assessment: breast, ovarian, and pancreatic, version 2.2021, NCCN clinical practice guidelines in oncology. J Natl Compr Canc Netw 2021;19:77–102.

11. Gilpin C, Carson N, Hunter A. A preliminary validation of a family history assessment form to select women at risk for breast or ovarian cancer for referral to a genetics center. Clin Genet 2000;58:299–308.
12. Cintolo-Gonzalez JA, Braun D, Blackford AL, et al. Breast cancer risk models: a comprehensive overview of existing models, validation, and clinical applications. Breast Cancer Res Treat 2017;164:263–84.
13. . https://bcrisktool.cancer.gov/.
14. Gail MH, Brinton LA, Byar DP, et al. Projecting individualized probabilities of developing breast cancer for white females who are being examined annually. J Natl Cancer Inst 1989;81:1879–86.
15. Matsuno RK, Costantino JP, Ziegler RG, et al. Projecting individualized absolute invasive breast cancer risk in asian and pacific islander american women. J Natl Cancer Inst 2011;103:951–61.
16. Gail MH, Costantino JP, Pee D, et al. Projecting individualized absolute invasive breast cancer risk in african american women. J Natl Cancer Inst 2007;99:1782–92.
17. Banegas MP, John EM, Slattery ML, et al. Projecting Individualized absolute invasive breast cancer risk in US hispanic women. J Natl Cancer Inst 2017;109: djw215.
18. Adams-Campbell LL, Makambi KH, Palmer JR, et al. Diagnostic accuracy of the Gail model in the Black Women's Health Study. Breast J 2007;13:332–6.
19. Pankratz VS, Hartmann LC, Degnim AC, et al. Assessment of the accuracy of the Gail model in women with atypical hyperplasia. J Clin Oncol 2008;26:5374–9.
20. Claus EB, Risch N, Thompson WD. Genetic analysis of breast cancer in the cancer and steroid hormone study. Am J Hum Genet 1991;48:232–42.
21. Evans DGR, Howell A. Breast cancer risk-assessment models. Breast Cancer Res 2007;9:213.
22. Kim G, Bahl M. Assessing risk of breast cancer: a review of risk prediction models. J Breast Imaging 2021;3:144–55.
23. Claus EB, Risch N, Thompson WD. Autosomal dominant inheritance of early-onset breast cancer. Implications for risk prediction. Cancer 1994;73:643–51.
24. Parmigiani G, Berry D, Aguilar O. Determining carrier probabilities for breast cancer-susceptibility genes BRCA1 and BRCA2. Am J Hum Genet 1998;62:145–58.
25. Mazzola E, Blackford A, Parmigiani G, et al. Recent enhancements to the genetic risk prediction model BRCAPRO. Cancer Inform 2015;14s2:CIN.S17292.
26. Antoniou AC, Pharoah PD, McMullan G, et al. A comprehensive model for familial breast cancer incorporating BRCA1, BRCA2 and other genes. Br J Cancer 2002; 86:76–83.
27. Antoniou AC, Pharoah PP, Smith P, et al. The BOADICEA model of genetic susceptibility to breast and ovarian cancer. Br J Cancer 2004;91:1580–90.
28. Valero MG, Zabor EC, Park A, et al. The tyrer–cuzick model inaccurately predicts invasive breast cancer risk in women with LCIS. Ann Surg Oncol 2020;27:736–40.
29. Boughey JC, Hartmann LC, Anderson SS, et al. Evaluation of the Tyrer-Cuzick (International Breast Cancer Intervention Study) model for breast cancer risk prediction in women with atypical hyperplasia. J Clin Oncol 2010;28:3591–6.
30. Maxwell KN, Wubbenhorst B, D'Andrea K, et al. Prevalence of mutations in a panel of breast cancer susceptibility genes in BRCA1/2-negative patients with early-onset breast cancer. Genet Med 2015;17:630–8.
31. Cosgrove J., Genetic services: information on genetic counselor and medical geneticist workforces, In: Office G.A., Online, 2019, United State Government Accountability Office, 1-45, Available at: https://www.gao.gov/assets/gao-20-593.pdf. Accessed January 4, 2022..

32. Plichta JK, Sebastian ML, Smith LA, et al. Germline genetic testing: what the breast surgeon needs to know. Ann Surg Oncol 2019;26:2184–90.

33. Hall JM, Lee MK, Newman B, et al. Linkage of early-onset familial breast cancer to chromosome 17q21. Science 1990;250:1684–9.

34. Wooster R, Neuhausen SL, Mangion J, et al. Localization of a breast cancer susceptibility gene, BRCA2, to chromosome 13q12-13. Science 1994;265:2088–90.

35. Supreme Court Decision in Association for Molecular Pathology v. Myriad Genetics, Inc. 2013. Available at: https://www.supremecourt.gov/opinions/12pdf/12-398_1b7d.pdf. Accessed September 11, 2016.

36. Plichta JK, Griffin M, Thakuria J, et al. What's new in genetic testing for cancer susceptibility? Oncology (Williston Park) 2016;30:787–99.

37. Welsh JL, Hoskin TL, Day CN, et al. Clinical decision-making in patients with variant of uncertain significance in BRCA1 or BRCA2 genes. Ann Surg Oncol 2017;24:3067–72.

38. Dillon J, Ademuyiwa FO, Barrett M, et al. Disparities in genetic testing for heritable solid-tumor malignancies. Surg Oncol Clin N Am 2022;31:109–26.

39. Ademuyiwa FO, Salyer P, Ma Y, et al. Assessing the effectiveness of the National Comprehensive Cancer Network genetic testing guidelines in identifying African American breast cancer patients with deleterious genetic mutations. Breast Cancer Res Treat 2019;178:151–9.

40. Chapman-Davis E, Zhou ZN, Fields JC, et al. Racial and ethnic disparities in genetic testing at a hereditary breast and ovarian cancer center. J Gen Intern Med 2021;36:35–42.

41. Forman AD, Hall MJ. Influence of race/ethnicity on genetic counseling and testing for hereditary breast and ovarian cancer. Breast J 2009;15(Suppl 1):S56–62.

42. Reid S, Cadiz S, Pal T. Disparities in genetic testing and care among black women with hereditary breast cancer. Curr Breast Cancer Rep 2020;12:125–31.

43. Cragun D, Weidner A, Lewis C, et al. Racial disparities in BRCA testing and cancer risk management across a population-based sample of young breast cancer survivors. Cancer 2017;123:2497–505.

44. Ademuyiwa FO, Salyer P, Tao Y, et al. Genetic counseling and testing in african american patients with breast cancer: a nationwide survey of US breast oncologists. J Clin Oncol 2021;39(36):4020–8.

45. Eichmeyer JN, Zuckerman DS, Beck TM, et al. The value of a genetic counselor for patient identification. J Clin Oncol 2012;30:97.

46. Pederson HJ, Hussain N, Noss R, et al. Impact of an embedded genetic counselor on breast cancer treatment. Breast Cancer Res Treat 2018;169:43–6.

47. Daly M.B., Pal T., Arun B., et al., NCCN Clinical Practice Guidelines in Oncology: Genetic/Familial High-Risk Assessment: Breast, Ovarian, and Pancreatic, Version 2022. Available online at: https://www.nccn.org/professionals/physician_gls/pdf/genetics_bop.pdf. Accessed January 4, 2022.

48. Bland KCE, Klimberg V, Gradishar W. The breast comprehensive management of benign and malignant diseases. 5th ed. Philadelphia, PA: Elsevier; 2018.

49. Vourtsis A, Berg WA. Breast density implications and supplemental screening. Eur Radiol 2019;29:1762–77.

50. Geisel J, Raghu M, Hooley R. The role of ultrasound in breast cancer screening: the case for and against ultrasound. Semin Ultrasound CT MR 2018;39:25–34.

51. Sung JS, Lebron L, Keating D, et al. Performance of dual-energy contrast-enhanced digital mammography for screening women at increased risk of breast cancer. Radiology 2019;293:81–8.

52. Vreugdenburg TD, Willis CD, Mundy L, et al. A systematic review of elastography, electrical impedance scanning, and digital infrared thermography for breast cancer screening and diagnosis. Breast Cancer Res Treat 2013;137:665–76.
53. Yao K, Liederbach E, Tang R, et al. Nipple-sparing mastectomy in BRCA1/2 mutation carriers: an interim analysis and review of the literature. Ann Surg Oncol 2015;22:370–6.
54. Carbine NE, Lostumbo L, Wallace J, et al. Risk-reducing mastectomy for the prevention of primary breast cancer. Cochrane Database Syst Rev 2018;4: Cd002748.
55. Heemskerk-Gerritsen BAM, Jager A, Koppert LB, et al. Survival after bilateral risk-reducing mastectomy in healthy BRCA1 and BRCA2 mutation carriers. Breast Cancer Res Treat 2019;177:723–33.
56. Gahm J, Wickman M, Brandberg Y. Bilateral prophylactic mastectomy in women with inherited risk of breast cancer–prevalence of pain and discomfort, impact on sexuality, quality of life and feelings of regret two years after surgery. Breast 2010; 19:462–9.
57. Jeffers L, Reid J, Fitzsimons D, et al. Interventions to improve psychosocial well-being in female BRCA-mutation carriers following risk-reducing surgery. Cochrane Database Syst Rev 2019;10:Cd012894.
58. van den Broek AJ, Schmidt MK, van 't Veer LJ, et al. Worse breast cancer prognosis of BRCA1/BRCA2 mutation carriers: what's the evidence? A systematic review with meta-analysis. PLoS One 2015;10:e0120189.
59. van den Broek AJ, Schmidt MK, van 't Veer LJ, et al. Prognostic impact of breast-conserving therapy versus mastectomy of BRCA1/2 mutation carriers compared with noncarriers in a consecutive series of young breast cancer patients. Ann Surg 2019;270:364–72.
60. van den Broek AJ, van 't Veer LJ, Hooning MJ, et al. Impact of age at primary breast cancer on contralateral breast cancer risk in BRCA1/2 mutation carriers. J Clin Oncol 2016;34:409–18.
61. Ludwig KK, Neuner J, Butler A, et al. Risk reduction and survival benefit of prophylactic surgery in BRCA mutation carriers, a systematic review. Am J Surg 2016;212:660–9.
62. Tutt ANJ, Garber JE, Kaufman B, et al. Adjuvant olaparib for patients with BRCA1- or BRCA2-mutated breast cancer. N Engl J Med 2017;377(6):523–33.
63. Robson M, Im SA, Senkus E, et al. Olaparib for metastatic breast cancer in patients with a germline BRCA mutation. N Engl J Med 2017;377:523–33.
64. Litton JK, Rugo HS, Ettl J, et al. Talazoparib in patients with advanced breast cancer and a germline BRCA mutation. N Engl J Med 2018;379:753–63.
65. Gradishar WJ, Moran MS, Abraham J, et al. NCCN Guidelines: Breast Cancer (version 1.2022) 2021;1. 2022. Available at: https://www.nccn.org/professionals/physician_gls/pdf/breast.pdf. Accessed December 13, 2021.
66. Berry DA, Iversen ES Jr, Gudbjartsson DF, et al. BRCAPRO validation, sensitivity of genetic testing of BRCA1/BRCA2, and prevalence of other breast cancer susceptibility genes. J Clin Oncol 2002;20:2701–12.
67. Antoniou AC, Cunningham AP, Peto J, et al. The BOADICEA model of genetic susceptibility to breast and ovarian cancers: updates and extensions. Br J Cancer 2008;98:1457–66.
68. https://ccge.medschl.cam.ac.uk/boadicea/boadicea-web-application/. [Accessed 4 January 2022].
69. https://ems-trials.org/riskevaluator/. [Accessed 4 January 2022].

Genomic Profiling and Liquid Biopsies for Breast Cancer

Clayton T. Marcinak, MD[a,b,1],
Muhammed Murtaza, MBBS, PhD[a,b,2], Lee G. Wilke, MD[a,c],*

KEYWORDS

• Breast cancer • Genomics • Sequencing • Liquid biopsy • Oncology

KEY POINTS

• Multiple gene-expression profiling assays are now commercially available. One assay, OncotypeDx, has been incorporated into staging and treatment guidelines, with high-level evidence supporting its use as a clinical decision-making tool.
• Next-generation sequencing of the cancer genome has led to a wealth of new information regarding potential pathways of treatment and resistance.
• Analysis of cell-free DNA is a promising avenue of research and development, including in the realm of early detection and monitoring of minimal residual disease.

INTRODUCTION

In the early 2000s, with the mapping of the human genome and The Cancer Genome Atlas (TCGA), great advances were made in understanding the genomic alterations underlying many diseases, inclusive of neoplasms.[1] In breast cancer, researchers and society in general had previously come to widely appreciate the genetic basis of cancer—that is, the inherited predisposition to the disease posed by somatic mutations such as *BRCA1*, *BRCA2*, *PALB2*, *CDH1*, and others.[2] In contrast, the cancer genome refers to those mutations identified in a malignancy, rather than germline mutations found in all of an individual's cells. These genomic alterations have shown utility as markers for both targeted therapy and patient-specific treatment plans, giving rise to the era of precision oncology.

[a] Department of Surgery, University of Wisconsin–Madison, Madison, WI, USA; [b] Center for Human Genomics and Precision Medicine, University of Wisconsin–Madison, Madison, WI, USA; [c] University of Wisconsin Carbone Cancer Center, Madison, WI, USA
[1] Present address: 600 Highland Avenue, MC 7375, Madison, WI 53792.
[2] Present address: 1111 Highland Avenue, WIMR West Wedge 2770, Madison, WI 53705.
* Corresponding author. 600 Highland Avenue, K4/624, Madison, WI 53792.
E-mail address: wilke@surgery.wisc.edu
Twitter: @ctmarcinak (C.T.M.); @LeeWilke (L.G.W.)

Surg Clin N Am 103 (2023) 49–61
https://doi.org/10.1016/j.suc.2022.08.003
0039-6109/23/© 2022 Elsevier Inc. All rights reserved.

surgical.theclinics.com

This paradigm shift has been particularly striking in breast cancer, starting with the use of tamoxifen for hormone-receptor-positive tumors.[3-5] The identification of the role of *HER2/neu* in the pathogenesis of breast cancer served as another landmark in the development of targeted therapy.[6,7] Perou and colleagues[8] described four different subtypes of breast cancer based on "molecular portraits." These discoveries marked the beginning of a series of breakthroughs that have rapidly changed our understanding and treatment of this disease. As of the 2020s, breast cancer is widely considered the malignancy with the most personalized treatment approach, incorporating a combination of clinical factors, histopathology, immunohistochemistry, genomic assays, and next-generation sequencing (NGS). In this article, we present the current established genomic approaches to breast cancer, as well as recent cutting-edge investigations that will guide the future of personalized therapy.

Gene-Expression Profiling

Introduction
Genomic-informed treatment of breast cancer began with the development of gene-expression assays. This technology is based on varied polymerase chain reaction (PCR) methods that provide a snapshot of a tumor's molecular aberrancy. In this section, we will discuss available gene-expression profile assays and their utility in clinical decision-making and prognostication.

Basic principles
Four gene-expression profiling assays are currently commercially available: OncotypeDx, MammaPrint, PAM50 (also called Prosigna), and EndoPredict (EP). Despite differences in their development, included genes, and target patient population, all four assays stratify a subset of patients with breast cancer using genomic information without requiring DNA or RNA sequencing.

OncotypeDx uses reverse-transcriptase polymerase chain reaction (RT-PCR) and a multigene panel composed of 16 cancer genes and 5 reference genes to provide a recurrence score between 0 (lowest risk) and 100 (highest risk) for patients with hormone receptor (HR)-positive, human epidermal growth factor receptor 2 (HER2)-negative tumors.[9] Using this score, patients are categorized as low, intermediate, or high risk for recurrence. Since 2016, the American Joint Commission on Cancer has incorporated OncotypeDx as a component of the breast cancer staging for patients with T1 or T2 tumors that are estrogen receptor (ER) positive and HER2 negative.[10]

MammaPrint incorporates a panel of 70 genes and mRNA microarrays. MammaPrint categorizes breast cancer patients with HER2-negative tumors as either low or high risk of distant metastases, regardless of ER or lymph node status.[11,12] Tumors must be less than or equal to 5 cm in greatest dimension, and a patient should have no more than three positive lymph nodes.

PAM50 (Prosigna) is a quantitative PCR (qPCR) assay of 50 genes that provides clinicians and patients with two pieces of information: a risk of recurrence score (ROR) and a molecular subtype according to the classification by Perou and colleagues[13-15] The ROR is then used to classify a patient as having a low, medium, or high risk of recurrence. This assay is also designed for patients with HR-positive tumors. The PAM50 test has been adapted to use the NanoString nCounter instrument to allow pathology labs within the broader community to run the assay.[13]

Finally, EP uses RT-PCR and a panel of 11 genes—eight cancer-related genes and three reference genes—to provide an EP score, which ranges from 0 to 15. The EP score, nodal status, and tumor size can be combined to calculate the EPclin (or EP clinical) score, which ranges from 0 to 8.[16] An EPclin score of 3.3 or greater indicates a high risk of distant recurrence.

Clinical utility of gene-expression assays

Several large studies have been conducted to evaluate the clinical utility of each of these four assays. For this article, we focus on the most relevant data with the highest level of evidence, which is available for OncotypeDx and MammaPrint.

The first compelling evidence concerning the OncotypeDx assay was published in 2004. In this validation study, the investigators performed the assay on 668 formalin-fixed, paraffin-embedded (FFPE) tissue blocks from patients with tamoxifen-treated, lymph node-negative tumors.[9] Their primary outcome was to determine if a larger proportion of patients in the low-risk category (ie, a recurrence score <18) were free of distant recurrence at 10 years than patients in the high-risk category (a recurrence score of 31 or higher). Of the 338 patients in the low-risk category, 93.2% were free of distant recurrence at 10 years, compared with 69.5% of the 151 patients in the high-risk category (P < 0.001). In addition, in a multivariate Cox regression, the OncotypeDx recurrence score proved to be a predictive marker of distance recurrence, independent of patient age and tumor size. Finally, the OncotypeDx recurrence score was correlated with both relapse-free survival and overall survival.

Approximately 10 years after this initial validation on FFPE, prospective data regarding the use of OncotypeDx as a clinical decision-making tool began to appear in the literature. Two large clinical trials, TAILORx and RxPONDER, provided the largest body of evidence. The first results from TAILORx were published in 2015.[17] Investigators enrolled 10,253 eligible patients with HR-positive, HER2-negative, and lymph node-negative cancer who met the clinicopathologic criteria for consideration of adjuvant chemotherapy. Patients with an OncotypeDx recurrence score between 0 and 10 (n = 1,626) were given endocrine therapy alone, whereas the patients with a recurrence score of 26 or higher (n = 1,730) were given both adjuvant endocrine therapy and chemotherapy. Patients with scores from 11 to 25 (n = 6,897) were randomly assigned to receive either endocrine therapy alone or both adjuvant treatments. Patients with a recurrence score from 0 to 10 showed the following event rates at 5 years: a 93.8% rate of invasive disease-free survival, a 99.3% rate of freedom from distant recurrence, a 98.7% rate of freedom from any recurrence, and a 98.0% rate of overall survival.

An analysis of the patients with an intermediate recurrence score (11–25)—who were randomized to either endocrine therapy only or both chemotherapy and endocrine therapy—was published in 2018. Ultimately, 6,711 patients were included in the final analysis.[18] Endocrine therapy alone was found to be non-inferior to combined chemotherapy plus endocrine therapy in both intention-to-treat and as-treated analyses. In the exploratory analysis, patients aged 50 years or younger with a recurrence score between 16 and 25 showed a higher rate of freedom from distant recurrence at both 5- and 9-year follow-up intervals with the addition of chemotherapy but had equivalent overall survival with either treatment approach.

Finally, an analysis of the high recurrence score (26+) patients in TAILORx was published in 2020.[19] Of the original high score cohort of 1,730 patients, data were available for 1,389, and adjuvant chemotherapy and endocrine therapy were administered to 1,300 patients. This final cohort showed the following event rates at 5 years: 87.6% rate of invasive disease-free survival, a 93.0% rate of freedom from distant recurrence, a 91.0% rate of freedom from any recurrence, and a 95.9% overall survival. The investigators used data from the National Surgical Adjuvant Breast and Bowel Project (NSABP) B-20 trial to estimate the rate of freedom from distant recurrence if the cohort had not received chemotherapy, with notably lower 5-year rates of 78.8% and 9-year rates of 65.4%. The aggregate evidence from the TAILORx trial suggests that the 21-gene OncotypeDx assay is a key tool to determine which patients with HR-positive, HER2-negative, and lymph node-negative disease would derive benefit from the addition of adjuvant chemotherapy.

By contrast, the RxPONDER trial sought to determine the role of the OncotypeDx assay in patients with lymph node-positive disease. A total of 5,083 women with HR-positive, HER2-negative, N1 disease (ie, between 1 and 3 positive lymph nodes), and a recurrence score between 0 and 25 were randomized to receive either adjuvant endocrine therapy alone or a combination of adjuvant chemotherapy plus endocrine therapy.[20] In the 3,353 postmenopausal patients, adjuvant chemotherapy showed no benefit in 5-year rates of invasive disease-free survival, a new primary cancer, or death. Meanwhile, in the 1,665 premenopausal patients, a slight benefit was shown in the chemotherapy group, with a hazard ratio of 0.60 (95% confidence interval [CI], 0.43–0.83) for 5-year rates of invasive disease-free survival, a new primary cancer, or death. In summary, RxPONDER showed that postmenopausal patients with N1 disease and low recurrence scores on the OncotypeDx assay do not benefit from adjuvant chemotherapy, whereas premenopausal patients likely derive a benefit that may be related to the temporary or permanent ovarian suppression provided by cytotoxic treatment. Owing to the high level of evidence from TAILORx and RxPONDER supporting its use, OncotypeDx has now incorporated into the National Comprehensive Cancer Network (NCCN) guidelines for breast cancer.[21]

The MINDACT trial is the largest randomized prospective study to assess the clinical utility of MammaPrint. Published in 2016 and updated in 2021, MINDACT enrolled 6,693 patients with early-stage breast cancer—defined as T1, T2, or operable T3—at over 100 European medical centers.[22,23] Unlike the TAILORx and RxPONDER studies, the MINDACT investigators enrolled patients regardless of HR or HER2 status; however, the cohort was restricted to patients with N0 or N1 disease. Each patient's risk was determined using two methods: genomic risk (high vs low) determined by MammaPrint, whereas the clinical risk was determined by a modified Adjuvant! Online risk assessment tool.[24] Those women with ER-positive breast cancer deemed to have both low genomic and low clinical risk received adjuvant endocrine therapy only, and those with both high genomic and high clinical risk received both chemotherapy and endocrine therapy. Those women with discordant risks (n = 2,142) were randomly assigned to either the chemotherapy or no-chemotherapy arm. The patients with low clinical risk and a high MammaPrint genomic risk did not derive benefit from chemotherapy in the four primary outcomes: distant metastasis-free survival, distant metastasis-free interval, disease-free survival, and overall survival. Ultimately, chemotherapy did not provide a disease-free or overall survival benefit in patients with a high clinical risk and low genomic risk, but it did provide a slight benefit in distant metastasis-free survival and distant metastasis-free interval in this risk group. Current American Society of Clinical Oncology (ASCO) guidelines do not recommend the use of MammaPrint for adjuvant therapy decisions in patients with HR-positive, HER2-negative, node-positive breast cancer at low clinical risk, or in patients with HER2-positive or triple-negative breast cancer, because of the lack of confirmatory studies in these patients.

Next-Generation Sequencing of Tumor Tissue

Introduction
Although gene-expression profiling assays rely on traditional PCR technologies, the field of molecular oncology is increasingly moving toward the use of NGS as a means

of genomic tumor analysis. NGS is an umbrella term used to describe various genomic sequencing methods developed as improvements on Sanger sequencing. Whereas Sanger sequencing uses chain termination and capillary electrophoresis for nucleotide identification, NGS technology allows the sequencing of millions of molecules simultaneously, thereby providing a tremendous amount of genomic data in a short period of time.[25] In this section, we will discuss the ongoing efforts to harness genomic sequencing of tumor tissue for targeted therapies in breast cancer.

Basic principles
Sequencing of nucleic acids from tumor tissue has shed light on many cellular pathways prevalent in breast cancer, increasing our understanding of both the tumor genome and mechanisms of neoplasia.[26] For example, amplification of HER2/neu — also referred to as ERBB2 — has long been a useful target for precision oncology. However, since the advent of NGS-based tumor genome studies, the increasingly complex nature of this gene has come into focus. Sequencing data of breast tumors has revealed that some patients deemed to have non-amplification of HER2 by traditional immunohistochemistry harbor targetable mutations in the gene.[27] Therefore, these patients may benefit from anti-HER2 monoclonal antibody therapy. Investigators have also made similar discoveries in the realm of tumor resistance. For instance, some tumors acquire mutations in ESR1, the gene that encodes the cellular ER, thereby making the tumor resistant to hormonal therapy.[28] These tumors are still deemed HR-positive by immunohistochemistry, but the ESR1 mutation may render hormonal therapy ineffective.

The powerful implications of NGS on diagnosis and treatment have led to gene panel-based investigations into the tumor genome.[29] Many institutions have created molecular tumor boards to review the NGS outputs and identify potential clinical trials and treatment options.[30] These efforts allow the enrollment of patients in genotype-matched trials, such as those involving PI3 kinase inhibitors for patients with PIK3CA mutations.[31,32] FoundationOne CDx is one such NGS-based assay of 324 cancer-related genes.[33,34] Using this assay, clinically actionable mutations were identified in 76% of samples. Another panel, known as MammaSeq, focuses on the identification of 79 gene targets, of which 25 are deemed actionable according to the OncoKB precision oncology knowledge base.[35] It is worth noting that the definition of clinical actionability varies widely, and many of the mutations implicated by MammaSeq are targetable only with precision therapeutics that are not broadly available. Currently, most clinical trials evaluating precision therapeutics for mutations identified by NGS are in patients with metastatic disease or in patients who have failed conventional standard-of-care treatment.[30] However, as the field advances within both NGS and precision medicine, these trials will begin to incorporate patients with early-stage cancer.

Challenges
Despite its many benefits and strengths, the use of NGS on tumor tissue has several drawbacks and challenges that have limited its broader implementation. One drawback to the use of tumor tissue for NGS-guided molecular classification is the issue of tumor heterogeneity. Typically, sequencing is performed on DNA or RNA extracted from either a core biopsy or a small sample of resected tumor. Although genomic alterations may be detected, the tissue sample may not best represent the mutational burden of the tumor. This heterogeneity exists both spatially and temporally. First, an unsampled subsection of tumor with more genomic perturbations may exist, therefore representing a more aggressive clonal population. These more aggressive clones

may ultimately be responsible for the development of metastatic disease. Second, in a heterogenous tumor, a clonal population with a high number of mutations may ultimately replace the remaining tumor cells. If sequencing is based on tissue obtained before this replacement, patients and providers may have an inaccurate portrait of the tumor's mutational burden.[36] If the need for further biopsy-driven NGS arises, obtaining a repeat sample of tumor tissue requires subjecting the patient to an invasive procedure.

Another issue arising from the sequencing of tumor tissue is the quality of the tissue. Most tissue sequencing is performed on FFPE tissue. Although this method of tissue preservation is convenient for the preparation of histology slides, formalin fixation has a known detrimental effect on DNA quality.[37] Beyond preservation methods, the presence of cells from non-neoplastic sources can affect the results of genomic sequencing by lowering the fraction of tumor cells in the sample, thereby making mutations more difficult to detect.

Finally, although NGS has become a more streamlined process in recent years, the turn-around time for results is still far longer than from traditional immunohistochemistry or gene-expression assays. To meaningfully impact treatment decisions, sample processing, sequencing, and bioinformatic analysis of the subsequent data must all be performed in an appropriate time frame. Creating an efficient analytical pipeline increases the possibility that NGS results are clinically actionable. Currently, patient-level NGS data are primarily used in patients with metastatic disease or to enroll patients in clinical trials.[38]

Liquid Biopsies in Breast Cancer

Introduction

The analysis of peripheral blood for tumor-derived components has generated a tremendous amount of interest in the realm of oncology, giving rise to the term "liquid biopsy." Unlike acquiring tumor tissue, collection of peripheral blood is minimally invasive, which makes it an ideal method for serial monitoring of disease. The many approaches to liquid biopsies vary in terms of analyte (circulating tumor cells [CTCs], DNA, RNA, tumor-educated platelets, or exomes) and purpose (early detection or monitoring of residual disease). In this section, we will discuss the most recent advances in liquid biopsy technology for breast cancer.

Circulating tumor cells

As their name suggests, CTCs are cells released from a tumor that enter the bloodstream. A detection and enumeration system for these cells, known as CellSearch, is currently the only method approved by the US Food and Drug Administration (FDA).[39] CellSearch primarily uses the surface expression of the epithelial cell adhesion molecule (EpCAM) to detect carcinoma cells and their apoptotic remnants or cellular debris.[40] A CTC count of five cells per 7.5 mL of blood or higher has been shown to be associated with both shorter progression-free survival and shorter overall survival in patients with metastatic breast cancer.[41,42] In addition to reiterating these findings, a multicenter European examination using CellSearch found that adding CTC count to a clinicopathologic model increased the prognostic accuracy for both progression-free survival and overall survival.[43] A more recent study added further nuance to CTC count by proposing the metric of CTC trajectory, divided into four groups: negative, low, intermediate, and high.[44] These investigators showed significant statistical discrimination between these four groups in terms of progression-free and overall survival in patients with metastatic disease. Furthermore, they showed that detection of CTCs throughout treatment portended a worse prognosis.

Like sequencing of tumor tissue, CTC detection also presents unique challenges. One notable challenge is the relative scarcity of CTC targets in the bloodstream in comparison to other cell types, particularly leukocytes.[40] This challenge is particularly important in nonmetastatic disease, when the threshold of five CTCs per 7.5 mL of blood is difficult to achieve in any patient. Indeed, one study speculated that a CTC enumeration method would need to be 100-fold more sensitive than the current threshold to detect pre-metastatic disease.[45] They further hypothesized that a CTC threshold of 9 ± 6 cells per liter of blood would be required to reduce the risk of developing metastatic disease from 9.2% to 1%.[45]

Nucleic acids (DNA and RNA): basic principles

Before discussing the current and future directions of DNA- and RNA-based liquid biopsies for breast cancer, we will discuss some general considerations for this technology. Cell-free nucleic acids, especially DNA, have been studied with increasing interest in multiple fields of medicine. In the realm of prenatal testing, detection of plasma cell-free DNA (cfDNA) has been widely adopted as a means of screening pregnant women for genetic syndromes in the fetus.[46] Circulating nucleic acids are released from cells through multiple mechanisms, namely apoptosis, necrosis, and exocytosis.[47] The sources for these nucleic acids are myriad: the majority originate in leukocytes, whereas a minority arise from solid organ tissues. In patients with cancer, tumors are noted to shed genetic material in the bloodstream, which can be analyzed for early detection, prognostication, and monitoring of minimal residual disease. Like the enumeration of CTCs, collecting plasma for cfDNA analysis is minimally invasive and can be deployed in a serial manner for disease monitoring.

The most broadly adopted cell-free nucleic acid analysis is that of plasma cfDNA sequencing. In comparison to RNA, DNA is a more stable analyte that is more easily isolated from plasma. Enzymatic degradation of DNA in the bloodstream begins immediately and is completed within a matter of hours, making its detection useful as a real-time liquid biopsy.[48] Similar to the tissue-based NGS assays, many research groups have focused on the detection of oncogenic mutations within the plasma landscape to discern circulating tumor DNA (ctDNA) from the remainder of cfDNA. By searching for mutations in driver mutations in genes such as *TP53, PTEN, KRAS,* or *PIK3CA*, investigators and oncologists can gain useful insight into a patient's disease. Unlike in sequencing of tumor tissue, plasma cfDNA more accurately depicts tumoral heterogeneity in patients with metastatic disease, which may have an impact on treatment decisions.[49-51]

Mutation-based ctDNA sequencing assays have their own obstacles. First, although the variant allele frequency (VAF)—that is, the percentage total cfDNA that can be attributed to the neoplasm—is often 10% or greater in patients with metastatic disease, the localized disease may have a VAF of 0.1% or lower.[52] At these frequencies, distinguishing tumor mutations from background sequencing noise becomes extremely challenging. To add to the complexity of this process, benign leukocytes often carry mutations that are deemed "oncogenic."[53] Therefore, early detection and monitoring of minimal residual disease in this setting rely heavily on sophisticated computational pipelines to delineate ctDNA from the background.

Another obstacle faced by mutation-based ctDNA sequencing assays is their inability to detect large structural variants. Most of these detection methods rely on the identification of single nucleotide variants, thereby missing pathogenic insertions, deletions, and duplications that may be 1000 base pairs or longer. This problem is sometimes referred to as the depth versus breadth tradeoff: by sequencing a given set of mutations enough times to distinguish signal from noise (depth), information about genome-wide changes is sacrificed (breadth).

Cell-free DNA: novel methods in early detection

To address these obstacles, several novel techniques have been developed to differentiate tumor from non-tumor DNA in plasma. One assay, known as CancerSEEK, uses several strategies to improve the possibility of early cancer detection. First, CancerSEEK combines mutation-based ctDNA detection with the detection of eight cancer-associated proteins to improve sensitivity. Second, the investigators modified the pre-sequencing PCR reactions in a unique manner to reduce both PCR errors and sequencing noise.[54] The assay was deployed on plasma samples from 1,005 patients with nonmetastatic disease across eight different cancer types, including breast. At >99% specificity, CancerSEEK was 62% sensitive overall, with the lowest sensitivity—33%—in breast cancer.[54]

Novel methods for early detection are not limited to mutation-based approaches. For instance, the Circulating Cell-free Genome Atlas (CCGA) Study was performed through a large collaboration of medical centers throughout the United States, Canada, and the United Kingdom. As opposed to deep sequencing of oncogenic mutations in cfDNA, the CCGA investigators performed targeted bisulfite sequencing to examine >100,000 selected cancer-related methylation changes from across the genome. In addition, the CCGA study compared individuals with over 50 cancer types to a healthy cohort, thereby striving to create an assay that is tumor-agnostic.[55] The study showed an assay specificity of 99.3%, with sensitivities between 18% and 93% depending on stage. Furthermore, the CCGA assay was able to predict tissue of origin with 93% accuracy.[55] One downside to this method is the bisulfide sequencing process, which is expensive and degrades DNA. Efforts are being made to overcome these challenges by creating a bisulfite-free methylation sequencing technique.[56]

A further effort to differentiate between patients with cancer and healthy controls involves a genome-wide assessment of DNA fragmentation patterns. One method, nicknamed DELFI (DNA Evaluation of Fragments for Early Interception), examined fragmentation patterns between 236 patients with seven cancer types, including breast, and compared them to fragmentation patterns in 245 healthy adults. For patients with breast cancer ($n = 54$), they were able to reach a sensitivity of 70% at 95% specificity for disease detection.[57] By combining their technique with a mutation-based approach, the assay was able to detect 82% of patients with cancer, including 80% of those with a VAF of <1%.[57]

Cell-free DNA: monitoring of minimal residual disease

Although many research groups have focused their efforts on early detection, the monitoring of minimal residual disease after therapy represents an equally difficult barrier to overcome. Not only would a sensitive and specific liquid biopsy be useful for serial monitoring after surgical resection, but it may also lead to a fundamental paradigm shift in treating patients with a pathologic complete response to neoadjuvant therapy. In other words, those with a complete response to neoadjuvant therapy may be able to avoid surgery if a liquid biopsy indicated no residual disease.

One study, published in 2017, sought to determine if tumor mutations found in a surgical resection specimen could be detected in ctDNA as a biomarker for recurrent disease in patients treated for triple-negative breast cancer. Of the 33 patients with mutations identified in tumor tissue, only 4 patients eventually had the same mutation identified in ctDNA.[58] All four patients experienced a recurrence in a short time frame; however, nine additional patients also ultimately had recurrent disease, yielding a sensitivity of 31%.[58] This study highlights the enormous challenge of detecting residual disease after treatment due to a scarcity of mutated ctDNA fragments in circulation. Although additional blood samples could increase sensitivity, collecting large volumes of blood from these patients or combining multiple serial samples are both invasive and impractical.[59]

Like the developers of CancerSEEK, the research group behind the Targeted Digital Sequencing (TARDIS) assay optimized the pre-sequencing PCR reactions to boost the number of DNA fragments available for analysis. In addition, they sought to detect multiple mutations simultaneously to increase sensitivity. First, whole exome sequencing on each patient's tumor biopsy was performed to identify founder somatic mutations.[60] In a cohort of 33 patients, they identified between 9 and 286 mutations, with a mean of 65.8 mutations per patient. Before neoadjuvant treatment, each patient's personalized TARDIS mutation panel was able to detect these oncogenic mutations in the ctDNA of every patient. These samples had a VAF between 0.002% and 1.1%, with a median of 0.11%.[60] Additionally, after neoadjuvant therapy, ctDNA was detected in 17 of 22 patients, and those with a pathologic complete response had a 5.7-fold lower ctDNA VAF compared with those with residual disease (means of 0.003% and 0.018%, respectively).[60] This assay shows a remarkably low limit of detection for ctDNA, thanks to both PCR optimization and a multi-mutation approach, although larger clinical studies are needed to evaluate the clinical validity, relevance, and potential utility of such findings.

SUMMARY

The field of genomic profiling in oncology has progressed markedly in recent years and continues to do so at lightning speed. With the advent of gene-expression assays, providers have been able to determine more accurately which patients are at highest risk of recurrence, and therefore may benefit from additional treatment. Furthermore, advances in NGS have transformed the landscape of molecular oncology, providing invaluable insights into cancers for each individual patient. Although challenges remain, particularly in terms of early detection and minimal residual disease monitoring, genomic technology is only expected to improve and become more affordable. As it becomes more accessible, the cancer genome will likely play an increasingly large role in the care of each patient.

CLINICS CARE POINTS

- Clinical trials have validated the use of the 21-gene OncotypeDx assay for use in hormone receptor-positive, human epidermal growth factor receptor 2-negative patients to help determine the benefit of adjuvant chemotherapy.
- Next-generation sequencing assays are increasingly used to match patients to clinical trials of precision therapeutics, especially for those patients with advanced disease or failure of conventional therapy.
- A rapidly enlarging body of evidence suggests that liquid biopsies will play an increasingly large role diagnosis and treatment of patients with cancer.

DISCLOSURE

L.G. Wilke: Founder and Minority Stock Owner Elucent Medical (not discussed in this publication). M. Murtaza: Licensing relationships with Exact Sciences and Inivata. Advisor with stock options PetDx. Consulting relationships with AstraZeneca and Castle Biosciences. C.T. Marcinak: nothing to disclose.

C.T Marcinak is funded by grant 5T32HG002760-19 from the National Institutes of Health/National Human Genome Research Institute.

REFERENCES

1. Sjöblom T, Jones S, Wood LD, et al. The Consensus Coding Sequences of Human Breast and Colorectal Cancers. Science 2006;314(5797):268–74.
2. Cazier JB, Tomlinson I. General lessons from large-scale studies to identify human cancer predisposition genes. J Pathol 2010;220(2):255–62.
3. Adjuvant Chemotherapy for Breast Cancer. JAMA 1985;254(24):3461–3.
4. Fisher B, Redmond C, Brown A, et al. Treatment of Primary Breast Cancer with Chemotherapy and Tamoxifen. N Engl J Med 1981;305(1):1–6.
5. Fisher B, Costantino J, Redmond C, et al. A Randomized Clinical Trial Evaluating Tamoxifen in the Treatment of Patients with Node-Negative Breast Cancer Who Have Estrogen-Receptor–Positive Tumors. N Engl J Med 1989;320(8):479–84.
6. Baselga J, Norton L, Albanell J, et al. Recombinant Humanized Anti-HER2 Antibody (Herceptin™) Enhances the Antitumor Activity of Paclitaxel and Doxorubicin against HER2/neu Overexpressing Human Breast Cancer Xenografts1. Cancer Res 1998;58(13):2825–31.
7. Cobleigh MA, Vogel CL, Tripathy D, et al. Multinational Study of the Efficacy and Safety of Humanized Anti-HER2 Monoclonal Antibody in Women Who Have HER2-Overexpressing Metastatic Breast Cancer That Has Progressed After Chemotherapy for Metastatic Disease. J Clin Oncol 1999;17(9):2639.
8. Perou CM, Sørlie T, Eisen MB, et al. Molecular portraits of human breast tumours. Nature 2000;406(6797):747–52.
9. Paik S, Shak S, Tang G, et al. A Multigene Assay to Predict Recurrence of Tamoxifen-Treated, Node-Negative Breast Cancer. N Engl J Med 2004;351(27): 2817–26.
10. Giuliano AE, Connolly JL, Edge SB, et al. Breast Cancer-Major changes in the American Joint Committee on Cancer eighth edition cancer staging manual. CA Cancer J Clin 2017;67(4):290–303.
11. van 't Veer LJ, Dai H, van de Vijver MJ, et al. Gene expression profiling predicts clinical outcome of breast cancer. Nature 2002;415(6871):530–6.
12. van de Vijver MJ, He YD, van 't Veer LJ, et al. A Gene-Expression Signature as a Predictor of Survival in Breast Cancer. N Engl J Med 2002;347(25):1999–2009.
13. Nielsen T, Wallden B, Schaper C, et al. Analytical validation of the PAM50-based Prosigna Breast Cancer Prognostic Gene Signature Assay and nCounter Analysis System using formalin-fixed paraffin-embedded breast tumor specimens. BMC Cancer 2014;14(1):177.
14. Wallden B, Storhoff J, Nielsen T, et al. Development and verification of the PAM50-based Prosigna breast cancer gene signature assay. BMC Med Genomics 2015; 8:54.
15. Parker JS, Mullins M, Cheang MC, et al. Supervised risk predictor of breast cancer based on intrinsic subtypes. J Clin Oncol 2009;27(8):1160–7.
16. Filipits M, Rudas M, Jakesz R, et al. A new molecular predictor of distant recurrence in ER-positive, HER2-negative breast cancer adds independent information to conventional clinical risk factors. Clin Cancer Res 2011;17(18):6012–20.
17. Sparano JA, Gray RJ, Makower DF, et al. Prospective Validation of a 21-Gene Expression Assay in Breast Cancer. N Engl J Med 2015;373(21):2005–14.
18. Sparano JA, Gray RJ, Makower DF, et al. Adjuvant Chemotherapy Guided by a 21-Gene Expression Assay in Breast Cancer. N Engl J Med 2018;379(2):111–21.

19. Sparano JA, Gray RJ, Makower DF, et al. Clinical Outcomes in Early Breast Cancer With a High 21-Gene Recurrence Score of 26 to 100 Assigned to Adjuvant Chemotherapy Plus Endocrine Therapy: A Secondary Analysis of the TAILORx Randomized Clinical Trial. JAMA Oncol 2020;6(3):367–74.

20. Kalinsky K, Barlow WE, Gralow JR, et al. 21-Gene Assay to Inform Chemotherapy Benefit in Node-Positive Breast Cancer. N Engl J Med 2021;385(25):2336–47.

21. NCCN Clinical Practice Guidelines in Oncology (NCCN Guidelines®); Guideline Breast Cancer 4.2022. National Comprehensive Cancer Network, Inc. 2022.

22. Cardoso F, van't Veer LJ, Bogaerts J, et al. 70-Gene Signature as an Aid to Treatment Decisions in Early-Stage Breast Cancer. N Engl J Med 2016;375(8):717–29.

23. Piccart M, van 't Veer LJ, Poncet C, et al. 70-gene signature as an aid for treatment decisions in early breast cancer: updated results of the phase 3 randomised MINDACT trial with an exploratory analysis by age. Lancet Oncol 2021; 22(4):476–88.

24. Ravdin PM, Siminoff LA, Davis GJ, et al. Computer Program to Assist in Making Decisions About Adjuvant Therapy for Women With Early Breast Cancer. J Clin Oncol 2001;19(4):980–91.

25. Metzker ML. Sequencing technologies - the next generation. Nat Rev Genet 2010;11(1):31–46.

26. Ellis MJ, Ding L, Shen D, et al. Whole-genome analysis informs breast cancer response to aromatase inhibition. Nature 2012;486(7403):353–60.

27. Bose R, Kavuri SM, Searleman AC, et al. Activating HER2 mutations in HER2 gene amplification negative breast cancer. Cancer Discov 2013;3(2):224–37.

28. Reinert T, Saad ED, Barrios CH, et al. Clinical Implications of ESR1 Mutations in Hormone Receptor-Positive Advanced Breast Cancer. Front Oncol 2017;7:26.

29. Gurda GT, Ambros T, Nikiforova MN, et al. Characterizing Molecular Variants and Clinical Utilization of Next-generation Sequencing in Advanced Breast Cancer. Appl Immunohistochem Mol Morphol 2017;25(6):392–8.

30. Larson KL, Huang B, Weiss HL, et al. Clinical Outcomes of Molecular Tumor Boards: A Systematic Review. JCO Precis Oncol 2021. https://doi.org/10.1200/PO.20.00495. 5doi:.

31. Pezo RC, Chen TW, Berman HK, et al. Impact of multi-gene mutational profiling on clinical trial outcomes in metastatic breast cancer. Breast Cancer Res Treat 2018;168(1):159–68.

32. Stockley TL, Oza AM, Berman HK, et al. Molecular profiling of advanced solid tumors and patient outcomes with genotype-matched clinical trials: the Princess Margaret IMPACT/COMPACT trial. Genome Med 2016;8(1):109.

33. Frampton GM, Fichtenholtz A, Otto GA, et al. Development and validation of a clinical cancer genomic profiling test based on massively parallel DNA sequencing. Nat Biotechnol 2013;31(11):1023–31.

34. Kawaji H, Kubo M, Yamashita N, et al. Comprehensive molecular profiling broadens treatment options for breast cancer patients. Cancer Med 2021; 10(2):529–39.

35. Smith NG, Gyanchandani R, Shah OS, et al. Targeted mutation detection in breast cancer using MammaSeq. Breast Cancer Res 2019;21(1):22.

36. Yates LR, Gerstung M, Knappskog S, et al. Subclonal diversification of primary breast cancer revealed by multiregion sequencing. Nat Med 2015;21(7):751–9.

37. Do H, Dobrovic A. Sequence artifacts in DNA from formalin-fixed tissues: causes and strategies for minimization. Clin Chem 2015;61(1):64–71.

38. Zardavas D, Piccart-Gebhart M. Clinical trials of precision medicine through molecular profiling: focus on breast cancer. Am Soc Clin Oncol Educ Book 2015;35: e183–90.

39. Kagan M, Howard D, Bendele T, et al. A sample preparation and analysis system for identification of circulating tumor cells. J Clin Ligand Assay 2002;25:104–10.

40. Andree KC, van Dalum G, Terstappen LW. Challenges in circulating tumor cell detection by the CellSearch system. *Mol Oncol* Mar 2016;10(3):395–407.

41. Cristofanilli M, Budd GT, Ellis MJ, et al. Circulating Tumor Cells, Disease Progression, and Survival in Metastatic Breast Cancer. N Engl J Med 2004;351(8): 781–91.

42. Cristofanilli M, Hayes DF, Budd GT, et al. Circulating Tumor Cells: A Novel Prognostic Factor for Newly Diagnosed Metastatic Breast Cancer. J Clin Oncol 2005; 23(7):1420–30.

43. Bidard F-C, Peeters DJ, Fehm T, et al. Clinical validity of circulating tumour cells in patients with metastatic breast cancer: a pooled analysis of individual patient data. Lancet Oncol 2014;15(4):406–14.

44. Magbanua MJM, Hendrix LH, Hyslop T, et al. Serial Analysis of Circulating Tumor Cells in Metastatic Breast Cancer Receiving First-Line Chemotherapy. J Natl Cancer Inst 2021;113(4):443–52.

45. Coumans FAW, Siesling S, Terstappen LWMM. Detection of cancer before distant metastasis. BMC Cancer 2013;13(1):283.

46. Wong FCK, Lo YMD. Prenatal Diagnosis Innovation: Genome Sequencing of Maternal Plasma. Annu Rev Med 2016;67(1):419–32.

47. Wan JCM, Massie C, Garcia-Corbacho J, et al. Liquid biopsies come of age: towards implementation of circulating tumour DNA. Nat Rev Cancer 2017;17(4): 223–38.

48. Yao W, Mei C, Nan X, et al. Evaluation and comparison of in vitro degradation kinetics of DNA in serum, urine and saliva: A qualitative study. Gene 2016;590(1): 142–8.

49. Murtaza M, Dawson SJ, Pogrebniak K, et al. Multifocal clonal evolution characterized using circulating tumour DNA in a case of metastatic breast cancer. Nat Commun 2015;6:8760.

50. Coto-Llerena M, Benjak A, Gallon J, et al. Circulating Cell-Free DNA Captures the Intratumor Heterogeneity in Multinodular Hepatocellular Carcinoma. JCO Precis Oncol 2022;6:e2100335.

51. Garcia-Murillas I, Schiavon G, Weigelt B, et al. Mutation tracking in circulating tumor DNA predicts relapse in early breast cancer. Sci Transl Med 2015;7(302): 302ra133.

52. Abbosh C, Birkbak NJ, Wilson GA, et al. Phylogenetic ctDNA analysis depicts early-stage lung cancer evolution. Nature 2017;545(7655):446–51.

53. Chan HT, Nagayama S, Chin YM, et al. Clinical significance of clonal hematopoiesis in the interpretation of blood liquid biopsy. Mol Oncol 2020;14(8):1719–30.

54. Cohen JD, Li L, Wang Y, et al. Detection and localization of surgically resectable cancers with a multi-analyte blood test. Science 2018;359(6378):926–30.

55. Liu MC, Oxnard GR, Klein EA, et al. Sensitive and specific multi-cancer detection and localization using methylation signatures in cell-free DNA. Ann Oncol 2020; 31(6):745–59.

56. Siejka-Zielińska P, Cheng J, Jackson F, et al. Cell-free DNA TAPS provides multimodal information for early cancer detection. Sci Adv 2021;7(36):eabh0534.

57. Cristiano S, Leal A, Phallen J, et al. Genome-wide cell-free DNA fragmentation in patients with cancer. Nature 2019;570(7761):385–9.

58. Chen YH, Hancock BA, Solzak JP, et al. Next-generation sequencing of circulating tumor DNA to predict recurrence in triple-negative breast cancer patients with residual disease after neoadjuvant chemotherapy. NPJ Breast Cancer 2017;3:24.
59. Garcia-Murillas I, Chopra N, Comino-Mendez I, et al. Assessment of Molecular Relapse Detection in Early-Stage Breast Cancer. JAMA Oncol 2019;5(10): 1473–8.
60. McDonald BR, Contente-Cuomo T, Sammut S-J, et al. Personalized circulating tumor DNA analysis to detect residual disease after neoadjuvant therapy in breast cancer. Sci Transl Med 2019;11(504). https://doi.org/10.1126/scitranslmed. aax7392.

Breast Cancer Screening Modalities, Recommendations, and Novel Imaging Techniques

Sarah Nielsen, DO[a], Anand K. Narayan, MD, PhD[b],*

KEYWORDS

- Cancer screening guidelines • Health care providers • Mammography • Screening
- Breast neoplasm

KEY POINTS

- Screening mammography reduces breast cancer mortality.
- The American Society of Breast Surgeons recommends that average-risk women undergo breast cancer screening every year starting at age 40.
- Women with risk factors for breast cancer may benefit from earlier, supplemental screening.
- Black, Hispanic, and Asian women are more likely to be diagnosed with breast cancer before the age of 50.

INTRODUCTION

Breast cancer remains the second leading cause of cancer death for women in the United States.[1] In the United States in 2022, the American Cancer Society (ACS) estimates that 290,560 will be diagnosed with breast cancer. Approximately 43,780 Americans will die from this disease.[2] Roughly 1 in 1000 American men (.01%) will develop breast cancer. Owing to the increased availability of screening and treatment, breast cancer mortality has significantly declined in the United States. Mammography remains the only validated screening tool for breast cancer and is the gold standard for breast imaging. The goal of any mammography screening program is the detection of small, node-negative tumors with the least amount of morbidity to the patient and cost

---

[a] Section Head – Breast Imaging, Department of Radiology, Marshfield Clinic Health System, Marshfield Clinic – Wausau Center, 2727 Plaza Drive, Wausau, WI 54401, USA; [b] Equity, Department of Radiology, University of Wisconsin-Madison, 600 Highland Avenue, F6/178C, Madison, WI 53792-3252, USA
* Corresponding author.
E-mail address: anarayan@uwhealth.org
Twitter: @AnandKNarayan (A.K.N.)

Surg Clin N Am 103 (2023) 63–82
https://doi.org/10.1016/j.suc.2022.08.004
0039-6109/23/© 2022 Elsevier Inc. All rights reserved.

surgical.theclinics.com

to society. However, there are limitations to mammography, one of which is the variable sensitivity based on breast density. Supplemental screening modalities using digital breast tomosynthesis (DBT), screening ultrasound (US), breast MRI, and molecular breast imaging (MBI) may be considered based on the patient's risk level and breast density. Higher-risk women should start mammographic screening earlier and may benefit from supplemental screening modalities. This article reviews the fundamentals of mammography screening and current age-based mammography screening recommendations, supplemental breast cancer screening recommendations in women at higher-than-average risk, and novel imaging technologies.

DISCUSSION
Breast Cancer Screening

Mammography
Technique and physics. A mammogram is a radiographic examination of the breast, either displayed on film or on a digital computer monitor. Since 2000, full-field digital mammography (FFDM) has largely replaced film-screen mammography. When a digital mammogram is performed, the patient's breast is placed in compression and X-rays travel through the breast and onto a detector. The detector converts X-rays into electrical signals. The electrical signals are sent to a computer for processing and to the radiologist for interpretation. When looking at a mammogram one will see various shades of gray based on the differential attenuation characteristics of the tissue. Specifically, fat attenuates fewer X-rays than fibroglandular tissue and appears darker gray. Fibroglandular and stromal tissue appear lighter white, as do mineral deposits such as calcifications within a malignant lesion appearing bright white. With the invention of digital mammography came improved contrast resolution. As cancer is radiopaque, good contrast resolution is necessary to be able to discern the subtle differences between a cancer and the normal surrounding fibroglandular tissue. Compression also helps with finding abnormalities by spreading out the tissues and minimizing motion artifacts.

There are two standard views in screening mammography named for the direction of the X-ray beam from the source to the detector: craniocaudal (CC) and mediolateral oblique (MLO) (**Fig. 1**).

For the CC view, the patient's breast is positioned on the image detector with the paddle compressing the breast in the superior to inferior direction. The image should ideally include the cleavage area and some of the pectoralis muscle (seen in roughly 30%). These landmarks help to ensure that an adequate amount of tissue is included and that a portion of tissue harboring a malignancy is not excluded. When looking at a CC view on a monitor, the lateral breast is placed superior to the screen, and the medial breast is inferior.

For the MLO view, the machine is angled generally 40 to 60° to image as much of the pectoralis muscle as possible. A line drawn from the nipple to the chest wall should be within 1 cm of the same line drawn on the CC view to ensure adequate tissue inclusion. Breast cancers may develop within the axillary tail and it is essential to include as much tissue from this region as possible. When looking at an MLO view on a monitor, superior is superior, and inferior is inferior.

The radiation dose is very low in mammography. Compression decreases the radiation dose by decreasing the number of photons needed to penetrate the breast tissue. One screening FFDM is about equivalent to simply living for approximately 7 weeks (background radiation),[3] or flying for roughly 13,000 miles.[4] Combining both FFDM with three-dimensional (tomosynthesis) images increases the dose

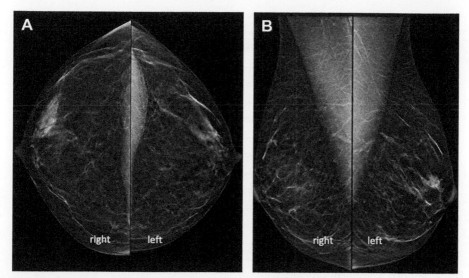

Fig. 1. (*A*) Standard craniocaudal (CC) mammographic views. (*B*) Standard mediolateral oblique (MLO) mammographic views.

to ~ 2.5 mGy, which is well below the American College of Radiology's (ACR) 3 mGy per film cutoff. New technology allows the two-dimensional (2D) images to be reconstructed from the 3D images that drop the dose by an estimated 43%.[5] Regardless if your facility performs 2D ± tomosynthesis ± reconstructed 2D views, mammography is a very low dose radiation procedure.

Radiation dose and image quality in mammography are heavily regulated under the Mammography Quality Standards Act (MQSA) Program passed in 1992. All facilities performing mammography in the United States must be certified by the Food and Drug Administration (FDA) or an FDA-approved Certifying State. Certification requires standards to be met in the quality of mammographic equipment, personnel who perform and interpret mammography, and reporting. MQSA requires that all facilities have a procedure in place for following abnormal findings and tracking pathologic results from biopsy procedures. The facility is inspected annually by trained FDA or state inspectors. In addition, the ACR evaluates both phantom and patient images from each machine that performs mammography to ensure minimum quality standards are met. If your facility is an ACR Breast Imaging Center of Excellence it means it has received full accreditation by the ACR in all imaging modalities.

Interpretation of a Mammogram

When interpreting a mammogram, the radiologist uses the Breast Imaging Reporting and Data System (BI-RADS) lexicon.[6] The BI-RADS lexicon is used to describe and classify findings, and each mammogram is given a final BI-RADS assessment category (0–6) (**Fig. 2**) The BI-RADS lexicon serves to standardize reports, and allow for clear communication between the clinicians and radiologists, and what, if anything, needs to be done next. Screening mammograms are performed on the asymptomatic breast. Screening mammograms with potential abnormalities are typically given a BI-RADS category 0 assessment and are subsequently evaluated with a diagnostic mammogram or US at the discretion of the radiologist.

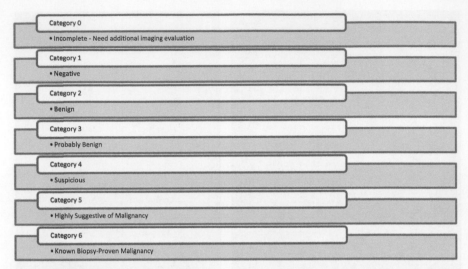

Category 0
• Incomplete - Need additional imaging evaluation

Category 1
• Negative

Category 2
• Benign

Category 3
• Probably Benign

Category 4
• Suspicious

Category 5
• Highly Suggestive of Malignancy

Category 6
• Known Biopsy-Proven Malignancy

Fig. 2. BI-RADS assessment categories.

On mammograms, cancers present as masses, asymmetries, calcifications, or architectural distortions. A mass is 3-dimensional and occupies space. It is seen on two different mammographic projections. The shape of a mass is described as oval, round or irregular, whereas the margins are described as circumscribed, obscured, microlobulated, indistinct, and spiculated. The density of a mass can be reported as high, equal, low, or fat-containing density. The several different types of asymmetry involve a spectrum of mammographic findings that represent unilateral deposits of fibroglandular tissue not conforming to the definition of a radiodense mass. The asymmetry is visible on only one projection. Focal (involving less than a quadrant), global (involving at least one quadrant), and developing (new, increasing) asymmetries have concave-outward borders, whereas a radiodense mass displays completely or partially convex-outward borders. Architectural distortion, which can occur with our without a central mass, is used to describe speculations radiating from a point and focal retraction at the edge of the parenchyma. In the absence of a history of trauma or surgery, architectural distortion is suspicious of malignancy or radial scar and should be biopsied. Typically benign calcifications are generally larger than those associated with malignancy (coarse, round, rod-like, rim, dystrophic, or "layering" milk of calcium on 90° medial-lateral images). The morphology of calcifications associated with malignancy are usually very small requiring the use of magnification and are described as amorphous, coarse heterogeneous, fine pleomorphic, and fine linear or fine linear branching. The distribution is used to describe the arrangement of calcifications in the breast. Distribution descriptors are diffuse, regional, grouped, linear, and segmental. It should be noted that in evaluating the likelihood of malignancy for calcifications, the distribution is at least as important as the morphology. The radiologists generally report the location of abnormal findings either as a clock position or by quadrant and include the distance from the nipple.

Using the BI-RADS lexicon and assessment system, a quality audit is generated. The current BI-RADS atlas establishes clear definitions for how to determine whether findings in a screening mammogram are true-positive (TP), true-negative (TN), false-positive (FP), or false-negative (FN). From these outcomes, the metrics of sensitivity (TP/TP + FN), specificity (TN/TN + FP), and positive predictive value

(PPV) (TP/TP + FN) are calculated.[6] PPV is a measure of how likely it is that a positive test result indicates presence of disease with three subtypes: PPV1, PPV2, and PPV3 (**Fig. 3**). The commonly used performance metrics for screening mammography are recall rate, cancer detection rate (CDR), and PPVs.

The National Mammography Database (NMD) is a component of the ACR National Radiology Data Registry established in 2008. The NMD is a robust automated data collection process that accrues screening mammography interpretation and biopsy results in addition to other clinical practice data from over 200 volunteer facilities across 30 states. For quality improvement purposes, the NMD was designed to enable mammographic facilities and radiologists to compare their mammography performance with that of their peers locally, regionally, and nationally. The screening performance metrics (CDR, recall, and PPVs) are calculated for all facilities by use of the standard BI-RADS audit procedures, and provide practice-based screening performance benchmark data.[7]

Benefits of Early Detection Through Mammography Screening

Early detection of breast cancer with screening mammography significantly reduces the risk of death from the disease.[8,9] The strongest evidence is provided by randomized controlled studies (RCTs) and pooled estimates from eight RCTs showing that mammography can reduce breast cancer mortality by at least 20%.[10] Meta-analyses of RCTs have been the primary source of evidence supporting the benefit of screening mammography in guideline development. Observational studies evaluating breast cancer screening must be interpreted with caution because of susceptibility to biases, including selection bias, lead time bias, length bias, and others.[11] However, RCTs were conducted decades ago with obsolete older film screen technology and protocols. With advances in digital mammography technology, the ACS concluded that large, methodologically rigorous observational studies can provide valuable information about the contemporary effectiveness of screening mammography.[10] Numerous observational studies have shown mortality reductions of 40% or greater with organized screening.[12–17]

PPV1	PPV2	PPV3
• PPV1 is the percentage of patients recalled from screening for additional imaging who receive a cancer diagnosis. PPV1 is a useful metric for monitoring the success of screening interpretations by incorporating both the cancer detection rate (CDR) and the recall rate in a single metric.	• PPV2 is the percentage of all diagnostic examinations recommended for biopsy or surgical consultation that result in a cancer diagnosis and is a useful metric representing the radiologist's interpretive recommendations.	• PPV3 is the percentage of all known biopsies performed after positive findings of diagnostic evaluations and is useful at the society level because it reflects clinical care actually delivered.

Fig. 3. Positive predictive value definitions.

BREAST CANCER SCREENING RECOMMENDATIONS FOR WOMEN OF AVERAGE RISK

Because screening mammography reduces breast cancer mortality, every major guideline-producing organization in the United States has recommended screening mammography in average-risk women.[18] However, recommendations differ about when women should start screening and how often they should undergo mammographic screening (**Fig. 4**). We describe the varying perspectives used to inform each screening guideline recommendation.

American Society of Breast Surgeons

The American Society of Breast Surgeons (ASBrS) published guidelines in 2019 derived from a literature review conducted by an expert panel. The ASBrS recommended that average-risk women undergo breast cancer screening every year starting at age 40. Although noting that there are disadvantages of starting annual screening mammography at the age of 40, the ASBrS noted that meta-analyses of randomized control trials found that screening mammography reduced breast cancer mortality.

They noted that USPSTF guidelines weighed the results from statistical models generated by the Cancer Intervention and Surveillance Modeling Network (CISNET). Analyses of CISNET models have confirmed that screening strategies starting every year beginning at age 40 yield the largest reductions in breast cancer mortality. The USPSTF opted to base their recommendations on efficiency frontiers evaluating the average gain in life-years per additional mammogram performed per 1000 women. The ASBrS guidelines prioritized mortality reduction benefits over efficiency frontiers.

In addition, they recommended that women with a life expectancy of at least 10 years should continue screening mammography every year. While noting that randomized control trials excluded women older than 74, the ASBrS noted that observational studies have found survival benefits of screening mammography in older women without severe co-morbidities[19] and that false positives would be expected to be lower compared with younger populations.

American Cancer Society

The ACS developed its recommendations using standardized methodologies derived from the Institute of Medicine,[20] supplemented by Breast Cancer Surveillance

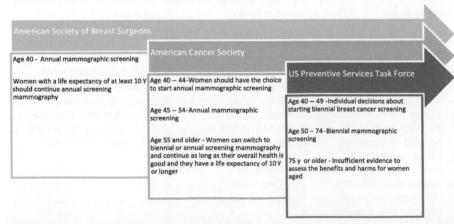

American Society of Breast Surgeons

Age 40 - Annual mammographic screening

Women with a life expectancy of at least 10 y should continue annual screening mammography

American Cancer Society

Age 40 – 44-Women should have the choice to start annual mammographic screening

Age 45 – 54-Annual mammographic screening

Age 55 and older - Women can switch to biennial or annual screening mammography and continue as long as their overall health is good and they have a life expectancy of 10 y or longer

US Preventive Services Task Force

Age 40 – 49 -Individual decisions about starting biennial breast cancer screening

Age 50 – 74-Biennial mammographic screening

75 y or older - Insufficient evidence to assess the benefits and harms for women aged

Fig. 4. Summary of breast cancer screening guidelines by Professional societies for average risk women.

Consortium (BCSC) data.[21] Compared with premenopausal women who underwent mammographic screening every year, premenopausal women who underwent mammographic screening every 2 years were more likely to be diagnosed with poorer prognosis breast cancers. In contrast, post-menopausal women undergoing screening every 2 years showed no statistically significant increases in advanced-stage breast cancers compared with women undergoing screening every year.

The ACS noted that women between the ages of 40 to 44 showed less morbidity and mortality from breast cancer compared with other 5-year age categories. Consequently, the ACS recommended that average-risk women start annual screening at the age of 45. If women between the ages of 40 to 44 year old chose to initiate breast cancer screening, the ACR recommended that they undergo annual screening. With comparatively fewer benefits of annual screening mammography in women after menopause, the ACS recommended that starting at age 55 (the age at which the majority of women are post-menopausal), average-risk women should transition to biennial screening or continue annual screening.

Beyond the age of 74, the ACS noted that age is one of the most important risk factors for breast cancer. Women between the ages of 75 to 79 show the highest breast cancer incidence rates. 26% of breast cancer deaths are attributable to breast cancer diagnoses after the age of 74. Consequently, the ACS recommended that women continue screening mammography as long as their overall health is good and they have a life expectancy of 10 years or longer.

US Preventive Services Task Force

The US Preventive Services Task Force (USPSTF) is a volunteer panel of 16 nationally recognized experts in primary care, prevention, and evidence-based medicine. Details regarding guideline development methods are described elsewhere.[22] In determining their recommendation, the USPSTF noted that most of the benefits of mammographic screening result from biennial screening during ages 50 to 74 years. While noting that mammographic screening between the ages of 40 to 49 may reduce breast cancer mortality, they noted that comparatively smaller numbers of breast cancer deaths were averted by starting screening at age 40 instead of age 50, whereas the number of FP results and unnecessary biopsies increased by starting screening at age 40.

The USPSTF found that current evidence is insufficient to assess the benefits and harms for women aged 75 years or older, citing a lack of randomized control trial data in women in this age group. However, they cited CISNET modeling studies suggesting that screening women older than 74 year old may be beneficial among women with no or low comorbidity.

Harms Associated with Mammographic Screening, Diagnosis, and Treatment

The USPSTF conducted a systematic review and meta-analysis to estimate potential harms of screening including FPs, overdiagnosed/overtreated breast cancers, anxiety, pain during procedures, and radiation exposure.[23] Of these harms, the USPSTF identified overdiagnosis/overtreatment and FPs as the two major potential harms associated with screening mammography.

Overdiagnosis/Overtreatment

Overdiagnosis/overtreatment refers to the diagnosis and treatment of breast cancers that would not cause harm during a patient's lifetime because these cancers would progress too slowly, not progress at all, or resolve spontaneously. According to the USPSTF, overdiagnosis/overtreatment is the principal harm associated with screening mammography.

The USPSTF systematic review found estimates of overdiagnosis/overtreatment ranging between 0% to 54% of breast cancer cases. A major methodological challenge associated with the quantitative estimation of over-diagnosis is that currently we do not have ways to identify or predict which cancers will progress.[24] Widely ranging estimates about the magnitude and extent of overdiagnosis/overtreatment present challenges for health care providers who are counseling their patients about the potential harms of mammographic screening.

False Positives

The USPSTF systematic review estimated the cumulative probability of FP results based on data from the BCSC[25,26] They found that FP results were highest among women receiving annual mammography, 40 to 49-year-old women, women with extremely dense breast tissue, and/or women using combination hormone therapy.

To evaluate the consequences of FP examinations, USPSTF identified four systematic reviews with varying conclusions about the impacts of FPs. One study was nested within the Digital Mammographic Imaging Screening Trial, a randomized control trial.[27] Tosteson and colleagues found that women with FP results were more likely to experience short-term anxiety however did not experience any differences in anxiety or health-related quality of life 1 year later. In addition, women with FP mammography results were more likely to state that they would undergo screening mammography in the future. Overall, the USPSTF concluded that the absolute magnitude and time course of anxiety experienced by individual women after FPs were difficult to estimate and varied widely.

Maximizing the Benefits and Reducing Potential Harms Associated with Screening Mammography

The ACS emphasized the need to minimize the harms of FP examinations from screening mammography.[28] Screening mammography recalls are common in the United States;[29] however, the vast majority of recalls turn out to be normal.[30] Framing recalls as part of a continuous portion of the screening process in which additional images are occasionally required to complete the imaging evaluation, health care providers can help reduce anxiety associated with recalls. In addition, radiology practices can implement strategies to reduce harm associated with FPs from mammographic screening.[31–33] Emerging technologies like artificial intelligence offer the prospect of reducing variation in mammography performance.[34] By adopting these interventions, radiology practices can maximize the benefits of screening mammography while reducing potential harms.

BREAST CANCER SCREENING RECOMMENDATIONS FOR HIGH-RISK WOMEN

The principal goal of breast cancer screening is to detect small, non-palpable, node-negative breast cancers to allow the least morbid treatments and mortality. Identifying women at the highest risk of disease can direct the use of supplemental screening in addition to screening mammography.

Population Subgroups at Increased Risk

The ASBrS cites the National Comprehensive Cancer Network (NCCN) guidelines for characterizing women as high risk for breast cancer including the following groups (**Fig. 5**)[35,36] In only 5% to 10% of women with breast cancer is a known genetic mutation identified.[37]

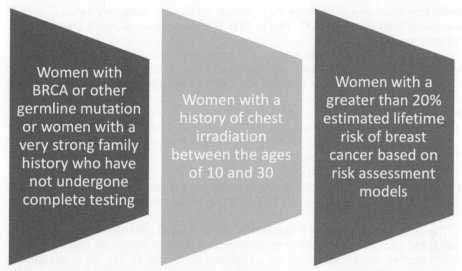

Fig. 5. Women categorized as high risk for breast cancer according to NCCN guidelines.

Breast Cancer Risk Assessment

Women with risk factors for breast cancer can benefit from earlier, supplemental screening. The ASBrS and NCCN recommend all women undergo a formal risk assessment at 25 year old.[38]

To determine whether a woman is at average or increased risk, the assessment begins with gathering patient genetic, familial, personal, reproductive, demographic, lifestyle factors, and factors such as the number of biopsies (especially those finding atypical hyperplasia, lobular carcinoma in situ, and flat epithelial atypia). The family history should be assessed for first-degree, second-degree, and third-degree relatives on both the maternal and paternal sides of the family.

Many statistical models have been developed to estimate the risk of developing breast cancer and the risk of carrying a heritable genetic mutation. Common models include Gail model, Claus, BRCAPRO, BOADICEA, and Tyrer-Cuzick. Each model incorporates and weighs different sets of risk factors. Hence, the models can give different estimates for the same woman. To improve discriminatory accuracy, a few models also include modifiable lifestyle risk factors such as body mass index, alcohol use, exercise, and non-modifiable mammographic breast density (MBD). The modified Tyrer-Cuzick 8 risk-assessment model includes MBD, which is an important risk factor. The Tyrer-Cuzick model is the most comprehensive but is also the most time intensive.[39] To determine eligibility for MRI screening, the ACS and NCCN recommend using models that are largely dependent on family history (eg, Claus, BRCAPRO and Tyrer-Cuzick) and recommend against using models with limited family history (eg, Gail or modified Gall).[40]

Implications of Breast Density

Breast density is a mammographic assessment of the ratio of fibroglandular tissue (white) to fat (gray) in the breast. The ACR BI-RADS atlas[6] requires reporting of breast density in every mammogram report as fatty (A), scattered (B), heterogeneously dense (C), or extremely dense (D). The fatty and scattered categories (A and B) are considered non-dense, whereas the heterogeneously and extremely dense (C and D) are considered dense (**Fig. 6**). Nearly 43% of women aged 40 to 74 year old have dense breasts.[41]

Mammographic density is one of the strongest risk factors for breast cancer. Women with extremely dense mammographic patterns show four to six times higher risk of developing breast cancer compared with those with fatty breasts[41,42] Another implication of dense breasts is the masking effect, or reduced sensitivity of mammography in detecting noncalcified cancers in women with dense breasts. The sensitivity of mammography in the detection of breast cancer is close to 90% for fatty breasts and drops to 60% for women with extremely dense breasts.[43] This masking effect can cause a delay in diagnosis, potentially resulting in an interval, clinically palpable tumor. An interval cancer is one that manifests within 1 year of a normal mammogram. Interval cancers typically have a worse prognosis than cancers detected by radiologic screening, and interval cancer rates increase with increasing breast density.[44]

The definition of "dense" is subjective by the radiologist and therefore inter-observer variability can be significant among radiologists. Improving the consistency of screening recommendations based on density assessments has led to the growth of automated software programs for reliable and reproducible quantitative and volumetric breast density assessment. Application of deep learning (DL) methods for density assessment is an emerging area of research.

In the United States, currently at least 38 states require patients to be notified about their breast density and what it means to have dense breasts.[43] Because of the limitations of mammography, supplemental screening has been advocated for women with dense breast tissue. In 2019, the FDA proposed a rule to the MQSA Act that would make it a national requirement that all mammography centers in all states communicate information about dense breast tissue to their patients. As of this date, this proposed rule is under review.

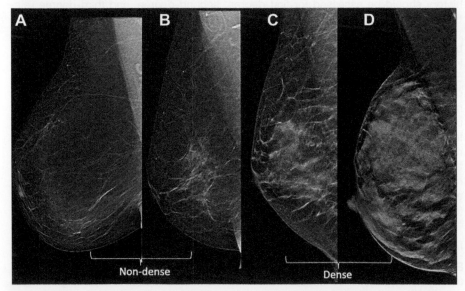

Fig. 6. BI-RADS Breast Density Categories: (*A*) Fatty (*B*) Scattered fibroglandular (*C*) Heterogeneously Dense (*D*) Extremely dense.

SUPPLEMENTAL SCREENING MODALITIES

As risk assessments become more comprehensive with the incorporation of breast density, more women are being notified of their lifetime risk for breast cancer. For women deemed high risk, the screening guidelines are relatively well-defined. For women with intermediate-risk and/or increased breast density, supplemental screening modalities should be discussed with these women. Available options include anatomic screening with DBT and whole-breast ultrasound (WBUS), and functional screening with breast MRI, contrast-enhanced digital mammography (CEDM), MBI, and fluorodeoxyglucose-PET dedicated breast imaging. The American College of Radiology Appropriateness Criteria are evidence-based guidelines for specific clinical conditions that are reviewed annually by a multidisciplinary expert panel. The ACR Appropriateness Criteria reviewed the evidence regarding supplemental Breast Cancer Screening based on Breast Density and lifetime risk.[45] (**Table 1**).

Digital Breast Tomosynthesis

DBT, approved by the FDA in 2011, is an X-ray mammography technique in which tomographic images of the breast are reconstructed from multiple low-dose projections acquired by moving the X-ray tube in an arc over a limited angular range (**Fig. 7**). DBT technique reduces the impact of overlapping breast tissue which ultimately increases the conspicuity of lesions while reducing FPs due to summation. The FDA has approved software for the reconstruction of 2D synthetic views from 3D acquired data, which allows the radiation dose to remain comparable to that of conventional FFDM and has permitted DBT with synthetic reconstruction to replace FFDM.[46]

The use of DBT is widespread and currently many facilities in the United States offer DBT as their primary screening modality. Two prospective European screening trials[44,47] showed an incremental CDR of 2.3 and 2.7 per 1000 screening examinations with DBT as compared with digital mammography alone. Friedwald and colleagues,[48] using a multi-institutional retrospective analysis, showed an incremental CDR of 1.2 cancers per 1000 screening examination with DBT. However, for extremely dense breasts, there was no improvement in cancer detection for DBT over DM.[49] Additional benefits of adding DBT to 2D mammography is the reduction in recall rate, with a meta-analysis showing an absolute reduction in recall rate of 0.8% to 3.6%.[50] The ACR Appropriateness criteria suggest that DBT is appropriate for all women regardless of breast density and risk status.[45]

Whole-Breast Ultrasound

Multiple studies confirm the incremental cancer detection capabilities of WBUS in women with higher risk. ACRIN 6666 was a prospective, multicenter trial, randomized to the sequence of mammography and US, designed to evaluate the performance of screening US in conjunction with mammography in high-risk women.[51] Screening US was associated with the detection of an additional 4.2 cancers per 1000 women screened. However, these additional cancers were balanced by a large increase in FP findings and reduce PPVs. In the Japan Strategic Anti-cancer Randomized Trial (J-START), asymptomatic women between the ages of 40 to 49 were randomized to undergo mammography and ultrasonography versus mammography alone twice in 2 years.[52] Women undergoing supplemental screening US had more cancers detected than those undergoing mammography alone; however, specificity was lower. With increased experience with screening-breast US and technological advances, some of the limitations associated with screening-breast US may diminish.[53]

Table 1
Summary of ACR recommendations for supplemental screening based on cancer risk and breast density

Modality	Average Risk		Intermediate Risk		High Risk	
	Non-dense	Dense	Non-dense	Dense	Non-dense	Dense
Digital breast tomosynthesis	Usually appropriate	Usually appropriate	Usually appropriate	Usually appropriate	Usually appropriate	Usually appropriate
Whole-breast ultrasound	Usually not appropriate	May be appropriate	Usually not appropriate	May be appropriate	May be appropriate	Usually appropriate
Breast MRI	Usually not appropriate	May be appropriate	May be appropriate	May be appropriate	Usually appropriate	Usually appropriate
Abbreviated breast MRI	Usually not appropriate	May be appropriate	May be appropriate	May be appropriate	May be appropriate	Usually appropriate
Molecular breast imaging	Usually not appropriate	Usually not appropriate	Usually not appropriate	Usually not appropriate	Usually not appropriate	Usually not appropriate
Contrast-enhanced mammography	Usually not appropriate	May be appropriate	May be appropriate	May be appropriate	May be appropriate	May be appropriate

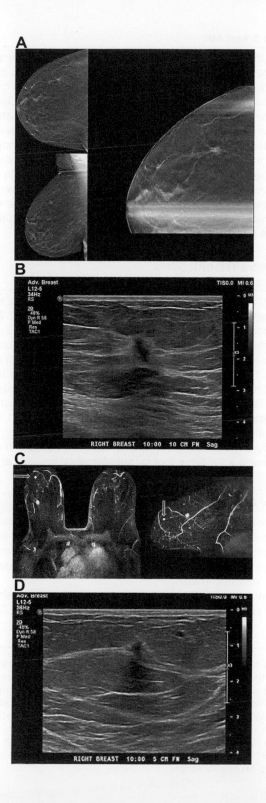

Contrast Enhanced Breast MRI

The ASBrS notes that contrast-enhanced breast MRI is more sensitive than either mammography and/or US.[54] In addition, cancers detected on breast MRI were more likely to be invasive carcinomas, whereas cancers detected on mammography were more likely to be in situ cancers.[55] Consequently, the ACS advocates MRI screening for women with an approximately 20% to 25% or greater lifetime risk of breast cancer, regardless of breast density.[40] The ASBrS recommends that these patients should be offered MR screening starting at age 25 and mammography at age 30, or 10 years before the first-degree relative was diagnosed, but no earlier than age 25. Emerging data suggest that MRI may be beneficial in women with extremely dense breast tissue, regardless of underlying breast cancer risk. A multicenter, randomized, controlled trial in the Netherlands found that supplemental MRI screening in women with extremely dense breast tissue resulted in the diagnosis of significantly fewer interval cancers than mammography alone.[56]

EMERGING SCREENING TECHNOLOGIES
Molecular Breast Imaging

MBI is a functional imaging technique involving the injection of a radiopharmaceutical agent (technetium-99m sestamibi) and obtaining CC and MLO projections (similar to mammography) using a dedicated breast imaging system with dual-head solid-state detectors. Studies evaluating MBI as a supplemental screening technique for women with dense breasts have shown an incremental CDR between 7.5 to 8 per 1000. The median tumor size of cancer detected by MBI only is 1 cm, with an additional recall rate of 5.9% to 8.4%[57–59] As Tc-99 sestamibi is systemically distributed, tissues outside the breast receive the largest radiation dose. The estimated whole-body dose for 8 mi of Tc-99 sestamibi is 2.1 to 2.6 mSv which is below annual natural background levels of $\sim$3 mSv.[60] Concerns regarding MBI radiation risk, though disputed, have led to it slow adoption in clinical practice. However, MBI remains a sensitive tool for supplemental imaging and further studies are needed.

Contrast-Enhanced Digital Mammography

By enhancing tumor vascularity, contrast-enhanced breast MRI screening substantially increases cancer detection compared with mammography and/or breast US. However, the dissemination of breast MRI has been limited by lack of widespread availability and high costs. CEDM uses CEDM platforms to leveraged enhanced cancer detection from vascular imaging.

Initial studies evaluating CEDM as a screening modality have yielded promising results.[61] Sung and colleagues[62] evaluated the performance of CEDM in 904 women

Fig. 7. (A) A 63-year-old woman presenting for screening mammogram with tomosynthesis. Patient was found to have a focal asymmetry in the right upper outer breast, which persisted on additional diagnostic spot compression views. (B) Focused ultrasound of the right breast found a 0.9-cm mass at 10:00, 10 cm from the nipple, which was subsequently biopsied revealing invasive lobular carcinoma, grade 2/3. (C) A pre-operative MRI evaluation showed the known malignancy in the right breast at 10:00, but also revealed a second smaller mass in the right breast at 10:00 at anterior depth (arrow). (D) MR-directed ultrasound showed a 0.6-cm mass at 10:00, 5 cm from the nipple, which revealed invasive lobular carcinoma grade 2/3 on needle biopsy.

undergoing screening CEDM for a variety of indications (dense breasts, family history of breast cancer in a first-degree relative, personal history of breast cancer) and found high CDRs (15.5 per 1000 women) and high sensitivity (87.5%). CEM may be an alternative for patients who are unable to undergo MRI, intermediate-risk patient populations who do not qualify for MRI screening, and as an alternative to breast MRI in settings with limited access to breast MRI.

Abbreviated Breast MRI

Abbreviated breast MRI examinations reduce image acquisition and interpretation times to increase access and decrease costs associated with breast MRIs. Chen and colleagues[63] found no statistically significant differences in sensitivity comparing full breast MRI protocols with abbreviated breast MRI protocols. The ECOG-ACRIN Cancer Research Group conducted a prospective, multicenter, study in the United States and Germany.[64] Among women with dense breasts undergoing screening, abbreviated breast MRI was associated with a higher rate of invasive breast cancer detection (incremental cancer detection increase of 7 cancers per 1000 women).

Generalizability of Screening Recommendations

A major limitation of the existing literature is that randomized control trials used for meta-analyses incorporated study populations with limited numbers of racial/ethnic minorities. As a result, observational studies and statistical models have been used to address gaps in randomized control trial data.

Using SEER population registries, Banegas and colleagues[65] found that Hispanic and Black women had a 10% to 50% greater risk of breast cancer-specific mortality compared with non-Hispanic white women. Stapleton and Oseni and colleagues[66] found that Black, Hispanic, and Asian women were more likely to be diagnosed with breast cancer before the age of 50. In part, due to the potential harms of delayed onset of screening mammography in racial/ethnic minority women, the ASBrS recommends annual screening mammography starting at age 40 in average-risk women.

For transgender patients who are at average risk, ACR recommendations for breast cancer screening were based on expert opinion derived from limited data.[67] For average-risk transgender patients, the ACR recommends annual screening starting at age 40 for male-to-female transgender patients who have used hormones for 5 years as well as female-to-male transgender patients who have not undergone mastectomy [99]. Individuals who identify as lesbian, gay, bisexual, or queer are less likely to present for cancer screening, emphasizing the importance of creating and fostering inclusive environments.[68]

SUMMARY

In summary, breast cancer is the second leading cause of cancer death among women in the United States. Mammography screening in average-risk women reduces breast cancer mortality. Black, Hispanic, and Asian women are more likely to be diagnosed with breast cancer before the age of 50. To reduce disparities and prevent the maximum number of breast cancer deaths, the ASBrS recommends that average-risk women undergo breast cancer screening every year starting at age 40. Women with risk factors for breast cancer can benefit from earlier, supplemental screening. Emerging technologies such as contrast-enhanced mammography and abbreviated breast MRI may facilitate early detection and improve patient outcomes in the appropriate clinical settings.

CLINICS CARE POINTS

- Screening mammography reduces breast cancer mortality
- The American Society of Breast Surgeons recommends that average-risk women undergo breast cancer screening every year starting at age 40
- Women with risk factors for breast cancer can benefit from earlier, supplemental screening
- Black, Hispanic, and Asian women are more likely to be diagnosed with breast cancer before the age of 50
- The American College of Radiology recommends annual screening starting at age 40 for male-to-female transgender patients who have used hormones for 5 years as well as female-to-male transgender patients who have not undergone mastectomy

---

DISCLOSURE

The authors have nothing to disclose.

REFERENCES

1. Smith RA, Andrews KS, Brooks D, et al. Cancer screening in the United States, 2019: A review of current American Cancer Society guidelines and current issues in cancer screening. CA Cancer J Clin 2019;69(3):184–210.
2. Siegel RL, Miller KD, Fuchs HE, et al. Cancer statistics, 2022. CA Cancer J Clin 2022;72(1):7–33.
3. Radiation Dose to Adults from Common Imaging Examinations. ACR Available at: https://www.acr.org/-/media/ACR/Files/Radiology-Safety/Radiation-Safety/Dose-Reference-Card.pdf Google Scholar.
4. Calculate Your Radiation Dose. EPA Available at: https://www.epa.gov/radiation/calculate-your-radiation-dose Google Scholar.
5. Garayoa J, Hernandez-Giron I, Castillo M, et al. In: Fujita H, Hara T, Muramatsu C, editors. Digital breast tomosynthesis: image quality and dose Saving of the Synthesized image. Breast imaging. IWDM 2014. Lecture notes in computer Science, 8539. Cham: Springer; 2014. https://doi.org/10.1007/978-3-319-07887-8_22.
6. Sickles EA, D'Orsi CJ. ACR BI-RADS Follow-up and Outcome Monitoring. In: D'Orsi CJ, Sickles EA, Mendelson EB, et al, editors. ACR BI-RADS atlas, breast imaging reporting and data system. Reston, VA: American College of Radiology; 2013 [Google Scholar].
7. Lee CS, Moy L, Friedewald SM, et al. Harmonizing Breast Cancer Screening Recommendations: Metrics and Accountability. AJR Am J Roentgenol 2018;210(2): 241–5.
8. Smith RA, Duffy SW, Gabe R, et al. The randomized trials of breast cancer screening: what have we learned? Radiol Clin North Am 2004;42(5):793-v.
9. Tabár L, Yen AM, Wu WY, et al. Insights from the breast cancer screening trials: how screening affects the natural history of breast cancer and implications for evaluating service screening programs. Breast J 2015;21(1):13–20.
10. Oeffinger KC, Fontham ET, Etzioni R, et al. Breast Cancer Screening for Women at Average Risk: 2015 Guideline Update From the American Cancer Society [published correction appears in JAMA. JAMA 2015;314(15):1599–1614, 1406.
11. Narayan AK, Lee CI, Lehman CD. Screening for Breast Cancer. Med Clin North Am 2020;104(6):1007–21.

12. Broeders M, Moss S, Nyström L, et al. The impact of mammographic screening on breast cancer mortality in Europe: a review of observational studies. J Med Screen 2012;19(Suppl 1):14–25.
13. Coldman A, Phillips N, Wilson C, et al. Pan-Canadian study of mammography screening and mortality from breast cancer [published correction appears in. J Natl Cancer Inst 2015;107(1):dju404.
14. Pocobelli G, Weiss NS. Breast cancer mortality in relation to receipt of screening mammography: a case-control study in Saskatchewan, Canada. Cancer Causes Control 2015;26(2):231–7.
15. Yen AM, Tsau HS, Fann JC, et al. Population-Based Breast Cancer Screening With Risk-Based and Universal Mammography Screening Compared With Clinical Breast Examination: A Propensity Score Analysis of 1 429 890 Taiwanese Women. JAMA Oncol 2016;2(7):915–21.
16. Morrell S, Taylor R, Roder D, et al. Mammography service screening and breast cancer mortality in New Zealand: a National Cohort Study 1999-2011. Br J Cancer 2017;116(6):828–39.
17. Moss SM, Nyström L, Jonsson H, et al. The impact of mammographic screening on breast cancer mortality in Europe: a review of trend studies. J Med Screen 2012;19(Suppl 1):26–32.
18. Narayan AK, Lehman CD. Mammography Screening Guideline Controversies: Opportunities to Improve Patient Engagement in Screening. J Am Coll Radiol 2020;17(5):633–6.
19. Badgwell BD, Giordano SH, Duan ZZ, et al. Mammography before diagnosis among women age 80 years and older with breast cancer. J Clin Oncol 2008; 26(15):2482–8.
20. Brawley O, Byers T, Chen A, et al. New American Cancer Society process for creating trustworthy cancer screening guidelines. JAMA 2011;306(22):2495–9.
21. Miglioretti DL, Zhu W, Kerlikowske K, et al. Breast Tumor Prognostic Characteristics and Biennial vs Annual Mammography, Age, and Menopausal Status. JAMA Oncol 2015;1(8):1069–77.
22. Harris RP, Helfand M, Woolf SH, et al. Current methods of the US Preventive Services Task Force: a review of the process. Am J Prev Med 2001;20(3 Suppl): 21–35.
23. Nelson HD, Pappas M, Cantor A, et al. Harms of Breast Cancer Screening: Systematic Review to Update the 2009 U.S. Preventive Services Task Force Recommendation. Ann Intern Med 2016;164(4):256–67 [published correction appears in Ann Intern Med. 2018 Nov 20;169(10):740].
24. Puliti D, Duffy SW, Miccinesi G, et al. Overdiagnosis in mammographic screening for breast cancer in Europe: a literature review. J Med Screen 2012;19(Suppl 1): 42–56.
25. Breast Cancer Surveillance Consortium. Breast Cancer Surveillance Consortium. Available at URL: https://www.bcsc-research.org/. Accessed July 09, 2020.
26. Hubbard RA, Kerlikowske K, Flowers CI, et al. Cumulative probability of false-positive recall or biopsy recommendation after 10 years of screening mammography: a cohort study. Ann Intern Med 2011;155(8):481–92 [published correction appears in Ann Intern Med. 2014 May 6;160(9):658].
27. Tosteson AN, Fryback DG, Hammond CS, et al. Consequences of false-positive screening mammograms. JAMA Intern Med 2014;174(6):954–61.
28. Lehman CD, Arao RF, Sprague BL, et al. National Performance Benchmarks for Modern Screening Digital Mammography: Update from the Breast Cancer Surveillance Consortium. Radiology 2017;283(1):49–58.

29. Nelson HD, O'Meara ES, Kerlikowske K, et al. Factors Associated With Rates of False-Positive and False-Negative Results From Digital Mammography Screening: An Analysis of Registry Data. Ann Intern Med 2016;164(4):226–35.
30. Berg WA. Benefits of screening mammography. JAMA 2010;303(2):168–9.
31. Burnside ES, Park JM, Fine JP, et al. The use of batch reading to improve the performance of screening mammography. AJR Am J Roentgenol 2005;185(3):790–6.
32. Froicu M, Mani KL, Coughlin B. Satisfaction With Same-Day-Read Baseline Mammography. J Am Coll Radiol 2019;16(3):321–6.
33. Dontchos BN, Narayan AK, Seidler M, et al. Impact of a Same-Day Breast Biopsy Program on Disparities in Time to Biopsy. J Am Coll Radiol 2019;16(11):1554–60.
34. Lehman CD, Yala A, Schuster T, et al. Mammographic Breast Density Assessment Using Deep Learning: Clinical Implementation. Radiology 2019;290(1):52–8.
35. NCCN Guidelines Version 1.2021 Breast Cancer Screening and Diagnosis.
36. NCCN Guidelines Version 1.2022 Breast Cancer Risk Reduction.
37. Claus EB, Schildkraut JM, Thompson WD, et al. The genetic attributable risk of breast and ovarian cancer. Cancer 1996;77(11):2318–24.
38. The American Society of Breast Surgeons website. Position statement on screening mammography. Available at: www.breastsurgeons.org/docs/statements/Position Statement-on-Screening-Mammography.pdf.
39. Monticciolo DL, Newell MS, Moy L, et al. Breast Cancer Screening in Women at Higher-Than-Average Risk: Recommendations From the ACR. J Am Coll Radiol 2018;15(3 Pt A):408–14.
40. Saslow D, Boetes C, Burke W, et al. American Cancer Society guidelines for breast screening with MRI as an adjunct to mammography. CA Cancer J Clin 2007;57(2):75–89 [published correction appears in CA Cancer J Clin. 2007 May-Jun;57(3):185].
41. McCormack VA, dos Santos Silva I. Breast density and parenchymal patterns as markers of breast cancer risk: a meta-analysis. Cancer Epidemiol Biomarkers Prev 2006;15(6):1159–69.
42. Yaghjyan L, Colditz GA, Rosner B, et al. Mammographic breast density and breast cancer risk: interactions of percent density, absolute dense, and non-dense areas with breast cancer risk factors. Breast Cancer Res Treat 2015; 150(1):181–9.
43. DenseBreast-Info. Legislation and regulation. 2015. Available at. https://dense breast-info.org/legislation.aspx. Google Scholar.
44. Ciatto S, Houssami N, Bernardi D, et al. Integration of 3D digital mammography with tomosynthesis for population breast-cancer screening (STORM): a prospective comparison study. Lancet Oncol 2013;14(7):583–9.
45. Expert Panel on Breast Imaging, Weinstein SP, Slanetz PJ, et al. ACR Appropriateness Criteria® Supplemental Breast Cancer Screening Based on Breast Density. J Am Coll Radiol 2021;18(11S):S456–73.
46. Svahn TM, Houssami N, Sechopoulos I, et al. Review of radiation dose estimates in digital breast tomosynthesis relative to those in two-view full-field digital mammography. Breast 2015;24(2):93–9.
47. Skaane P, Bandos AI, Gullien R, et al. Comparison of digital mammography alone and digital mammography plus tomosynthesis in a population-based screening program. Radiology 2013;267(1):47–56.
48. Friedewald SM, Rafferty EA, Rose SL, et al. Breast cancer screening using tomosynthesis in combination with digital mammography. JAMA 2014;311(24): 2499–507.

49. Rafferty EA, Durand MA, Conant EF, et al. Breast Cancer Screening Using Tomosynthesis and Digital Mammography in Dense and Nondense Breasts. JAMA 2016;315(16):1784–6.

50. Houssami N. Digital breast tomosynthesis (3D-mammography) screening: data and implications for population screening. Expert Rev Med Devices 2015; 12(4):377–9.

51. Berg WA, Blume JD, Cormack JB, et al. Combined screening with ultrasound and mammography vs mammography alone in women at elevated risk of breast cancer. JAMA 2008;299(18):2151–2163 [published correction appears in JAMA. 2010 Apr 21;303(15):1482].

52. Ohuchi N, Suzuki A, Sobue T, et al. Sensitivity and specificity of mammography and adjunctive ultrasonography to screen for breast cancer in the Japan Strategic Anti-cancer Randomized Trial (J-START): a randomised controlled trial. Lancet 2016;387(10016):341–8.

53. Weigert J, Steenbergen S. The connecticut experiments second year: ultrasound in the screening of women with dense breasts. Breast J 2015;21(2):175–80.

54. Kuhl CK, Schrading S, Leutner CC, et al. Mammography, breast ultrasound, and magnetic resonance imaging for surveillance of women at high familial risk for breast cancer. J Clin Oncol 2005;23(33):8469–76.

55. Sung JS, Stamler S, Brooks J, et al. Breast Cancers Detected at Screening MR Imaging and Mammography in Patients at High Risk: Method of Detection Reflects Tumor Histopathologic Results. Radiology 2016;280(3):716–22.

56. Bakker MF, de Lange SV, Pijnappel RM, et al. Supplemental MRI Screening for Women with Extremely Dense Breast Tissue. N Engl J Med 2019;381(22): 2091–102.

57. Rhodes DJ, Hruska CB, Phillips SW, et al. Dedicated dual-head gamma imaging for breast cancer screening in women with mammographically dense breasts. Radiology 2011;258(1):106–18.

58. Rhodes DJ, Hruska CB, Conners AL, et al. Journal club: molecular breast imaging at reduced radiation dose for supplemental screening in mammographically dense breasts. AJR Am J Roentgenol 2015;204(2):241–51.

59. Shermis RB, Wilson KD, Doyle MT, et al. Supplemental Breast Cancer Screening With Molecular Breast Imaging for Women With Dense Breast Tissue. AJR Am J Roentgenol 2016;207(2):450–7.

60. Hruska CB. Let's Get Real about Molecular Breast Imaging and Radiation Risk. Radiol Imaging Cancer 2019;1(1):e190070. Published 2019 Sep 27.

61. Jochelson MS, Lobbes MBI. Contrast-enhanced Mammography: State of the Art. Radiology 2021;299(1):36–48. https://doi.org/10.1148/radiol.2021201948.

62. Sung JS, Lebron L, Keating D, et al. Performance of Dual-Energy Contrast-enhanced Digital Mammography for Screening Women at Increased Risk of Breast Cancer. Radiology 2019;293(1):81–8.

63. Chen SQ, Huang M, Shen YY, et al. Application of Abbreviated Protocol of Magnetic Resonance Imaging for Breast Cancer Screening in Dense Breast Tissue. Acad Radiol 2017;24(3):316–20.

64. Comstock CE, Gatsonis C, Newstead GM, et al. Comparison of Abbreviated Breast MRI vs Digital Breast Tomosynthesis for Breast Cancer Detection Among Women With Dense Breasts Undergoing Screening. JAMA 2020;323(8):746–56 [published correction appears in JAMA. 2020 Mar 24;323(12):1194].

65. Banegas MP, Li CI. Breast cancer characteristics and outcomes among Hispanic Black and Hispanic White women. Breast Cancer Res Treat 2012;134(3): 1297–304.

66. Stapleton SM, Oseni TO, Bababekov YJ, et al. Race/Ethnicity and Age Distribution of Breast Cancer Diagnosis in the United States. JAMA Surg 2018;153(6): 594–5.
67. Monticciolo DL, Malak SF, Friedewald SM, et al. Breast Cancer Screening Recommendations Inclusive of All Women at Average Risk: Update from the ACR and Society of Breast Imaging. J Am Coll Radiol 2021;18(9):1280–8.
68. Perry H, Fang AJ, Tsai EM, et al. Imaging Health and Radiology Care of Transgender Patients: A Call to Build Evidence-Based Best Practices. J Am Coll Radiol 2021;18(3 Pt B):475–80.

De-Escalating Breast Cancer Therapy

Mary A. Varsanik, MD, Sarah P. Shubeck, MD, MS*

KEYWORDS

• Breast cancer therapy • De-escalation • Chemotherapy • Surgical management

DE-ESCALATION OF BREAST CANCER THERAPY

Patients with breast cancer, including those with early-stage disease, have historically been subject to invasive surgical procedures, medical therapies, and radiation therapy. However, the reporting of large-scale, randomized controlled trial results has led to significant paradigm shifts in the management of patients with breast cancer allowing for decreased morbidity, increased patient choice, and improved survival.[1–6] This significant progress in appropriate patient selection for procedures, such as axillary lymph-node dissection (ALND), and the opportunity to selectively tailor medical management, such as identifying those most likely to benefit from chemotherapy, have resulted in significant therapeutic de-escalation. These changes to standard treatment options can reduce morbidity for patients without compromising breast cancer-specific survival.[4,7]

This article highlights the significant breast cancer therapy de-escalation across diagnoses and treatment modalities and recent changes in the overall care for patients with breast cancer. The article also explores the current and future potential de-implementation of low-value practices in breast cancer therapy.

SURGICAL DE-ESCALATION

Breast conservation. De-escalation in the surgical management of invasive breast cancer has allowed for the omission of mastectomy in a large proportion of patients in recent years.[8,9] When performed in combination with adjuvant radiotherapy, breast-conserving surgery affords similar survival to mastectomy. The rate of local recurrence is decreased with the addition of radiotherapy, but the retained tissue has been found to have a slightly increased risk of local recurrence. Several large-scale trials and their long-term follow-up data allowed breast conservation to be an acceptable alternative to mastectomy for the treatment of early-stage breast cancer amenable to local excision.[10,11]

Department of Surgery, University of Chicago, 5841 South Maryland Avenue, Chicago, IL 60637, USA
* Corresponding author.
E-mail address: Shubeck@bsd.uchicago.edu

Surg Clin N Am 103 (2023) 83–92
https://doi.org/10.1016/j.suc.2022.08.005
0039-6109/23/© 2022 Elsevier Inc. All rights reserved.

surgical.theclinics.com

The management of ductal carcinoma in situ (DCIS), Stage 0 breast cancer, has also changed significantly in the last few decades. Currently, there are no studies comparing breast conservation to mastectomy in the management of DCIS. However, several randomized trials compared partial mastectomy alone to partial mastectomy followed by radiation for DCIS. For example, the National Surgical Adjuvant Breast and Bowel Project (NSABP) B-17 trial showed that radiation after partial mastectomy reduced invasive Ipsilateral Breast Tumor Recurrence (IBTR) by 52% compared with those who did not receive adjuvant radiation. In addition, radiation provided a 10-year risk reduction of IBTR of 15%.[12] European Organisation for Research and Treatment of Cancer (EORTC) 10853 achieved similar results with a reduction in local recurrence rates as a result of adjuvant radiation after local excision of DCIS.[13] These studies and others inferred the safety of partial mastectomy for DCIS, but required more frequent adjuvant radiation to achieve the above-described oncologic outcomes.

The use of neoadjuvant chemotherapy, or systemic therapy before surgery, has served to further increase the success of de-escalation in breast surgery for invasive cancer through the potential to downstage breast malignancies over 2 cm. By decreasing tumor volume, neoadjuvant medical therapy can allow for improved candidacy for breast conservation and avoidance of mastectomy. The NSABP B-18 and EORTC 10902 trials showed that patients receiving preoperative chemotherapy were more likely to receive breast-conserving surgery secondary to downstaging of the primary tumor with no difference in overall survival, disease-free survival, or local regional recurrence compared with similar patients receiving adjuvant chemotherapy.[14,15] Furthermore, in a review of a larger set of randomized control trials comparing neoadjuvant to adjuvant therapy, patients receiving neoadjuvant therapy consistently had increased breast conservation rates without impacting the rate of local control.[16]

Another significant opportunity for de-escalation in surgical therapy for invasive breast cancer occurred in response to the Society of Surgical Oncology and American Society of Radiation Oncology (SSO-ASTRO) guideline for surgical margins specifying "no tumor on ink" in 2014. In patients undergoing breast conservation for an early-stage malignancy with adjuvant whole breast radiation, margins wider than "no tumor on ink" did not significantly decrease breast recurrence.[17] Upon release of this guideline, the initial rate of partial mastectomy for patients remained unchanged; however, the rate of surgery after index partial mastectomy decreased by approximately 40% with reduced subsequent conversion to mastectomy.[18,19] After this change in standard recommendations, the rates of re-excision and conversion to mastectomy following index excision decreased significantly.[19–21] This clarity in the definition of acceptable surgical margin led to a de-escalation of surgical therapy for invasive breast cancer, decreased surgical morbidity for patients, and reduced resource utilization.

Axillary surgery. One of the most significant shifts in breast cancer surgery occurred in response to the results of the American College of Surgeons Oncology Group (ACOSOG) Z0011. This randomized controlled trial compared completion ALND to sentinel lymph-node biopsy (SLNB) alone for patients with micrometastasis or macrometastasis in 1 or 2 sentinel lymph nodes at the time of breast-conserving surgery for clinical T1-2 N0 breast cancer. Patients undergoing a partial mastectomy and SLNB with subsequent whole breast radiation had no difference in overall survival or local, regional, or distant recurrence with long-term follow-up compared with those undergoing ALND.[3] Before the release of these results, ALND was the standard surgical approach in patients with positive sentinel nodes. After these findings were presented at national meetings and published in 2011, the percentage of patients undergoing ALND decreased significantly from 63% in 2004 to 14% in 2016. The greatest period of change from 62% to 31% between 2010 to 2011 corresponded with the release and dissemination of trial findings.[18]

Further axillary surgical de-escalation for older women with early-stage estrogen receptor-positive cancer occurred after the publication of the findings of CALGB 9343.[22] This study randomized women over the age of 70 with estrogen receptor-positive, clinical stage I breast cancer to tamoxifen with radiation therapy or tamoxifen alone after partial mastectomy. Radiation provided a small benefit in locoregional recurrence, but had no impact on survival. In addition, the authors reported no difference in survival for patients who underwent SLNB compared with those who did not. In the long-term data, there was a very minimal increase in axillary recurrence in patients who avoided post-partial mastectomy radiation and SLNB.[6,22] These findings suggest the limited role of SLNB in this population and in adjuvant therapy decision-making. These findings informed a national guideline recommending avoidance of SLNB in this population as part of the Choosing Wisely campaign (www.choosingwisely.org). However, in spite of clear evidence supporting the avoidance of this practice, SLNB continues to be performed at an elevated rate in this population with 88% in 2013 and 87% in 2016.[18]

The use of SLNB for axillary assessment in pre-neoadjuvant, clinically node-negative breast surgery patients is well established.[23–25] The reliability of axillary assessment allowed for the omission of routine ALND and therefore reduction in morbidity reduction with low false negative rates. Axillary surgery has been further de-escalated in patients undergoing neoadjuvant chemotherapy with the demonstration of the safety and reliability of SLNB for axillary assessment in previously node-positive patients. ACOSOG Z1071 and SENTINA (SENTinel NeoAdjuvant) showed the feasibility and appropriately low false negative rate of less than 10% in patients with previously positive axillae after neoadjuvant chemotherapy when performed with dual tracer mapping and removal of three or more lymph nodes.[26,27] The ability to assess axillary involvement with a sufficient success rate allowed for patients who would previously have been required to undergo ALND to be candidates for SLNB.[28,29] This allowed the identification of patients who achieved a nodal pathologic complete response after neoadjuvant therapy to avoid the more morbid completion of axillary dissection.

Mastectomy. Another area of surgical de-escalation in the current era of breast cancer treatment addresses women of average risk with unilateral breast cancer who opt to undergo a bilateral mastectomy. Although contralateral prophylactic mastectomy does decrease the risk of contralateral breast cancer, it offers no survival compared with unilateral breast surgery in patients of average risk without a genetic predisposition to breast cancer.[30] In 2007, the SSO issued a consensus guideline recommending against routine contralateral prophylactic mastectomy in average-risk women, yet rates of this procedure continued to increase from 11% in 2004 to 26% in 2016.[18] However, a more recent study evaluated patient likelihood to undergo bilateral mastectomy before and after receiving a negative genetic testing result. In this study cohort, patients were much less likely to choose bilateral breast surgery when aware of their negative genetics before finalizing a surgical plan.[31]

Surveillance versus surgery. There are several areas of an ongoing investigation for continued surgical de-escalation. Recently, exploration of the overdiagnosis and therefore associated potential overtreatment of DCIS have led to studies evaluating the potential safety in the omission of surgery in DCIS.[32] These protocols include active surveillance alone or active surveillance with the addition of endocrine therapy for patients with biopsy-proven DCIS.[33] These ongoing trials include the COMET (Comparison of Operative versus Monitoring and Endocrine Therapy), LORIS (the

LOw RISk DCIS Trial), and LORD (LOw Risk DCIS) trials.[34,35] These trials most often include patients with DCIS with low-risk features to explore how often the diagnosis will actually impact oncologic outcomes in the absence of surgical resection. The safety and effectiveness of these active surveillance protocols will be determined after the completion of these trials and final analysis. Importantly, the outcome of these trials has the potential to significantly de-escalate the role of surgical resection, medical treatment, and adjuvant radiation for DCIS and could result in significant changes to standard treatment recommendations. Additional areas of potential surgical de-escalation include ongoing evaluation for the potential omission of surgery in women with exceptional responses to chemotherapy.[36,37]

DE-ESCALATION OF MEDICAL THERAPY

Recent developments in breast cancer therapeutics, release of large-scale trials assessing appropriate candidates for chemotherapy benefit, and improved understanding of breast cancer biology have allowed for significant de-escalation in medical therapy. For example, the Oncotype DX assay is a 21-gene analysis that is widely used in the assessment of recurrence risk for hormone receptor-positive breast cancer. This was used in the TAILORx study (Trial Assigning Individualized Options for Treatment) to determine the likelihood of benefit for receipt of chemotherapy.[4,38] The findings of this trial allowed for patients with Hormone Receptor Positive (HR+)/HER2-, axillary node-negative breast cancer to be stratified by Oncotype DX recurrence score. Those patients over age 50 with a score less than 26 were found to be less likely to benefit from chemotherapy, whereas those under age 50 with a score less than 16 received little to no benefit from chemotherapy.[39] These patients instead went on to endocrine therapy without enduring the added toxicity and potential complications of adjuvant chemotherapy.

These findings then were extended with RxPONDER (a Clinical Trial Rx for Positive Node, Endocrine Responsive Breast Cancer) to include women with HR+/HER2- breast cancers with one to three positive lymph nodes.[5,40] In this trial, patients with recurrence scores 0 to 25 were randomized to adjuvant chemotherapy and endocrine therapy compared with endocrine therapy alone. In the interim analysis, for postmenopausal (age greater than 50) women, there was no benefit to adding chemotherapy with invasive disease-free survival of 91.9% versus 91.6% with and without chemotherapy, respectively. However, in premenopausal women, the RxPONDER interim analysis showed a benefit of chemotherapy with invasive disease-free survival of 94.2% versus 89.0% in those with and without chemotherapy, respectively.[41]

Additional trials to improve the selective administration of chemotherapy for patients are ongoing. Specifically, the CompassHER2 (COMprehensive use of Pathologic response ASSessment to optimize therapy in HER2 positive breast cancer) Trial is currently evaluating the omission of additional adjuvant therapy for patients with HER2+ Stage II-IIIa breast cancer who achieve a pathologic complete response after neoadjuvant therapy.[42] Although ongoing innovation and drug discovery may escalate chemotherapy recommendations for some patient populations with breast cancer, the CompassHER2 trial, and other studies will likely further tailor the identification of candidates for chemotherapy benefit in addition to potentially reducing the toxicity of recommended regimens.

DE-ESCALATION OF RADIOTHERAPY

Opportunities for de-escalation of radiotherapy include strategies to decrease associated toxicity and burden of care for patients through reducing the duration and frequency of treatment.[43,44] Efforts to avoid adjuvant radiotherapy entirely have been limited to older patients with low-risk breast cancer diagnoses. Specifically, CALGB 9343 evaluated the impact of radiotherapy on women over 70 with early-stage estrogen receptor-positive breast cancer undergoing a partial mastectomy followed by radiotherapy with endocrine therapy or endocrine therapy alone as described above.[22] Radiotherapy reduced the rate of local recurrence but did not affect survival or potential future need for mastectomy. This suggests omission of radiotherapy may be considered in appropriate patients.

Additional support for the omission of adjuvant radiotherapy in older women with low-risk breast cancer (estrogen receptor positive, node negative, and T1-2 tumors) is found in the results of the PRIME II trial.[6] This trial randomized participants to whole breast radiotherapy versus omission of radiotherapy following breast-conserving surgery and in combination with endocrine therapy. This study showed that whole breast radiotherapy provided a small reduction in local recurrence for patients over 65 at 5 years, but that this reduction in breast tumor recurrence was low enough that it is reasonable to omit radiotherapy in certain patients with low-risk oncologic features.

DIAGNOSES NOT AMENABLE TO DE-ESCALATION

There are several diagnoses and clinical scenarios where de-escalation of breast cancer therapy does not currently have a role. For example, patients with inflammatory breast cancer have been found to have worse survival after breast-conserving therapy and therefore continue to require mastectomy.[45] Efforts to de-escalate axillary evaluation and management with SLNB in inflammatory breast cancer have also proven unsuccessful leading to the persistence of ALND and its associated morbidity in this population.[46] Certain pregnancy-associated breast cancer scenarios are also not amenable to de-escalation efforts. For example, patients in early pregnancy with nodal disease are often required to undergo more invasive surgical intervention given the interaction of potential neoadjuvant medical therapies with their pregnancy.[47,48]

DISCUSSION

Breast cancer therapy is particularly well suited to de-escalation given the large population of patients diagnosed with early-stage, curable disease as a result of screening recommendations and broad access.[49] However, de-implementing, or "reducing or stopping the use of a health service or practice provided to patients," is often a challenging prospect when traditional treatment practices, such as those in breast cancer therapy, are well engrained.[50]

Efforts to effectively de-implement medical practices with demonstrated little to no benefit to certain patient populations often rely on the development and release of national guidelines and recommendations in addition to the education of providers and patients.[17,51] The surgical de-escalation trends are reflected in current national breast cancer treatment recommendations, most notably the Choosing Wisely Campaign. The Choosing Wisely Campaign which focuses on breast cancer therapy encourages the avoidance of completion ALND in selected patients, routine contralateral prophylactic mastectomy in patients with unilateral breast cancer who are not gene carriers, SLNB in patients aged over 70 years with estrogen receptor-positive early-stage breast cancer, and re-excisions for previously considered positive surgical margins (www.choosingwisely.org).[17] Beyond the above examples, ongoing efforts to successfully de-escalate surgical therapy for breast cancer will rely on continued education for providers, integration of new trial results and therapeutic options into National Comprehensive Cancer Network (NCCN) Guidelines, and continued support and educational efforts of national organizations, including the Society of Surgical Oncology (SSO), the American Society of Clinic Oncology (ASCO), and the American Society of Breast Surgeons (ASBrS).

Whether opting for a less invasive surgery or omission of chemotherapy or radiation, patient or provider perceptions may rely on prior experience or social expectations rather than current data and guidelines in decision making.[52] To this point, patients must be educated about the benefits of de-escalation including reduced toxicity and morbidity, improved higher quality of life, and decreased complication risk, rather than on the potential perception of receiving less than the standard of care.[53] Therefore efforts to de-implement low-value practices may require targeted educational initiatives for patients and providers to understand the goal and data supporting de-escalated practices.

Further, given the multidisciplinary nature of breast cancer treatment, de-escalation in one treatment domain, such as surgery, may have significant impacts on decision-making for medical therapies and adjuvant radiation.[1] Attempts at de-escalation of single treatment modalities may inadvertently cause increased utilization of other therapies. This interdependence of treatment modalities sets up potentially competing de-escalation which may ultimately prevent the successful improvement in breast cancer-specific outcomes and survival noted in randomized control trials. To continue de-escalation of breast cancer therapy to proceed, the significant multidisciplinary collaboration will be required.

SUMMARY

The potential value of de-escalation in breast cancer therapy cannot be overstated. From reducing complications and morbidity of surgical therapy to the avoidance of chemotherapy in certain populations, the benefits of eliminating low-value therapies are significant. Further, those interventions that have minimal to no benefit may also further low-risk care cascades resulting in additional treatments or interventions without associated value, with increased financial toxicity, and resulting excess health care expenditures.[54,55]

The recent changes in breast cancer management have resulted in many evidence-based opportunities to de-escalate breast cancer therapy and span all aspects of the multidisciplinary treatment of breast cancer including surgery, medical therapies, and radiation therapy. Ongoing studies will likely serve to continue to move de-escalation of breast cancer forward. The ability to continue to successfully de-implement low-value practices will require multidisciplinary provider collaboration, patient education, and a clear understanding of the value in breast cancer care.

CLINICS CARE POINTS

- De-escalation in breast cancer therapy is occurring across the whole multidisciplinary care spectrum.
- Successful de-implementation of low-value breast cancer therapies will require educational interventions for providers and patients and multidisciplinary collaboration.

DISCLOSURE

The authors have nothing to disclose.

REFERENCES

1. Shubeck SP, Morrow M, Dossett LA. De-escalation in breast cancer surgery. NPJ Breast Cancer 2022;8(1):25.
2. Morrow M, Winer EP. De-escalating breast cancer surgery-where is the tipping point? JAMA Oncol 2020;6(2):183–4.
3. Giuliano AE, Hunt K, Blalman K, et al. Axillary dissection vs no axillary dissection in women with invasive breast cancer and sentinel node metastasis: a randomized clinical trial. JAMA 2011;305(6):569–75.
4. Sparano JA, Gray RJ, Makower D, et al. Adjuvant chemotherapy guided by a 21-gene expression assay in breast cancer. N Engl J Med 2018;379(2):111–21.
5. Kalinsky K, Barlow W, Gralow J, et al. 21-gene assay to inform chemotherapy benefit in node-positive breast cancer. N Engl J Med 2021;385(25):2336–47.
6. Kunkler IH, Williams L, Jack W, et al. Breast-conserving surgery with or without irradiation in women aged 65 years or older with early breast cancer (PRIME II): a randomised controlled trial. Lancet Oncol 2015;16(3):266–73.
7. Wang T, Baskin AS, Dossett LA. Deimplementation of the choosing wisely recommendations for low-value breast cancer surgery: a systematic review. JAMA Surg 2020;155(8):759–70.
8. Veronesi U, Luini A, Galimberti V, et al. Conservation approaches for the management of stage I/II carcinoma of the breast: milan cancer institute trials. World J Surg 1994;18(1):70–5.
9. Effects of radiotherapy and surgery in early breast cancer. An overview of the randomized trials. N Engl J Med 1995;333(22):1444–55.
10. Fisher B, Anderson S, Bryant J, et al. Twenty-year follow-up of a randomized trial comparing total mastectomy, lumpectomy, and lumpectomy plus irradiation for the treatment of invasive breast cancer. N Engl J Med 2002;347(16):1233–41.
11. Veronesi U, Cascinelli N, Mariani L, et al. Twenty-year follow-up of a randomized study comparing breast-conserving surgery with radical mastectomy for early breast cancer. N Engl J Med 2002;347(16):1227–32.
12. Wapnir IL, Dignam J, Fisher B, et al. Long-term outcomes of invasive ipsilateral breast tumor recurrences after lumpectomy in NSABP B-17 and B-24 randomized clinical trials for DCIS. J Natl Cancer Inst 2011;103(6):478–88.
13. Donker M, Litiere S, Werutsky G, et al. Breast-conserving treatment with or without radiotherapy in ductal carcinoma In Situ: 15-year recurrence rates and outcome after a recurrence, from the EORTC 10853 randomized phase III trial. J Clin Oncol 2013;31(32):4054–9.
14. Wolmark N, Wang J, Mamounas E, et al. Preoperative chemotherapy in patients with operable breast cancer: nine-year results from National Surgical Adjuvant Breast and Bowel Project B-18. J Natl Cancer Inst Monogr 2001;(30):96–102.
15. van der Hage JA, Van de Velde C, Julien J, et al. Preoperative chemotherapy in primary operable breast cancer: results from the European Organization for Research and Treatment of Cancer trial 10902. J Clin Oncol 2001;19(22):4224–37.
16. Mieog JS, van der Hage JA, van de Velde CJ. Neoadjuvant chemotherapy for operable breast cancer. Br J Surg 2007;94(10):1189–200.
17. Moran MS, Schnitt S, Giuliano A, et al. Society of Surgical Oncology-American Society for Radiation Oncology consensus guideline on margins for breast-conserving surgery with whole-breast irradiation in stages I and II invasive breast cancer. Ann Surg Oncol 2014;21(3):704–16.

18. Wang T, Bredbeck B, Sinco B, et al. Variations in persistent use of low-value breast cancer surgery. JAMA Surg 2021;156(4):353–62.
19. Morrow M, Abrahamse P, Hofer T, et al. Trends in reoperation after initial lumpectomy for breast cancer: addressing overtreatment in surgical management. JAMA Oncol 2017;3(10):1352–7.
20. Bhutiani N, Mercer M, Bachman K, et al. Evaluating the effect of margin consensus guideline publication on operative patterns and financial impact of breast cancer operation. J Am Coll Surg 2018;227(1):6–11.
21. Marinovich ML, Noguchi N, Morrow M, et al. Changes in reoperation after publication of consensus guidelines on margins for breast-conserving surgery: a systematic review and meta-analysis. JAMA Surg 2020;155(10):e203025.
22. Hughes KS, Schnaper K, Berry D, et al. Lumpectomy plus tamoxifen with or without irradiation in women age 70 years or older with early breast cancer: long-term follow-up of CALGB 9343. J Clin Oncol 2013;31(19):2382–7.
23. Kim T, Giuliano AE, Lyman GH. Lymphatic mapping and sentinel lymph node biopsy in early-stage breast carcinoma: a metaanalysis. Cancer 2006;106(1):4–16.
24. Veronesi U, Viale G, Paganelli G, et al. Sentinel lymph node biopsy in breast cancer: ten-year results of a randomized controlled study. Ann Surg 2010;251(4):595–600.
25. Krag DN, Anderson S, Julian T, et al. Sentinel-lymph-node resection compared with conventional axillary-lymph-node dissection in clinically node-negative patients with breast cancer: overall survival findings from the NSABP B-32 randomised phase 3 trial. Lancet Oncol 2010;11(10):927–33.
26. Boughey JC, Suman V, Mittendorf E, et al. Sentinel lymph node surgery after neoadjuvant chemotherapy in patients with node-positive breast cancer: the ACOSOG Z1071 (Alliance) clinical trial. JAMA 2013;310(14):1455–61.
27. Kuehn T, Bauerfeind I, Fehm T, et al. Sentinel-lymph-node biopsy in patients with breast cancer before and after neoadjuvant chemotherapy (SENTINA): a prospective, multicentre cohort study. Lancet Oncol 2013;14(7):609–18.
28. Tan VK, Goh B, Fook-Chong S, et al. The feasibility and accuracy of sentinel lymph node biopsy in clinically node-negative patients after neoadjuvant chemotherapy for breast cancer–a systematic review and meta-analysis. J Surg Oncol 2011;104(1):97–103.
29. Tee SR, Devane L, Evoy D, et al. Meta-analysis of sentinel lymph node biopsy after neoadjuvant chemotherapy in patients with initial biopsy-proven node-positive breast cancer. Br J Surg 2018;105(12):1541–52.
30. Pesce C, Liederback E, Wang C, et al. Contralateral prophylactic mastectomy provides no survival benefit in young women with estrogen receptor-negative breast cancer. Ann Surg Oncol 2014;21(10):3231–9.
31. Metcalfe KA, Gershman S, Ghadirian P, et al. Frequency of contralateral prophylactic mastectomy in breast cancer patients with a negative BRCA1 and BRCA2 rapid genetic test result. Ann Surg Oncol 2021;28(9):4967–73.
32. Francis A, Fallowfield L, Rea D. The LORIS trial: addressing overtreatment of ductal carcinoma in situ. Clin Oncol (R Coll Radiol) 2015;27(1):6–8.
33. Kanbayashi C, Thompson A, Hwang E, et al. The international collaboration of active surveillance trials for low-risk DCIS (LORIS, LORD, COMET, LORETTA). J Clin Oncol 2019;37(15_suppl):TPS603.
34. Hwang ES, Hyslop T, Lynch T, et al. The COMET (Comparison of Operative versus Monitoring and Endocrine Therapy) trial: a phase III randomised controlled clinical trial for low-risk ductal carcinoma in situ (DCIS). BMJ Open 2019;9(3):e026797.

35. Francis A., Bartlett J., Billingham L., et al., Abstract OT2-3-01: The LORIS trial: A multicentre, randomized phase III trial of standard surgery versus active monitoring in women with newly diagnosed low risk ductal carcinoma in situ. San Antonio Breast Symposium, San Antonio, TX. 2013.

36. Sun S, Van la Parra R, Rauch G, et al. Patient selection for clinical trials eliminating surgery for HER2-positive breast cancer treated with neoadjuvant systemic therapy. Ann Surg Oncol 2019;26(10):3071–9.

37. Heil J, Pfob A, Kuerer HM. De-escalation towards omission is the tipping point of individualizing breast cancer surgery. Eur J Surg Oncol 2020;46(8):1543–5.

38. Sparano JA, Gray R, Makower D, et al. Prospective validation of a 21-gene expression assay in breast cancer. N Engl J Med 2015;373(21):2005–14.

39. Andre F, Ismaila N, Henry N, et al. Use of biomarkers to guide decisions on adjuvant systemic therapy for women with early-stage invasive breast cancer: ASCO clinical practice guideline update-integration of results from TAILORx. J Clin Oncol 2019;37(22):1956–64.

40. Kalinsky K, B.W., Meric-Bernstam F et al., SWOG S1007: Adjuvant trial randomized ER+ patients who had a recurrence score <25 and 1–3 positive nodes to endocrine therapy (ET) versus ET + chemotherapy. Presented at the 2020 San Antonio Breast Cancer Symposium (SABCS): San Antonio, TX, December 8–11, 2020. Abstract GS3-01.

41. Postmenopausal Women with HR+/HER2- Early Breast Cancer, 1-3 Positive Nodes, and a Low Risk of Recurrence Can Safely Forego Chemotherapy. Oncologist 2021;26(Suppl 2):S11–2.

42. CompassHER2-pCR: Decreasing Chemotherapy for Breast Cancer Patients After Pre-surgery Chemo and Targeted Therapy. 2022.

43. Wang SL, Fang H, Song Y, et al. Hypofractionated versus conventional fractionated postmastectomy radiotherapy for patients with high-risk breast cancer: a randomised, non-inferiority, open-label, phase 3 trial. Lancet Oncol 2019;20(3):352–60.

44. Liu L, Yang Y, Guo Q, et al. Comparing hypofractionated to conventional fractionated radiotherapy in postmastectomy breast cancer: a meta-analysis and systematic review. Radiat Oncol 2020;15(1):17.

45. Dawood S, Lei X, Dent R, et al. Survival of women with inflammatory breast cancer: a large population-based study. Ann Oncol 2014;25(6):1143–51.

46. Stearns V, Ewing C, Slack R, et al. Sentinel lymphadenectomy after neoadjuvant chemotherapy for breast cancer may reliably represent the axilla except for inflammatory breast cancer. Ann Surg Oncol 2002;9(3):235–42.

47. Macdonald HR. Pregnancy associated breast cancer. Breast J 2020;26(1):81–5.

48. Case AS. Pregnancy-associated breast cancer. Clin Obstet Gynecol 2016;59(4):779–88.

49. Katz SJ, Jagsi R, Morrow M. Reducing overtreatment of cancer with precision medicine: just what the doctor ordered. JAMA 2018;319(11):1091–2.

50. Norton WE, Chambers DA, Kramer BS. Conceptualizing de-implementation in cancer care delivery. J Clin Oncol 2019;37(2):93–6.

51. Giuliano AE, Boolbol S, Degnim A, et al. Society of Surgical Oncology: position statement on prophylactic mastectomy. Approved by the Society of Surgical Oncology Executive Council, March 2007. Ann Surg Oncol 2007;14(9):2425–7.

52. Smith ME, Vitous C, Hughes T, et al. Barriers and Facilitators to De-Implementation of the Choosing Wisely(®) Guidelines for Low-Value Breast Cancer Surgery. Ann Surg Oncol 2020;27(8):2653–63.

53. Andrews C, Childers T, Wiseman K, et al. Facilitators and barriers to reducing chemotherapy for early-stage breast cancer: a qualitative analysis of interviews with patients and patient advocates. BMC Cancer 2022;22(1):141.
54. Greenup RA, Rushing C, Fish L, et al. Financial costs and burden related to decisions for breast cancer surgery. J Oncol Pract 2019;15(8):e666–76.
55. Berlin NL, Skolarus T, Kerr E, et al. Too much surgery: overcoming barriers to de-implementation of low-value surgery. Ann Surg 2020;271(6):1020–2.

Operative Management in Stage IV Breast Cancer

Sudheer R. Vemuru, MD[a], Sarah E. Tevis, MD[b],*

KEYWORDS

- De novo metastatic breast cancer
- Locoregional management of metastatic breast cancer
- Surgery for stage IV breast cancer

KEY POINTS

- Although the prognosis for metastatic breast cancer is poor, survival has improved in recent decades with advancement in diagnostic and treatment methods.
- Traditionally, surgery has been reserved for palliative purposes in patients with metastatic breast cancer.
- Retrospective studies have demonstrated an association between improved survival and receipt of locoregional therapy in patients with stage IV breast cancer.
- Three out of 4 randomized controlled trials to date with published results have not demonstrated improved survival in patients with stage IV breast cancer undergoing locoregional therapy.
- Comprehensive local therapy may be associated with improved survival in patients with metastatic inflammatory breast cancer or when no evidence of disease may be achieved but no randomized controlled trials have evaluated outcomes in these populations.

INTRODUCTION

Stage IV breast cancer, as defined by the eighth edition of the American Joint Committee on Cancer (AJCC) Staging Manual, is characterized by metastasis of tumor cells beyond the breast, chest wall, and regional lymph nodes.[1] As of 2017, an estimated 154,000 patients were living with metastatic breast cancer, which accounts for approximately 6% of breast cancer diagnoses in the United States.[2,3] Approximately 1 in 4 patients with distant metastases are diagnosed with de novo disease, which is characterized by the presence of distant metastases at the time of the initial

a Department of Surgery, University of Colorado Denver, 12631 East 17th Avenue, Room: 6111, Aurora, CO 80045, USA; b Division of Surgical Oncology, Department of Surgery, University of Colorado Denver, 12631 East 17th Avenue, Room: C-313, Aurora, CO 80045, USA
* Corresponding author.
E-mail address: sarah.tevis@cuanschutz.edu
Twitter: @sudheervemuru (S.R.V.); @SarahTevisMD (S.E.T.)

Surg Clin N Am 103 (2023) 93–106
https://doi.org/10.1016/j.suc.2022.08.006
0039-6109/23/© 2022 Elsevier Inc. All rights reserved.
surgical.theclinics.com

diagnosis of a cancer in the breast. Although the prognosis for stage IV disease is poor, survival has improved in recent decades.[2,4]

Traditionally, the focus of treatment of breast cancer with distant metastatic disease has been to reduce disease progression and promote quality of life.[5] Therefore, surgery in this population has been limited for palliation of symptoms. In patients with de novo stage IV disease, there has historically been little to no role for surgery for the purpose of locoregional control of the primary tumor and any axillary disease given no clear survival benefit.

More recently, the pendulum has begun to swing toward favoring aggressive local therapy in other malignancies with distant metastases.[6,7] This paradigm shift has led to a new effort to investigate the potential benefit of locoregional control of the primary breast tumor in patients with de novo stage IV disease. Although several retrospective studies showed improved outcomes in patients with metastatic disease who underwent surgical treatment of the primary tumor, prospective trials have not replicated these results. Currently, the National Comprehensive Cancer Network (NCCN) suggests an individualized approach for consideration of locoregional therapy in patients with de novo stage IV disease, recommending that "surgery should be undertaken only if complete local clearance of tumor may be obtained and if other sites of disease are not immediately threatening to life."[8] This article summarizes the myriad studies that have examined the outcomes of operative management in de novo stage IV breast cancer and have detailed populations that may receive maximum benefit from early locoregional therapy.

INCIDENCE AND MORTALITY ASSOCIATED WITH STAGE IV BREAST CANCER

Despite advances in treatment modalities, breast cancer with distant metastasis carries a worse prognosis compared with breast cancer diagnosed in the local and regional stages. Among all patients diagnosed with breast cancer, 64% were diagnosed at the early stage, 27% at the loco-regional advanced stage, and 6% at the distant (metastatic) stage, and within this group, 5-year overall survival rate of early, loco-regional advanced, and metastatic stages were 99%, 86%, and 27%, respectively.[3] Moreover, mortality among patients diagnosed with stage IV breast cancer is even worse among older patients and patients of African-American race.[3,9] Similarly, new cancers staged according to the Eighth Edition AJCC Breast Cancer Staging System show a similar decrease in overall survival as stage increases. The AJCC staging system also considers tumor biology and relevant prognostic factors and classifies breast cancer with any distant metastatic lesion including those in contralateral lymph nodes as stage IV disease. The 5-year survival associated with AJCC stage I, II, III, and IV disease has been reported as 94.4%, 85.0%, 56.6%, and 28.3%, respectively.[10] Stage, and more specifically presence of distant metastases, is a paramount prognostic factor for patients with breast cancer and thus, plays a key role in determining what treatment options are appropriate for each patient.

HISTORICAL APPROACH TO OPERATIVE MANAGEMENT FOR STAGE IV BREAST CANCER

A number of previously chronicled theories posited that surgical removal of the primary tumor may lead to more robust metastatic proliferation.[11] For example, angiotensin, an angiogenesis inhibitor secreted by the primary tumor, may be suppressed after primary tumor removal and lead to increased angiogenesis and proliferation of the metastatic lesion.[12] Additionally, surgical stress occurring within the immunologically compromised state of malignancy has been shown in animal models to induce the activity of growth factors that may increase metastatic proliferation in some malignancies.[13] Finally, surgical injury has been shown to upregulate activity of genes that promote breast cancer metastases to the lungs.[14]

Historically, the goal of treatment of metastatic breast cancer has been palliation. Therapies offering benefit with minimal detriment to the patient were preferred, and the goal of operative management was to ease the burden of symptoms rather than to achieve a cure. Surgical therapy for the primary breast lesions may address pain, bleeding, ulceration, and fungating masses, whereas therapy for metastatic lesions may address spinal cord compression, pathologic fractures, pleural or pericardial effusions, and localized bony pain among other symptoms.[5] Although the impact of surgical resection of the primary tumor on survival in patients with de novo stage IV breast cancer has been widely debated, recent data have suggested the oncologic outcomes may be improved after aggressive local therapy in other malignancies with distant metastases. For example, nephrectomy plus systemic therapy (ST) was shown to be superior to ST alone for the treatment of metastatic renal cell carcinoma in 2 randomized controlled trials published in 2001.[6,7] Primary tumor resection has also shown survival benefit in prospective randomized controlled trials of metastatic colorectal cancer.[15] This paradigm shift has led to a new effort to investigate the potential benefit of locoregional control of the primary breast tumor in patients with stage IV disease. Although several retrospective studies showed improved outcomes in patients with metastatic disease who underwent surgical treatment of the primary tumor, prospective trials have not replicated these results. These studies will be explored in depth in the coming sections of this article.

RETROSPECTIVE STUDIES ON SURGERY IN STAGE IV BREAST CANCER

The primary evidence base favoring aggressive local therapy in stage IV breast cancer comes from several retrospective analyses (**Tables 1** and **2**) beginning with a study published by Khan and colleagues in 2002.[16] In this review of 16,023 patients with stage IV disease isolated from the National Cancer Database from 1990 to 1993, the authors compared the outcomes of the 6861 patients who received no surgery to the 9162 patients who underwent either partial or total mastectomy. Mean survival for the group who received no surgical intervention was significantly lower at 19.3 months compared with 26.9 months for the partial mastectomy group and 31.9 months for the mastectomy group. Similarly, the authors found significant differences in 3-year overall survival among the groups with 17.3%, 27.7%, and 31.8% of the no surgery, partial mastectomy, and mastectomy groups alive at 3 years, respectively. Independent prognostic factors associated with improved survival in this analysis were negative margins on surgical pathology specimen, receipt of ST, number of metastatic sites, and presence of visceral metastases.

Subsequently, Rapiti and colleagues[17] published a review of 300 patients with distant metastases at diagnosis from the Geneva Registry from 1977 to 1996. Of these patients, 173 did not undergo surgery, whereas 87 underwent mastectomy, and 40 underwent partial mastectomy. The 5-year breast cancer–specific survival in this cohort was 27% for women who had surgery with negative margins, 16% for women who had surgery with positive margins, 12% for women who had surgery with unknown margin status, and 12% for women who did not have surgery. Notably, patients in the surgery cohort were younger, had lower T and N stage at diagnosis, more likely to have single site of metastasis, less likely to have visceral metastases, more likely to receive radiation, and less likely to receive chemotherapy. Notably, compared with other sites of metastasis, bone-only metastatic lesions were associated with improved survival with surgery.

Table 1
Summary of retrospective studies evaluating survival after surgery for stage IV breast cancer

		N	Survival Outcome	
Khan,[16] 2002	Total	16,023	3-y survival	Median survival
	No surgery	6861 (43%)	17.3%	19.3 mo
	Lumpectomy	3513 (22%)	27.7%	26.9 mo
	Total mastectomy	5649 (35%)	31.8%	31.9 mo
Rapiti et al,[17] 2006	Total	300	5-y disease-specific survival	
	No surgery	173 (58%)	12%	
	Surgery	127 (42%)		
	Negative margin	61 (48%)	27%	
	Positive margin	33 (26%)	16%	
	Unknown margin	33 (26%)	12%	
Babiera et al,[19] 2006	Total	224	Improved metastatic PFS, hormone receptor (HR) 0.54 (95% CI 0.38–0.77) with surgery; Trend toward improved OS	
	No surgery	142 (63%)		
	Surgery	82 (37%)		
Gnerlich et al,[18] 2007	Total	9734	Median survival	Overall survival
	No surgery	5156 (53%)	21 mo	HR 0.63 with surgery (95% CI 0.60–0.66)
	Surgery	4578 (47%)	36 mo	
Fields et al,[21] 2007	Total	409	Median survival	
	No Surgery	222 (54%)	12.6 mo	
	Surgery	187 (46%)	26.8 mo	
Bafford et al,[23] 2008	Total	147	Median survival	
	No surgery	86 (59%)	2.36 y	
	Surgery	61 (41%)	3.52 y	
Blanchard et al,[22] 2008	Total	395	Median survival	
	No surgery	153 (39%)	16.8 mo	
	Surgery	242 (61%)	27.1 mo	
Ruiterkamp et al,[24] 2009	Total	728	Median survival	5-y survival
	No surgery	440 (60%)	14 mo	24.5%
	Surgery	288 (40%)	31 mo	31.1%
Dominici et al,[27] 2011	Total	551	Median survival	
	No surgery	497 (90%)	3.4 y	
	Surgery	54 (10%)	3.5 y	
Lang et al,[20] 2013	Total	208	Median survival	
	No surgery	134 (64%)	37.2 mo	
	Surgery	74 (36%)	56.1 mo	
Thomas et al,[4] 2016	Total	21,372	Median survival	10-y survival
	No surgery	13,042 (61%)	19 mo	2.9%
	Surgery	8330 (39%)	28 mo	9.6%
Stahl et al,[26] 2021	Total	12,838	5-y survival	
	Systemic therapy only	6650 (51.8%)	21%	
	Systemic therapy and radiation therapy	2901 (22.6%)	19%	
	Systemic therapy and surgery (13.2%)	1695 (13.2%)	32%	
	Trimodality	1592 (12.4%)	38%	

Gnerlich and colleagues[18] reviewed 9734 patients with stage IV disease in the Surveillance, Epidemiology, and End Results (SEER) database from 1988 to 2003, of whom 4578 (47%) had surgery on their breast tumor and 5156 (53%) had no surgery.

Table 2
Summary of randomized controlled studies evaluating survival after surgery for stage IV breast cancer

	N	Survival Outcome		
Badwe et al,[31] 2015	Total 350	Median overall survival	2-y survival	Locoregional progression
No surgery	177 (51%)	20.5 mo	43%	10.6%
Surgery	173 (49%)	19.2 mo	41%	5.3%
• Patients with de novo metastatic breast cancer randomized after initial systemic therapy				
• Minimal use of taxanes, neoadjuvant endocrine therapy, or trastuzumab for HER2-positive disease				
• Improved survival if hormone receptor positive, fewer distant metastases				
Soran et al,[32] 2016	Total 274	3-y survival	5-y survival	Locoregional progression
No surgery	136 (55%)	51%	24%	11%
Surgery	138 (50%)	60%	42%	1%
• Patients with de novo metastatic breast cancer randomized upfront to receive either locoregional therapy plus systemic therapy or systemic therapy alone				
• Surgery group more likely to be ER positive, less likely to have triple-negative breast cancer				
• Improved survival if hormone receptor positive, HER2 negative, age less than 55 y, solitary bone metastases				
Fitzal et al,[33] 2019	Total 90	Median overall survival	Time to distant progression	Local progression
No surgery	45 (50%)	54.8 mo	29.0 mo	17.8%
Surgery	45 (50%)	34.6 mo	13.9 mo	8.9%
• Randomized upfront to receive either locoregional therapy followed by systemic therapy or systemic therapy alone				
• Surgery group with higher proportion of cT3 and cN2 tumors, more likely to receive RT				
• Luminal A subtype associated with worse outcomes with surgery				
• Quality of life improved after treatment in both groups				
Khan et al,[34] 2022	Total 256	Median overall survival	3-y survival	Disease Progression
No surgery	125 (49%)	53.1 mo	67.9%	39.8%
Surgery	131 (51%)	54.9 mo	68.4%	16.3%
• Patients with no disease progression after receipt of initial systemic therapy randomized to locoregional therapy or no locoregional therapy				
• 14.4% in LRT group did not receive surgery while 16.8% in non-LRT group received surgery				
• Triple-negative disease associated with worse survival, no differences in survival for oligometastatic disease				
• HRQoL superior in non-LRT group at 18 months after diagnosis, but similar at all other timepoints				

Patients who had surgery were more likely to be younger, Caucasian, married, and diagnosed before 1996, and their tumors were more likely to be smaller, higher grade, and with positive estrogen receptor (ER) and progesterone receptor (PR) markers compared with women who did not undergo surgery. In their univariate analysis, the authors identified older age, black race, being unmarried, larger tumor size, higher or unknown tumor grade, and negative or unknown ER and PR status to be associated with an increased risk of death, whereas recent year of diagnosis and receipt of radiation treatment were associated with a decreased risk of death. To account for the potential confounding effects of these factors, the authors used a propensity scoring method to match patients between groups and used a multivariate model incorporating tumor size, grade, year of diagnosis, and radiation receipt. They found that surgery was associated with a 37% lower risk of death during the study period.

In an institutional review of 224 patients treated at MD Anderson Cancer Center for stage IV breast cancer from 1997 to 2002, Babiera and colleagues[19] compared the outcomes of 142 patients treated without surgery and 82 treated with either partial mastectomy or mastectomy. In this analysis, the surgery group was younger, had less nodal involvement, had fewer sites of metastases, was more likely to have metastases to the liver, was more frequently positive for Her2/neu, and was more likely to receive chemotherapy as first-line ST. There was no effect of surgery on overall survival at 32.1 months median follow-up but surgery did improve progression-free survival even excluding patients undergoing surgery for curative intent; however, on multivariate analysis, the effect on progression-free survival was only significant in patients who were ER positive. Lang and colleagues[20] reported the longer-term results from this patient cohort. At a median follow-up time of 74.2 months, median survival for surgery group was 56.1 months and 37.2 months for no surgery group. In this analysis, surgery improved both overall survival and progression-free survival.

Multiple subsequently published retrospective studies continued to demonstrate improved survival in patients with stage IV breast cancer who underwent surgical excision of the primary tumor.[21–24] Furthermore, 2 large cohort analyses of outcomes in patients with stage IV breast cancer suggested improved outcomes after surgery.[4,25] Notably, Thomas and colleagues reviewed 21,372 diagnosed with stage IV breast cancer between 1988 and 2011 who did not have radiation therapy as part of their initial treatment. Thirty-nine percent underwent surgery of the primary tumor and these patients were on average younger, more likely to have hormone receptor negative tumors, and less likely to be African American or have tumors greater than 5 cm in size. Median survival of all patients regardless of receipt of surgery improved from 20 months (1988–1991) to 26 months (2007–2011), whereas the proportion of patients receiving surgery declined over time from 68% in 1988 to 25% in 2011. Despite these trends, receipt of surgery was associated with improved survival after adjusting for patient and clinical characteristics and time period. However, as a whole, improvements in overall survival despite declining proportions of patients receiving surgery to treat their primary tumor may be attributable to improvements in systemic therapies over time.

Finally, Stahl and colleagues[26] published a retrospective review of 12,838 patients in the National Cancer Database between 2010 and 2015 with stage IV breast cancer and known hormone receptor and HER2/neu status. The patients were divided based on whether they received ST only (51.8%), ST and radiation therapy (22.6%), ST and surgery (13.2%), or ST, radiation therapy, and surgery (trimodality therapy [12.4%]). Five-year overall survival was significantly higher in the 2 surgery groups compared with the other groups with the trimodality group at 38%, surgery and ST group at 32%, ST only group at 21%, and the ST and radiation therapy group at 19%. Notably, survival was higher in patients with HER2-positive tumors across all groups. In terms of baseline demographic and clinicopathologic factors, surgery was more likely to be performed in the earlier years of the analysis, at community-based cancer programs rather than academic cancer programs, for tumors with high-grade histology, and in patients with single metastatic lesions rather than oligometastatic disease. In the multivariable Cox proportional hazard model, the hazard ratio for mortality risk in the trimodality group and ST plus surgery group were 0.645 ($P < .0001$) and 0.732 ($P < .0001$) compared with ST alone, whereas the hazard ratio for ST plus radiation therapy was 1.10 ($P = .002$). Other factors that were associated with worse overall survival were African American race, aged older than 65 years at the time of diagnosis, receipt of treatment at a community cancer hospital or in a comprehensive community cancer program versus an academic medical center, and multiple comorbidities, high histologic grade; ER negative, PR negative, or HER2 negative status; and brain, lung, or liver metastases. Notably, in the subgroup analysis for patients who underwent surgery, neoadjuvant chemotherapy receipt was associated with improved survival compared with adjuvant chemotherapy receipt, suggesting that responders to neoadjuvant chemotherapy may have seen the most survival benefit from surgery.

Among the notable retrospective studies that did not show more favorable survival outcomes with surgical treatment of stage IV cancer was a case-matched analysis published by Dominici and colleagues in 2011.[27] Using the NCCN Breast Cancer Outcomes Database, they isolated 551 patients diagnosed with breast cancer who had distant metastases at the time of diagnosis from 1997 to 2007. Of these patients, 54 underwent surgery, whereas 497 did not undergo surgery. The 54 patients in the surgery group were matched with 236 in the no surgery group, although the surgery group was more likely to have been diagnosed earlier in the study period. Patients undergoing surgery did not have better rates of overall survival compared with those who did not undergo surgery in both the matched and nonmatched samples.

Further evidence to suggest limited role for surgery in stage IV breast cancer includes a review of 622 patients with stage IV breast cancer treated at the Massachusetts General Hospital and Brigham and Women's Hospital between 1970 and 2002.[28] In this case-matched analysis of 388 patients who did not undergo surgical treatment and 234 patients who did undergo surgical treatment, the authors identified that the survival benefit of surgery compared with no surgery was most evident in group that was administered chemotherapy before surgery. Notably, there was a substantial delay before the first precipitous drop in survival in the Cox proportional hazard model for the surgery group, which could be attributed to significant case selection bias suggesting that patients underwent surgery when they were responding to chemotherapy and tended not to be given surgery when they were nonresponders. Selection bias may also contribute significantly to the effects seen in the previously described studies and is a major limitation of all of these retrospective studies. When patients who are responders to ST or have more favorable tumor characteristics are the same patients most likely to undergo surgery on the primary tumor, the effect of that aggressive local therapy on Improved outcomes may be overstated. Thus, well-controlled, randomized prospective trials, which are less susceptible to these same biases, are needed to adequately assess the impact of surgery on survival in patients with stage IV breast cancer.

PROSPECTIVE STUDIES ON SURGERY IN STAGE IV BREAST CANCER

The Translational Breast Cancer Research Consortium 013 trial is a multi-institutional prospective registry evaluating 128 patients with stage IV disease, 112 of whom had metastases at initial presentation and 16 of whom developed metastases within 3 months of surgery. In the group with metastases at initial presentation, patients were offered resection of the primary tumor if they had a response to upfront ST. Among all patients, 2-year overall survival was 96% among those who underwent surgery and 74% in those who did not have surgery ($P = .002$). However, among those with de novo stage IV disease who had a clinical response to initial ST, 2-year overall survival was 94% for the surgery group and 92% for the nonsurgery group ($P = .5$).[29] Patients who underwent surgery had larger tumors, were more likely to have single organ metastatic disease, more likely to have received first-line chemotherapy. In the follow-up analysis of this cohort, 3 year overall survival was superior in responders to initial ST compared with nonresponders (78% vs 24%, respectively; $P < .001$).[30] Similar to the earlier analysis, 3-year overall survival among responders to initial ST was not different for the group pursuing surgery compared with the group electing to proceed without surgery (77% vs 76%, respectively; $P = .85$). Furthermore, survival outcomes for those undergoing surgery did not vary based on receptor status. These results suggest that improved survival may be more attributable to response to initial ST rather than to surgery.

To date, 5 randomized controlled trials have been initiated to evaluate the benefit of surgery in stage IV breast cancer, 4 of which have published results. The first published trial investigating this topic was NCT00193778, an open labeled, prospective, randomized controlled trial of 350 patients treated for de novo metastatic breast cancer at Tata Memorial Center in Mumbai, India from 2005 to 2013 randomized to receive locoregional therapy or no locoregional therapy.[31] This well-randomized cohort had a median follow-up of 23 months with median overall survival of 19.2 months for the locoregional treatment group and 20.5 months in the no locoregional treatment group, a nonsignificant difference. Two-year overall survival was 41.9% in the locoregional treatment group and 43.0% in the no locoregional treatment group, which was also a nonsignificant difference. In the subgroup analysis, there was no difference in the difference between bone only metastatic disease and visceral metastatic disease. Notably, most ST regimens excluded taxanes, neoadjuvant endocrine therapy was not routinely administered, and HER2-directed therapy was not administered for most patients with HER2-positive disease. Furthermore, overall survival was far lower in this cohort than in any of the other randomized cohorts.

The MF01-01 trial in Turkey accrued patients from 2007 to 2012 and was the second randomized controlled trial evaluating the impact of locoregional treatment.[32] In this trial, 274 patients were randomized to receive either locoregional therapy plus ST (LRT) or ST alone. However, despite randomization, patients in the ST group were more likely to have triple-negative disease and more likely to be ER negative. There were also more patients in the LRT group who had solitary bone metastases and fewer patients in this group had visceral metastases. At a median follow-up time of 55 months, hazard ratio of death for the locoregional therapy group was 0.66 (95% confidence interval 0.49–0.88). There was no difference in overall survival at 3 years (60% for LRT ad 51% for ST) but at 5 years, overall survival was higher in the LRT group (42%) compared with the ST group (24%). In the subgroup analysis, factors favoring surgery were ER/PR-positive status, HER2-negative status, younger age, and solitary bone metastasis. However, due to differences in the aforementioned factors between the 2 study arms, selection bias may contribute to the effect seen in the main group analysis.

The phase III ABCSG-28 POSYTIVE trial, published in 2019, was the third randomized controlled trial evaluating primary surgical therapy in de novo stage IV breast cancer.[33] In this Austrian trial, which was stropped early due to poor recruitment, 90 previously untreated patients with stage IV breast cancer were randomly assigned to surgical resection of the primary tumor followed by ST (Arm A) or primary ST (Arm B). Fifteen percent of patients in Arm B decided to undergo surgery, whereas

7% in Arm A decided not to have surgery. Patients in Arm A had a higher proportion of cT3 and cN2 tumors and were more likely to receive breast or chest wall radiotherapy than patients in Arm B but both arms were well-matched in terms of age, tumor subtype, metastasis location, and first-line ST regimen. An R0 resection was attained in 76% of patients undergoing surgery in Arm A and in 5 of the 7 patients who underwent surgery in Arm B. At a median follow-up of 37.5 months, median overall survival was 34.6 months for Arm A and 54.8 for Arm B (HR for nonsurgery 0.691; 95% CI 0.358–1.333). Time to distant progression was 13.9 months in the Arm A and 29 months in Arm B (HR for nonsurgery 0.598; 95% CI 0.343–1.043). Time to local progression including breast and regional lymph nodes was similar between the 2 arms (HR for nonsurgery 0.933; 95% CI 0.375–2.322). The post hoc subgroup analysis suggested a survival benefit of surgery in tumors with a luminal B subtype (ER positive, PR negative, HER2 positive), although this did not achieve statistical significance. Tumors with a luminal A subtype (ER positive, PR positive, HER2 negative) were associated with significantly worse survival with surgery. Quality of life was also evaluated and both arms demonstrated temporal improvements in global health status and emotional functioning as well as future perspective and breast symptoms, although the authors did not report any differences in these measures between the groups.

The Eastern Cooperative Oncology Group E2108 trial was the last of the 4 published randomized controlled trials investigating outcomes after early local therapy for the primary site in metastatic breast cancer.[34,35] In this multicenter trial, 390 patients with stage IV breast cancer and an intact primary tumor were administered 4 to 8 months of optimal ST, and those with no disease progression after receipt of ST (n = 256) were randomized to either locoregional therapy (n = 131) or no locoregional therapy (n = 125). Of the patients randomized to the locoregional therapy group, 14.4% decided not to undergo surgery, whereas 16.8% of patients in the ST alone group decided to undergo surgery. Of patients who underwent surgery, 91.6% had tumor-free margins. Median overall survival for the locoregional therapy group was 54.9 months versus 53.1 months for the ST alone group, a nonsignificant difference. Overall survival at 3 years was also similar between the 2 groups at 67.9% for the ST group and 68.4% for the locoregional therapy group. Subgroup analysis did not demonstrate a survival benefit of surgery in patients with oligometastatic disease, defined here as 3 or fewer site metastatic lesions at the time of diagnosis. Triple-negative tumor subtype was associated with worse overall survival (HR 3.33; 95% CI 1.09–10.12). There was a significantly higher rate of disease progression in the ST group (39.8%) compared with the locoregional therapy group (16.3%). Furthermore, health-related quality of life was superior in the ST alone group at baseline and at 18 months but there were no differences between the groups at any other time point.

The ongoing JCOG1017 PRIM-BC[36] trial, similar to the EA2108, enrolled patients with stage IV breast cancer and an intact primary tumor who receive primary ST up front. Patients who are responders to primary ST at 3 months will be randomized to primary tumor resection or ST alone. Primary outcomes being measured in this trial are overall survival and secondary outcomes being measured include proportion without disease progression and yearly recurrence-free survival. The study has achieved its target accrual and the results are forthcoming.

SPECIFIC POPULATIONS WITH POTENTIAL SURVIVAL BENEFIT OF LOCOREGIONAL CONTROL FOR STAGE IV BREAST CANCER

Patients with metastatic breast cancer may exhibit a variety of responses to treatment: some tumors are extremely aggressive and remain unresponsive to ST, whereas others may have robust responses and may be controlled for years. A subset of patients with stage IV breast cancer may present with oligometastatic disease, typically defined as 5 or fewer deposits of tumor cells within distant sites. Retrospective studies have suggested that limited metastatic disease burden including patients with singular metastases or oligometastatic disease is associated with improved survival outcomes both in patients undergoing primary tumor resection.[25,26,37,38] Furthermore, some studies have demonstrated superior survival outcomes following primary tumor resection in patients with solitary bone metastases compared with those with visceral metastases.[17,37] However, prospective studies have not shown locoregional therapy to be associated with improved survival in patients with oligometastatic disease[34] nor in patients with solitary bone metastases,[31,33,34] although the small sizes of the subgroups in these trials may limit the ability to detect differences. The Turkish MF01-01 trial did suggest solitary bone metastases were associated with improved survival but these results should be interpreted within the context of the limitations of this study highlighted in the previous section.

Local therapy as part of a multimodal treatment approach may also play a role in achieving no evidence of disease (NED) status in stage IV breast cancer. In an institutional review of 570 patients with stage IV breast cancer evaluated between 2003 and 2005, Bishop and colleagues found that 16% achieved NED. Overall survival at 3 and 5 years was 96% and 78%, respectively, if NED compared with 44% and 24%, respectively, for the overall study cohort. Achieving NED associated with local treatment of the breast primary, de novo stage IV disease, a single metastatic site, whereas triple-negative disease and obese or overweight classification based on body mass index were negatively associated with achieving NED. Moreover, 1 in 3 patients with NED remained in remission at their most recent follow-up.[39]

Improved survival has also been demonstrated in patients with stage IV disease who underwent metastatectomy. Among patients who underwent resection of bone, lung, liver, or brain metastases, positive survival outcomes were seen in patients with good performance status, long disease-free interval after treatment of the primary tumor, complete resection of the metastatic lesions, and single sites of metastasis.[40] A recent meta-analysis demonstrated an association between pulmonary metastatectomy and a relatively high 5-year overall survival of 46%. Positive hormone receptor status in the metastatic lesion, single metastatic lesions, disease-free interval of greater than 3 years, and complete resection of the metastases were positive prognostic factors for those undergoing pulmonary metastatectomy.[41] The NRG BR002 trial is actively accruing patients with limited metastatic disease treated with ST and definitive local therapy to the breast primarily to evaluate whether surgical resection or stereotactic body radiation therapy to the metastatic site affects progression-free survival and overall survival in oligometastatic breast cancer.[42]

Inflammatory breast cancer (IBC) is an aggressive form of breast cancer characterized by dermal lymphatic invasion leading to edema, thickening of the skin, erythema, and the classic peau d'orange appearance of the skin overlying the breast. Approximately 30% of patients with IBC will be diagnosed with de novo stage IV disease, which carries a shorter median survival of 2.3 years when compared with 3.4 years for stage IV non-IBC ($P = .013$).[43,44] In an institutional review of 172 patients with stage IV IBC treated between 1997 and 2002, investigators found that overall survival was 47% with surgery compared with 10% without surgery, whereas distant progression-free survival was 30% versus 3%, respectively. Surgery with or without radiation therapy and response to initial ST were independent predictors of improved survival and distant progression-free survival. Furthermore, local control was achieved in 81% of patients undergoing surgery compared with 8% in those who went without surgery.[45] Another study suggested that local failure was less common among stage IV IBC patients undergoing locoregional therapy versus ST alone (17% vs 57%).[46] Finally, among stage IV IBC patients undergoing trimodal therapy, 5-year locoregional control rate and overall survival were 86% and 54%, respectively.[47] Although selection bias likely affected the observed outcomes, these findings suggest a role for comprehensive local therapy in metastatic IBC both in terms of gaining local control and potentially improving survival, although prospective trials are needed to further evaluate the benefit of operative management in stage IV IBC.

SUMMARY

Distant metastases are associated with worse prognoses in patients with breast cancer. Although some evidence from early retrospective studies suggested a possible survival benefit of surgical resection of the primary tumor in patients with distant metastases, they were subject to significant selection bias. To date, the preponderance of evidence from prospective, randomized controlled trials suggests that locoregional control provides no clear survival advantage in patients with stage IV breast cancer and is not associated with improvement in quality of life outcomes. Thus, primary tumor resection may not have a role in treatment of stage IV breast cancer apart from providing palliation for women with severe symptoms and complications of local tumor infiltration, particularly as systemic therapies for the treatment of breast cancer advance. Further areas for exploration include the evaluation of quality of life measures in patients with stage IV breast cancer receiving definitive operative management, and identification and prospective evaluation of populations with stage IV disease who may experience maximal benefit from early locoregional treatment such as those who may achieve NED status with surgery or those with IBC.

CLINICS CARE POINTS

- All patients with de novo metastatic breast cancer should be evaluated for first-line systemic therapy.
- Patients with symptoms associated with local tumor infiltration, which may negatively influence quality of life should be evaluated for local therapy for palliative purposes.
- In select patients with stage IV breast cancer who have responded to systemic therapy and who may achieve no evidence of disease, surgical resection of the primary breast tumor should be discussed as part of a multidisciplinary approach to treatment.
- When discussing surgical treatment options for metastatic breast cancer, surgeons should disclose to patients that the best evidence base suggests that surgery to achieve local control is not associated with improved survival.

DISCLOSURE

The authors have nothing to disclose.

REFERENCES

1. Giuliano AE, Edge SB, Hortobagyi GN. Eighth edition of the AJCC cancer staging manual: breast cancer. Ann Surg Oncol 2018;25(7):1783–5.

2. Mariotto AB, Etzioni R, Hurlbert M, et al. Estimation of the number of women living with metastatic breast cancer in the united states. Cancer Epidemiol Biomarkers Prev 2017;26(6):809–15.

3. American Cancer Society. Breast Cancer Facts & Figures 2019-2020. https://www.cancer.org/content/dam/cancer-org/research/cancer-facts-and-statistics/breast-cancer-facts-and-figures/breast-cancer-facts-and-figures-2019-2020.pdf. [Accessed 12 May 2022].

4. Thomas A, Khan SA, Chrischilles EA, et al. Initial surgery and survival in stage IV Breast cancer in the united states, 1988-2011. JAMA Surg 2016;151(5):424–31.

5. Teshome M. Role of operative management in stage IV breast cancer. Surg Clin North Am 2018;98(4):859–68. https://doi.org/10.1016/j.suc.2018.03.012.

6. Flanigan RC, Salmon SE, Blumenstein BA, et al. Nephrectomy followed by interferon Alfa-2b compared with interferon Alfa-2b alone for metastatic renal-cell cancer. N Engl J Med 2001;345(23):1655–9.

7. Mickisch GHJ, Garin A, van Poppel H, et al. Radical nephrectomy plus interferon-alfa-based immunotherapy compared with interferon alfa alone in metastatic renal-cell carcinoma: a randomised trial. Lancet 2001;358(9286):966–70.

8. National Comprehensive Cancer Network. NCCN clinical practice guidelines in oncology: breast cancer, Version 1.2022. Available at: https://www.nccn.org/guidelines/guidelines-detail?category=1&id=1419.

9. Freedman RA, Keating NL, Lin NU, et al. Breast cancer-specific survival by age: worse outcomes for the oldest patients. Cancer 2018;124(10):2184–91.

10. Chitapanarux I, Sripan P, Somwangprasert A, et al. Stage-specific survival rate of breast cancer patients in northern thailand in accordance with two different staging systems. Asian Pac J Cancer Prev 2019;20(9):2699–706.

11. Rashid OM, Takabe K. Does removal of the primary tumor in metastatic breast cancer improve survival? J Womens Health (Larchmt) 2014;23(2):184–8.

12. Folkman J. New perspectives in clinical oncology from angiogenesis research. Eur J Cancer 1996;32(14):2534–9.

13. Fisher ER, Fisher B. Experimental studies of factors influencing the development of hepatic metastases: XIII. Effect of hepatic trauma in parabiotic pairs. Cancer Res 1963;23(6 Part 1):896–900.

14. Al-Sahaf O, Wang JH, Browne TJ, et al. Surgical injury enhances the expression of genes that mediate breast cancer metastasis to the lung. Ann Surg 2010; 252(6):1037–43.

15. Ferrand F, Malka D, Bourredjem A, et al. Impact of primary tumour resection on survival of patients with colorectal cancer and synchronous metastases treated by chemotherapy: Results from the multicenter, randomised trial Fédération Francophone de Cancérologie Digestive 9601. Eur J Cancer 2013;49(1):90–7.

16. Khan SA, Stewart AK, Morrow M. Does aggressive local therapy improve survival in metastatic breast cancer? Surgery 2002;132(4):620–6 [discussion: 626-7].

17. Rapiti E, Verkooijen HM, Vlastos G, et al. Complete excision of primary breast tumor improves survival of patients with metastatic breast cancer at diagnosis. J Clin Oncol 2006;24(18):2743–9.

18. Gnerlich J, Jeffe DB, Deshpande AD, et al. Surgical removal of the primary tumor increases overall survival in patients with metastatic breast cancer: analysis of the 1988–2003 SEER data. Ann Surg Oncol 2007;14(8):2187–94.

19. Babiera GV, Rao R, Feng L, et al. Effect of primary tumor extirpation in breast cancer patients who present with stage IV disease and an intact primary tumor. Ann Surg Oncol 2006;13(6):776–82.

20. Lang JE, Tereffe W, Mitchell MP, et al. Primary Tumor extirpation in breast cancer patients who present with stage IV disease is associated with improved survival. Ann Surg Oncol 2013;20(6):1893–9.

21. Fields RC, Jeffe DB, Trinkaus K, et al. Surgical resection of the primary tumor is associated with increased long-term survival in patients with stage IV breast cancer after controlling for site of metastasis. Ann Surg Oncol 2007;14(12):3345–51.

22. Blanchard DK, Shetty PB, Hilsenbeck SG, et al. Association of surgery with improved survival in stage IV breast cancer patients. Ann Surg 2008;247(5): 732–8.

23. Bafford AC, Burstein HJ, Barkley CR, et al. Breast surgery in stage IV breast cancer: impact of staging and patient selection on overall survival. Breast Cancer Res Treat 2009;115(1):7–12.

24. Ruiterkamp J, Ernst MF, van de Poll-Franse LV, et al. Surgical resection of the primary tumour is associated with improved survival in patients with distant metastatic breast cancer at diagnosis. Eur J Surg Oncol (EJSO) 2009;35(11):1146–51.

25. Vohra NA, Brinkley J, Kachare S, et al. Primary tumor resection in metastatic breast cancer: a propensity-matched analysis, 1988-2011 SEER data base. Breast J 2018;24(4):549–54.

26. Stahl K, Wong W, Dodge D, et al. Benefits of surgical treatment of stage IV breast cancer for patients with known hormone receptor and HER2 status. Ann Surg Oncol 2021;28(5):2646–58.

27. Dominici L, Najita J, Hughes M, et al. Surgery of the primary tumor does not improve survival in stage IV breast cancer. Breast Cancer Res Treat 2011; 129(2):459–65.

28. Cady B, Nathan NR, Michaelson JS, et al. Matched pair analyses of stage IV breast cancer with or without resection of primary breast site. Ann Surg Oncol 2008;15(12):3384–95.

29. King T, Lyman J, Gonen M, et al. Abstract P2-18-09: TBCRC 013: a prospective analysis of the role of surgery in stage IV breast cancer. Cancer Res 2013; 73(24_Supplement):P2, 18-09-P2-18-09.

30. King TA, Lyman J, Gonen M, et al. A prospective analysis of surgery and survival in stage IV breast cancer (TBCRC 013). J Clin Oncol 2016;34(15_suppl):1006.

31. Badwe R, Hawaldar R, Nair N, et al. Locoregional treatment versus no treatment of the primary tumour in metastatic breast cancer: an open-label randomised controlled trial. Lancet Oncol 2015;16(13):1380–8.

32. Soran A, Ozmen V, Ozbas S, et al. Randomized trial comparing resection of primary tumor with no surgery in stage IV breast cancer at presentation: protocol MF07-01. Ann Surg Oncol 2018;25(11):3141–9.

33. Fitzal F, Bjelic-Radisic V, Knauer M, et al. Impact of breast surgery in primary metastasized breast cancer: outcomes of the prospective randomized phase III ABCSG-28 POSYTIVE trial. Ann Surg 2019;269(6):1163–9.

34. Khan SA, Zhao F, Goldstein LJ, et al. Early local therapy for the primary site in de novo stage IV breast cancer: results of a randomized clinical trial (EA2108). J Clin Oncol 2022;40(9):978–87.

35. Khan SA, Zhao F, Solin LJ, et al. A randomized phase III trial of systemic therapy plus early local therapy versus systemic therapy alone in women with de novo stage IV breast cancer: a trial of the ECOG-ACRIN Research Group (E2108). J Clin Oncol 2020;38(18_suppl):LBA2.

36. Shien T, Mizutani T, Tanaka K, et al. A randomized controlled trial comparing primary tumor resection plus systemic therapy with systemic therapy alone in

metastatic breast cancer (JCOG1017 PRIM-BC). J Clin Oncol 2017; 35(15_suppl):TPS588.

37. Hotton J, Lusque A, Leufflen L, et al. Early locoregional breast surgery and survival in de novo metastatic breast cancer in the multicenter national ESME cohort. Ann Surg 2021. https://doi.org/10.1097/sla.0000000000004767.

38. Barinoff J, Schmidt M, Schneeweiss A, et al. Primary metastatic breast cancer in the era of targeted therapy – Prognostic impact and the role of breast tumour surgery. Eur J Cancer 2017;83:116–24.

39. Bishop AJ, Ensor J, Moulder SL, et al. Prognosis for patients with metastatic breast cancer who achieve a no-evidence-of-disease status after systemic or local therapy. Cancer 2015;121(24):4324–32.

40. Singletary SE, Walsh G, Vauthey J-N, et al. A Role for curative surgery in the treatment of selected patients with metastatic breast cancer. Oncologist 2003;8(3): 241–51.

41. Fan J, Chen D, Du H, et al. Prognostic factors for resection of isolated pulmonary metastases in breast cancer patients: a systematic review and meta-analysis. J Thorac Dis 2015;7(8):1441–51.

42. Chmura SJ, Winter KA, Al-Hallaq HA, et al. NRG-BR002: a phase IIR/III trial of standard of care therapy with or without stereotactic body radiotherapy (SBRT) and/or surgical ablation for newly oligometastatic breast cancer (NCT02364557). J Clin Oncol 2019;37(15_suppl):TPS1117.

43. Wingo PA, Jamison PM, Young JL, et al. Population-based statistics for women diagnosed with inflammatory breast cancer (United States). Cancer Causes & Control 2004;15(3):321–8.

44. Fouad TM, Kogawa T, Liu DD, et al. Overall survival differences between patients with inflammatory and noninflammatory breast cancer presenting with distant metastasis at diagnosis. Breast Cancer Res Treat 2015;152(2):407–16.

45. Akay CL, Ueno NT, Chisholm GB, et al. Primary tumor resection as a component of multimodality treatment may improve local control and survival in patients with stage IV inflammatory breast cancer. Cancer 2014;120(9):1319–28.

46. Warren LE, Guo H, Regan MM, et al. Inflammatory breast cancer: patterns of failure and the case for aggressive locoregional management. Ann Surg Oncol 2015;22(8):2483–91.

47. Takiar V, Akay CL, Stauder MC, et al. Predictors of durable no evidence of disease status in de novo metastatic inflammatory breast cancer patients treated with neoadjuvant chemotherapy and post-mastectomy radiation. Springerplus 2014;3:166.

New Technology for the Breast Surgeon

Michele Carpenter, MD[a,b,]*, Julie Le, MD[c,1]

KEYWORDS

- Localization • Oncoplasty • Nerve-sparing • Mastopexy • Robotic mastectomy
- LYMPHA

KEY POINTS

- Wireless localization devices are easy to use and have equivalent or lower re-excision rates compared with the wire technique.
- Intraoperative margin evaluation with spectroscopy, 3D recreation with micro-CT, and molecular imaging may reduce re-excision rates by 50%.
- Oncoplastic techniques can be used to improve aesthetics with equivalent oncological outcomes.
- Nerve-sparing and robotic mastectomies are emerging techniques that may improve the quality of life for patients.
- LYMPHA surgery is a promising approach to reduce primary lymphedema.

There are several new and exciting intraoperative tools and techniques for the breast surgeon. We will cover novel localization navigators and devices, margin imaging devices, and review surgical techniques for oncoplasty and lymphatic preserving to prevent lymphedema. In addition, we will also highlight the very emerging approaches of robotic mastectomy and nerve preservation for nipple-sparing mastectomy.

LOCALIZATION DEVICES AND NAVIGATORS

Many years ago localization devices were not common, and the surgeon relied solely on imaging to locate the abnormality in the breast. In the 1970s, 4 radiologists independently set up mammography screening programs with wire localization techniques. These men included Dr Ferris Hall (the hook wire), Dr Daniel Kopans (the spring hook wire), Dr Norman Sadowsky, and Dr Marc Homer (the J Wire).[1] Today,

---

[a] Center for Cancer Prevention and Treatment, St. Joseph Hospital, 1010 W. LaVeta suite 475, Orange, CA 92868, USA; [b] Department of Surgery, David Geffen School of Medicine at UCLA, Los Angeles, CA, USA; [c] UC San Diego Comprehensive Breast Health, 9400 Campus Point Drive, La Jolla, CA 92037, USA
[1] Present address: 3855 Health Sciences Drive, La Jolla, CA 92037
* Corresponding author. UCLA Breast Surgery Orange, 1010 W. LaVeta Avenue, Suite 475, Orange, CA 92868.
E-mail address: Mcarpenter@mednet.ucla.edu

Surg Clin N Am 103 (2023) 107–119
https://doi.org/10.1016/j.suc.2022.08.013
0039-6109/23/Published by Elsevier Inc.
surgical.theclinics.com

we have graduated to an array of choices for localization or navigations: radioactive (iodine) seeds, reflectors, magnetic seeds, and radiofrequency (RFID) tags.

SAVI scout from Merit Medical is a metallic reflector placed in the breast in the same manner as a biopsy clip placement. The reflector is detected with the use of nonradioactive radar waves during surgery (**Fig. 1**). The reflector is passive until it is activated by the guide and measures about 4 mm. The guide is connected to the computer which documents the distance from the guide to the scout which aids the surgeon in finding the area in question. As surgeons, we still must review the mammograms and see whereby the scout is placed to accurately remove the target. A downside of the SAVI scout is deactivation within proximity of the Bovie electrocautery, though Merit Medical is currently manufacturing devices that are impregnable to cautery disturbances. In at least one series, the SAVI scout localization system resulted in a lower rate of positive margins, reoperation, and surgical site occurrence.[2] Magseed is a tiny metallic "grain of rice-like" seed that is similarly inserted into the breast as a biopsy clip and is located by a "Sentimag" probe through its magnetic properties and the readout on the computer assists the surgeon in finding the target (**Fig. 2**). Magseed can cause MRI artifacts and metal instruments may interfere with the seed detection. In a multicenter nonrandomized control study, there were no significant differences between Wire localization and this newer technology.[3,4] There was no difference between the patients requiring re-excision, specimens by weight and volume were similar for both groups, and interactive identification and excision were successful in all patients.

Magtrace TM is the counterpart of Magseed for nonradionucleotide guided sentinel node detection using 60 NM organically coated iron oxide particle sized for retention in the nodes. It is injected into the subareolar region like blue dye, and detection is achieved with the same Sentimag probe used for Magseed. Risks of the magnetic tracer include injection and drainage site sensitivity. Magtrace can travel to areas away from the injection site such as liver, spleen, and other organs. Two studies comparing MagtraceTM to standard evaluation for axillary sentinel lymph nodes showed 96% to 98% overall concordance.[5,6]

LOCalizer by Hologic is another wire-free system that uses a miniature radiofrequency identification tag (RFID). Each tag has a unique identifier which allows for easier identification of multiple areas within the breast if needed. The system includes a single-use surgical probe with a small tip and a handheld reader that can be placed into a sterile cover in the field if desired (**Fig. 3**). The tags are 11 mm long and 2 mm in diameter. In a study of the LOCalize system, both radiologists and surgeons felt that this technology was as reliable as the wire and may contribute to lower re-excision rates.[7]

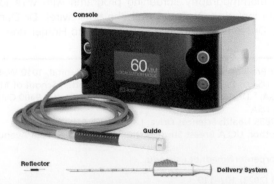

Fig. 1. SAVI Scout console with probe and delivery system. (Printed with permission © 2018 Merit Medical.)

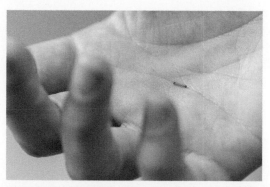

Fig. 2. Magseed "seed" sized to a penny held in hand for scale. (Printed with permission © 2017 Endomag.)

Elucent has the EnVisioTM Surgical navigation system which uses a SmartclipTM marker. This marker contains a unique electromagnetic signature that communicates with the navigation system during surgery. Depth, distance, and direction are triangulated between the clip, the navigator, and the tumor whereby the smart clip was placed. The image is displayed on a screen that can be attached to tools in the operating room that surgeons frequently use (**Fig. 4**). The EnVisioTM system is currently being evaluated in lungs, breast, and GI surgery. A major advantage of the Envision system is that up to 3 different markers can be placed into the breast.

CLINICS CARE POINT

1. Wireless localization devices seem to have a short learning curve, have a high success rate of identification of target lesions, and yield equivalent or lower re-excision rates compared with the wire approach.
2. Elucent navigation system displays the triangulation of the tumor with the SmartclipTM on commonly used intraoperative tools such as Bovie electrocautery.
3. Disadvantages of wireless localization tools include inadvertent deactivation with cautery or metal instruments.
4. Use of wireless devices still requires a thorough evaluation of imaging before surgery to ensure successful lesion excision.

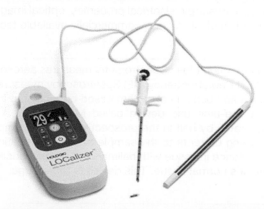

Fig. 3. Hologic LOCalizer Portable console with delivery system and marker. (Printed with permission ©2019 Hologic.)

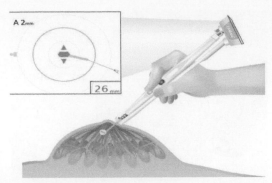

Fig. 4. EnVisio Surgical Navigator is placed on the Bovie electrocautery instrument for intra-operative navigation. (Printed with permission © 2019 Elucent Medical.)

INTRAOPERATIVE MARGIN IMAGING DEVICES

Margin assessment in breast cancer surgery has long been a point of discussion as well as a focal point of technological entrepreneurship. Delays in adjuvant therapy initiative and compromised cosmetic outcomes can be tied to re-excision rates, and therefore several new intraoperative options for margin assessment are under development and in use. In the past, gross examination with and without imaging such as ultrasound, intraoperative x-rays (in the form of self-contained radiology units such as Kubtec, Trident, and Faxitron), and intraoperative pathology assessments were the mainstay. With these methods, the re-excision rates ranged from under 10% to more than 20%. Due to the high variability in repeat surgery, newer technologies have been developed to establish consistency that would lower the re-excision rate.

Intraoperative assessment for decades has included discussions of radiography with and without newer 3D technology, gross pathology assessment by surgeon and pathologist, and "touch preparations." In one study looking at radiography versus pathology, "the negative predictive value was 97.4% for intraoperative assessment by radiography and 81.8% for intraoperative assessment by pathology. The re-operation rate among cases without intraoperative assessment was 23.6% compared with 7.3% among cases with intraoperative assessment."[8–10] Tumor size, histologic subtype, and multifocality were important factors that affect margin evaluation.[8–10]

So, what technology beyond these established ones can assist the breast surgeon? These devices use spectroscopy, electrical properties, optical imaging, and molecular imaging. We will limit this discussion to commercially available technologies.

Spectroscopy

Rapid Evaporative Ionization Mass Spectrometry measures aerosolized charged particles with the iKnife.[11] Radiofrequency (RF) Spectroscopy measures the RF waves at the specimen surface and uses an algorithm based on a dataset from malignant and healthy tissue in a one-time use device called Margin probe.[12] This device has reduced re-excision rates by half in the prospective study. Bioimpedance spectroscopy applies alternating currents to the sample to identify variations in extracellular and intracellular resistance in tissue with hallmarks of breast cancer but starts by first examining the patient's normal tissue. This device is Clear Edge.[13]

Optical Imaging

Optical coherence tomography (OCT) uses light waves to generate high-resolution images at the surface and just under the surface which mimic actual histopathology in the Perimeter Medical Device (**Fig. 5**). Other optical imaging systems have been tested and one of the areas that are important is "can the surgeon or radiologist be taught to identify abnormal imaging to correlate with cancer?"[14] Ha and colleagues reviewed OCT use on 63 excised specimens that were divided into training and testing groups. The authors showed it took approximately 3.4 hours for the physician to learn the technique and thereby made it possible to apply intraoperatively.

Microcomputed Tomography

Microcomputed tomography is an imaging technique that allows rapid digitization of the structures of a sample in 3D with great resolution. "The main principle is the generation of a series of radiographs, which are called projection images, of a rotating sample that is placed between an X-ray source and an Xray detector."[15] These projection images are then reconstructed with algorithms for image acquisition (**Fig. 6**). The primary advantage of this technology includes rapid acquisition with good resolution. The major disadvantage is a high amount of data is required for storage. The next direction of micro-CT involves improvement in details to include colors and reduction in the size of detection of the smallest elements.[16] Qiu and colleagues showed a 31% reduction in positive margins to 14% using this technology.[16]

Molecular Imaging

Small molecular fluorescent probes from Lumicell Imaging System use LUM015 dye which is administered before surgery. The molecule becomes fluorescent when cathepsin, a protease known to remodel a tumor's microenvironment, cleaves the

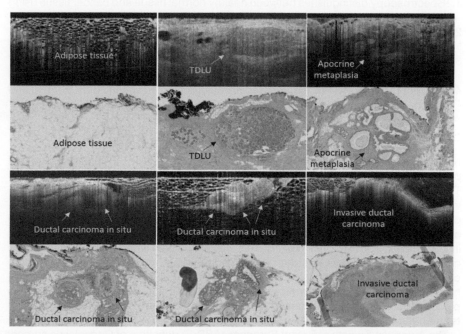

Fig. 5. Images of Perimeter OCT compared with histology slides outlining the underlying tissue and pathology samples. (Printed with permission. © 2022 Perimeter Medical Imaging AI. Images (IRB 16-01206) provided by Adriana Corben, M.D., Mount Sinai Hospital, New York, NY.)

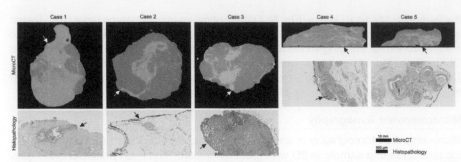

Fig. 6. Images of Micro CT with corresponding histology. (Printed with permission ©2021 Elsevier. *From* Qiu et al, Micro-computed tomography (micro-CT) for intraoperative surgical margin assessment of breast cancer: A feasibility study in breast conserving surgery. Eur J Surg Oncol. 11 2018;44(11):1708-1713.)

peptide. The signal can be detected by a probe used in the cavity but is limited to a maximum cavity dimension of 26 mm. These are just a few of the many ideas and technological advances that are coming to us in the future. There are no large-scale studies comparing these technologies to each other and most of the data surrounding each of these technologies is in single or multi-institutional studies comparing the technology to pathology.

CLINICS CARE POINTS

1. Spectroscopy distinguishes between healthy normal tissue and cancer tissue using radiofrequency waves.
2. Optical coherence tomography recreates simple surface images to provide a histopathology view that surgeons and radiologists can interpret.
3. Micro-CT recreates a 3D shape of the tumor that can be used to correlate with original imaging to identify close margins.
4. Many of these modalities require special equipment, high volume data storage, and preoperative training to interpret images which may make applicability difficult.

ONCOPLASTIC TECHNIQUES

National Surgical Adjuvant Breast and Bowel Project (NSABP) B-06 showed us that partial mastectomy is equivalent to total mastectomy in terms of overall survival.[17] The local recurrence rates were greater without radiation. In the 1980s, breast conservation surgery had more to do with the placement of the incisions and lacked approaches for tissue rearrangement to fill the defect beneath the skin. The resulting cosmetic result was fraught with empty quadrants after seromas were resorbed resulting in dimpling and retraction (**Fig. 7**). This was also a time when we performed partial mastectomies on tumors less than 4 cm. Today, armed with new techniques developed and promoted by our plastic as well as innovative breast surgeon colleagues, not only are we able to perform better partial resections of breast tumors but these pieces of tissue can be much larger and the final result in some cases can appear better than the original.

The American Society of Breast Surgeons (ASBrS) definition of Oncoplastic surgery is "a form of breast conservation surgery that includes oncologic resection with a partial mastectomy, ipsilateral reconstruction using volume displacement or volume replacement techniques with possible contralateral symmetry surgery when

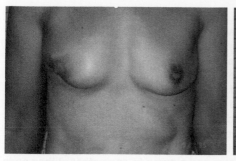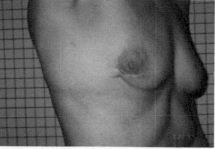

Fig. 7. Lumpectomy with no oncoplastic rearrangement 1995.

appropriate." Level 1 oncoplasty is when less than 20% of the overall breast tissue is removed, whereas Level 2 is when 20% to 50% of the breast tissue is removed and is called volume displacement. Reconstructive surgeons are usually needed for the replacement of volume when more than 50% of the breast tissue is removed. Some basic and more advanced techniques will be described here.

Crescent Mastopexy

The crescent mastopexy technique involves performing a crescent excision of the epithelium of the skin (this is described as "deepithelialization") superior to the areola so as to open a larger space for excision of the tissue as well as raising of the nipple. This can be conducted by itself or with a skin excision called "batwing" at the same time **(Fig. 8)**.

Donut Mastopexy

A variation of the crescent mastopexy is the donut mastopexy. A circular rim of epithelial tissue is removed around the areola concentrically or eccentrically and can include the pigmented areola **(Fig. 9)**. The eccentric version is utilized to change the position of the nipple if needed. The best reason to do a concentric donut is to be able to remove tumors from places that you may not be able to through a periareolar incision since the epithelium limits the ability to enlarge the incision. By keeping the dermis intact, the nipple will be viable.

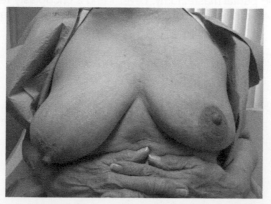

Fig. 8. One-year postoperative recovery following crescent mastopexy and "Batwing" extensions.

Inframammary Crescent Mammaplasty

The inframmary crescent mammaplasty involves de-epithelialization of skin along the inframammary ridge to create a "dermal flap" that can be fashioned to fill in a space left when a tumor is removed from the 6:00 position. This location of tumor excision is notorious for creating such an empty space that the nipple is pulled downwards resulting in a "bird peak deformity." The dermal pedicle is designed to resemble a fish tail where both ends of the fishtail are sutured together to fill in the space. An inframammary incision is designed with the blood supply to the pedicle coming from the abdominal portion at the center of the pedicle. The designed fishtail is de-epithelialized so it can be inserted into the lumpectomy cavity (**Fig. 10**A–C). The "fish-tails" are separated from the surrounding skin and sutured to each other at their ends to make a dermal flap that then can be anchored to the superior portion of the lumpectomy cavity to fill in the empty space (**Fig. 10**D, E). The skin at the superior aspect of the dermal flap is then brought down to the bottom of the deepithelialized dermal flap and sutured in place to reconstitute the inframammary ridge.

Reduction Mammaplasty

Lastly, the reduction mammoplasty constitutes the more advanced rearrangement of tissue for partial mastectomies. The breast and general surgeons in these cases will most of the time have more advanced training in plastic surgery techniques. Breast reduction started in the early 20th century for aesthetic purposes only. One of the first reports of combining breast reduction with cancer surgery was from Smith and colleagues in 1998 whereby the series described 10 women who received surgery between 1988 and 1996 with minimal complications.[18] Overall, patients who undergo combined reduction mammaplasty with cancer surgery have shown to have equivalent survival with good functional and cosmetic results. Breast reduction requires an understanding of the blood supply to the nipple-areolar complex (NAC) and the various pedicles that need to be preserved. The most useful, robust pedicle is the superomedial one, though, some plastic surgeons will use a combination of pedicles to ensure more than one blood supply to the NAC. The result is an inverted "T" scar no matter which pedicle is used (**Fig. 11**).

CLINICS CARE POINTS

1. Oncoplastic surgery is performing volume replacement or displacement techniques following partial mastectomy. Level 1 and 2 oncoplasty techniques are utilized when 20% or 20% to 50% of breast volume is removed, respectively.

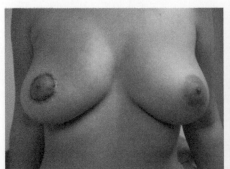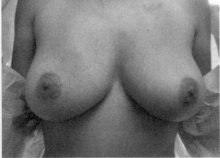

Fig. 9. Donut mastopexy in the immediate postoperative period and 1 year later.

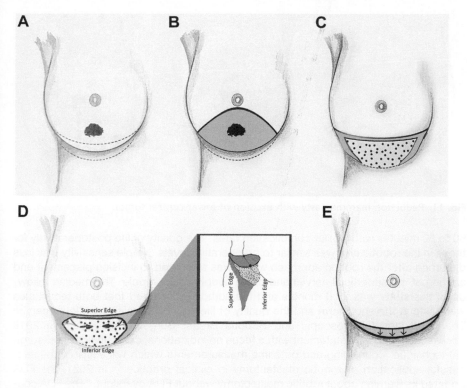

Fig. 10. Inframammary Crescent Mammaplasty. (*A*) Crescent lines are drawn 5 mm above and 10 mm below IMF (*B*) Incise superior line, create skin ap and excise tumor. (*C*) De-epithelialize the skin between the superior and inferior lines. Incise the inferior line but spare central skin and subcutaneous attachments to create a dermal ap Inframammary Crescent Mammaplasty. (*D*) Fish tails are separated from surrounding tissue and sutured together to create a dermal flap to fill lower cavity void. (*E*) Superior and inferior edges are sutured together to close defect.

2. Crescent mastopexy can lift the NAC through a more accessible peri- or circumareolar incision following tumor excision
3. Inframammary crescent mammaplasty is an excellent technique for volume replacement in the lower inner quadrant tumors.
4. More advanced techniques such as breast reduction require a thorough understanding of vascular pedicles and may require plastic surgery training.

ROBOTIC MASTECTOMY

Robotic-assisted mastectomy was first performed in 2015 in a case series of 3 BRCA mutation carriers.[19] Since then, there have been several case reports and series based on individual institution experience. The described technique uses both gas or gasless insufflation, and most of the cases involved immediate implant reconstruction. One randomized controlled trial from the European Institute of Oncology in Milan, Italy looked at complications and quality of life using validated questionnaires comparing robotic to open mastectomies in mutation carriers and patients with cancer.[20] A total of 80 patients were randomized to each group. The robotic procedure was longer by

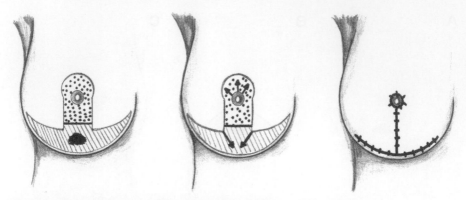

Fig. 11. Reduction mammaplasty with excision of lower central tumor.

60 to 80 minutes with similar complication rates. The quality of life postoperatively for those in the robotic arm was similar to preoperative levels. Nipple sensitivity was less disturbed after the robotic approach which was attributed to incision placement and sparing of the superficial nerves and blood supply to the nipple. The median follow-up of this study was 28.6 months and the authors concluded that both techniques were safe in the short term and the quality of life was better with robotic surgery.[20] The International Endoscopic and Robotic Breast Surgery Symposium in 2019 released a consensus statement with a focus on indications, contraindications, surgical technique, counseling and outcome measurements which will assist in the successful application of robotic mastectomy in clinical practice.[21] In 2021, the FDA updated its warning about robotic mastectomy without FDA oversight. "The FDA considers clinical studies performed in the United States involving RAS devices for mastectomy and the prevention and treatment of cancer to be significant risk studies. These clinical studies require FDA oversight under an approved investigational device exemption. There is little evidence on the safety and effectiveness of the use of RAS devices in patients undergoing mastectomy for the prevention or treatment of breast cancer, and the FDA has not granted any RAS system marketing authorization for mastectomy. For patients undergoing mastectomy, the surgical approach used with RAS devices differs from conventional surgical approaches. The impact of these differences on the prevention of cancer, overall survival, recurrence, and disease-free survival has not been established."[22]

NERVE PRESERVATION IN MASTECTOMY

Nerve preservation and allografting for sensory innervation following immediate reconstruction is a new approach to improving and restoring nipple sensation after mastectomy. Plastic surgeons have attempted the neurotization of breast reconstructive flaps and most recently this includes allografting and microsurgical techniques at the time of reconstruction. In 2019, Anne and Ziv Peled described their technique in 16 women who underwent nipple-sparing mastectomy with direct to preprectoral implant reconstruction.[23] In most of these cases, the nerves were able to be preserved. However, when nerve preservation was not possible, the surgeons used coapted transected T4 and T5 lateral intercostal nerves to the subareolar nerves.[23] NAC two-point discrimination was found to be preserved in 87%, decreased in 9%, and improved in 4%. The Peled surgeons concluded that this technique is safe and effective with a 90% sensation preservation rate.[23]

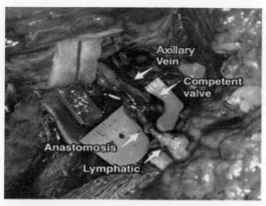

Fig. 12. Lymphatic microsurgical preventative healing approach. (Printed with permission ©2022 Springer Link. *From* Feldman S, Bansil H, Ascherman J, et al. Single Institution Experience with Lymphatic Microsurgical Preventive Healing Approach (LYMPHA) for the Primary Prevention of Lymphedema. Ann Surg Oncol. Oct 2015;22(10):3296-301.)

REVERSE LYMPHATIC MAPPING: LYMPHA

With the advent of sentinel lymph node biopsy as a safe and accurate alternative to completion dissection (ALND) for axillary staging, the incidence of secondary lymphedema has decreased. However, for women who undergo ALND, the rates of lymphedema remain high, with reports of up to 40%.[24] Management of secondary lymphedema focuses on symptom relief including lymphatic massage, compression sleeves, and physical therapy; yet none of these treatments reverse lymphedema. Lymphatic microsurgical preventative healing approach (LYMPHA) is a novel surgery for the primary prevention of lymphedema (**Fig. 12**). LYMPHA includes reverse mapping to identify the afferent lymphatics from the arm to allow for lymphatic-venous anastomosis performed between lymphatics and collateral branches of the axillary vein after standard level 1 to 2 ALND.[25,26] The lymphedema rate for patients with LYMPHA was 4% to 13% after 2 to 4 years of follow-up.[25–27] Additional surgical time added for LYMPHA completion was approximately 45 minutes.[27] LYMPHA represents a promising, safe method for the primary prevention of lymphedema.

DISCLOSURE OF ANY COMMERCIAL INTEREST

Authors have no conflict-of-interest disclosures to report.

REFERENCES

1. Hall FM, Kopans DB, Sadowsky NL, et al. Development of wire localization for occult breast lesions: Boston remembrances. Radiology 2013;268(3):622–7.

2. Tingen JS, McKinley BP, Rinkliff JM, et al. Savi Scout Radar Localization Versus Wire Localization for Breast Biopsy Regarding Positive Margin, Complication, and Reoperation Rates. Am Surg 2020;86(8):1029–31.

3. Zacharioudakis K, Down S, Bholah Z, et al. Is the future magnetic? Magseed localisation for non palpable breast cancer. A multi-centre non randomised control study. Eur J Surg Oncol 2019;45(11):2016–21.

4. Singh P, Scoggins ME, Sahin AA, et al. Effectiveness and Safety of Magseed-localization for Excision of Breast Lesions: A Prospective, Phase IV Trial. Ann Surg Open 2020;1(2). https://doi.org/10.1097/as9.0000000000000008.

5. Alvarado MD, Mittendorf EA, Teshome M, et al. SentimagIC: A Non-inferiority Trial Comparing Superparamagnetic Iron Oxide Versus Technetium-99m and Blue Dye in the Detection of Axillary Sentinel Nodes in Patients with Early-Stage Breast Cancer. Ann Surg Oncol 2019;26(11):3510–6.

6. Teshome M, Wei C, Hunt KK, et al. Use of a Magnetic Tracer for Sentinel Lymph Node Detection in Early-Stage Breast Cancer Patients: A Meta-analysis. Ann Surg Oncol 2016;23(5):1508–14.

7. DiNome ML, Kusske AM, Attai DJ, et al. Microchipping the breast: an effective new technology for localizing non-palpable breast lesions for surgery. Breast Cancer Res Treat 2019;175(1):165–70.

8. Manhoobi IP, Bodilsen A, Nijkamp J, et al. Diagnostic accuracy of radiography, digital breast tomosynthesis, micro-CT and ultrasound for margin assessment during breast surgery: A systematic review and meta-analysis. Acad Radiol 2022. https://doi.org/10.1016/j.acra.2021.12.006.

9. Koopmansch C, Noël JC, Maris C, et al. Intraoperative Evaluation of Resection Margins in Breast-Conserving Surgery for. Breast Cancer (Auckl) 2021;15. 1178223421993459.

10. Schwarz J, Schmidt H. Technology for Intraoperative Margin Assessment in Breast Cancer. Ann Surg Oncol 2020;27(7):2278–87.

11. St John ER, Balog J, McKenzie JS, et al. Rapid evaporative ionisation mass spectrometry of electrosurgical vapours for the identification of breast pathology: towards an intelligent knife for breast cancer surgery. Breast Cancer Res 2017; 19(1):59.

12. Allweis TM, Kaufman Z, Lelcuk S, et al. A prospective, randomized, controlled, multicenter study of a real-time, intraoperative probe for positive margin detection in breast-conserving surgery. Am J Surg 2008;196(4):483–9.

13. Dixon JM, Renshaw L, Young O, et al. Intra-operative assessment of excised breast tumour margins using ClearEdge imaging device. Eur J Surg Oncol 2016;42(12):1834–40.

14. Ha R, Friedlander LC, Hibshoosh H, et al. Optical Coherence Tomography: A Novel Imaging Method for Post-lumpectomy Breast Margin Assessment-A Multi-reader Study. Acad Radiol 2018;25(3):279–87.

15. Keklikoglou K, Arvanitidis C, Chatzigeorgiou G, et al. Micro-CT for Biological and Biomedical Studies: A Comparison of Imaging Techniques. J Imaging 2021;7(9). https://doi.org/10.3390/jimaging7090172.

16. Qiu SQ, Dorrius MD, de Jongh SJ, et al. Micro-computed tomography (micro-CT) for intraoperative surgical margin assessment of breast cancer: A feasibility study in breast conserving surgery. Eur J Surg Oncol 2018;44(11):1708–13.

17. Fisher B, Anderson S, Bryant J, et al. Twenty-year follow-up of a randomized trial comparing total mastectomy, lumpectomy, and lumpectomy plus irradiation for the treatment of invasive breast cancer. N Engl J Med 2002;347(16):1233–41.

18. Smith ML, Evans GR, Gurlek A, et al. Reduction mammaplasty: its role in breast conservation surgery for early-stage breast cancer. Ann Plast Surg 1998;41(3): 234–9.

19. Toesca A, Peradze N, Galimberti V, et al. Preliminary report of robotic nipple-sparing mastectomy and immediate reconstruction with implant. Eur J Cancer 2015;51(Suppl 3):S309.

20. Toesca A, Sangalli C, Maisonneuve P, et al. A Randomized Trial of Robotic Mastectomy versus Open Surgery in Women with Breast Cancer or BRCA Mutation. Ann Surg 2021. https://doi.org/10.1097/SLA.0000000000004969.
21. Lai HW, Toesca A, Sarfati B, et al. Consensus statement on robotic mastectomy – expert panel from International Endoscopic robotic breast surgery symposium (IERBS) 2019. Ann Surg 2020;271(6):1005–12.
22. UPDATE: Caution with Robotically-Assisted Surgical Devices in Mastectomy: FDA Safety Communication. https://www.fda.gov/medical-devices/safety-communications/update-caution-robotically-assisted-surgical-devices-mastectomy-fda-safety-communication. Accessed 26 March 2022.
23. Peled AW, Peled ZM. Nerve Preservation and Allografting for Sensory Innervation Following Immediate Implant Breast Reconstruction. Plast Reconstr Surg Glob Open 2019;7(7):e2332.
24. DiSipio T, Rye S, Newman B, et al. Incidence of unilateral arm lymphoedema after breast cancer: a systematic review and meta-analysis. Lancet Oncol 2013;14(6): 500–15.
25. Feldman S, Bansil H, Ascherman J, et al. Single Institution Experience with Lymphatic Microsurgical Preventive Healing Approach (LYMPHA) for the Primary Prevention of Lymphedema. Ann Surg Oncol 2015;22(10):3296–301.
26. Boccardo F, Casabona F, De Cian F, et al. Lymphatic microsurgical preventing healing approach (LYMPHA) for primary surgical prevention of breast cancer-related lymphedema: over 4 years follow-up. Microsurgery 2014;34(6):421–4.
27. Cook JA, Sasor SE, Loewenstein SN, et al. Immediate Lymphatic Reconstruction after Axillary Lymphadenectomy: A Single-Institution Early Experience. Ann Surg Oncol 2021;28(3):1381–7.

Postoperative Complications from Breast and Axillary Surgery

Sam Z. Thalji, MD[a], Chandler S. Cortina, MD, MS, FSSO[a],
Meng S. Guo, MD[b], Amanda L. Kong, MD, MS, FSSO[a],*

KEYWORDS

- Postoperative complications • Hematoma • Seroma • Nerve injury • Lymphedema

KEY POINTS

- Potential complications after breast and axillary surgery are numerous and vary in incidence and presentation.
- Risk profiles depend on the procedure performed, extent of axillary dissection, and the inclusion of various reconstructive techniques.
- Knowledge of potential complications and approaches for management are important components of the preoperative discussion with patients.
- Incidence, risk factors, presentation, implications to the patient, risk-reducing approaches, and management of postoperative complications after breast and axillary surgery (with or without reconstruction) are discussed herein.

INTRODUCTION

The prospective benefit of any operation must be weighed against the risk of its complications. Although surgery of the breast and axilla is generally well tolerated by patients, the breast surgeon recognizes that complications can occur even when operating with experience on the lowest risk patients. The operative repertoire ranges from breast conserving surgery (BCS), mastectomy (including skin-sparing and nipple-sparing types), to modified radical mastectomy (MRM), with each procedure carrying a different expected surgical morbidity. In the axilla, the majority of patients will only require a sentinel lymph biopsy (SLNB) with some for whom an axillary lymph node dissection (ALND) is still indicated. Select patients are candidates for omission of surgical nodal staging altogether. Each procedural component carries a unique risk

[a] Department of Surgery, Division of Surgical Oncology, Medical College of Wisconsin, Milwaukee, WI, USA; [b] Department of Plastic Surgery, Medical College of Wisconsin, Milwaukee, WI, USA
* Corresponding author. Department of Surgery/ Division of Surgical Oncology, 8701 Watertown Plank Road, Milwaukee, WI 53226.
E-mail address: akong@mcw.edu

Surg Clin N Am 103 (2023) 121–139
https://doi.org/10.1016/j.suc.2022.08.007
0039-6109/23/© 2022 Elsevier Inc. All rights reserved.

surgical.theclinics.com

profile that the surgeon must be well versed in explaining to patients in a practical format. Patients and families who are fully informed of potential complications before their operation describe greater trust in their surgeon and are better able to comanage complications with the surgical team, when they occur.[1]

EARLY COMPLICATIONS
Postoperative hematoma

Clinically significant hematoma formation after breast and axillary surgery is an uncommon complication that requires early recognition and urgent management. The incidence of postoperative hematoma requiring operative evacuation after breast surgery is estimated at less than 2% and seems to be higher among patients who receive mastectomy alone compared with patients who undergo immediate reconstruction or BCS.[2] Vessels arising from the pectoralis muscle are the most common primary source of postoperative bleeding while axillary hematomas are rare and are usually not associated with an identifiable source.[3] Postoperative hematomas generally accumulate within 12 to 24 hours after the initial operation and present as a palpable firm mass or fluid collection with spreading ecchymosis overlying the resection site and continued sanguineous output from surgical drains, when present. Skin tightness and eventually hemodynamic changes may occur if the hematoma is not recognized promptly and bleeding continues. The risk of postoperative hematoma after mastectomy is not altered by operative or oncologic factors and is higher among patients receiving anticoagulation.[4] Aside from sequelae of continued bleeding after surgery, hematomas may compromise the cosmetic outcome after reconstruction, threaten skin flaps or grafts, and are associated with the development of capsular contracture after implant-based reconstruction.[5]

Postoperative hematomas that present with jeopardized skin flaps, expansion, or hemodynamic instability must immediately return to the operating room for evacuation and exploration. Small minimally symptomatic hematomas are not uncommon and can be safely observed for evidence of stability and resolution. Vacuum-assisted percutaneous evacuation is being studied for delayed hematomas without the above alarm signs as a means to avoid reoperation.[6] Hematoma formation is minimized by practicing the fundamental surgical principle of diligent intraoperative hemostasis. Compressive dressings are commonly applied to decrease hematoma and seroma formation; however, this practice has not been definitively shown to reduce these unwanted complications.[7] Ancillary surgical techniques such as anchoring sutures and tissue sealants do not prevent hematoma formation.[8] Patients on anticoagulation should be managed following current guidelines (see "Venous Thromboembolism" section) and counseled regarding the increased risk of hematoma formation both immediately after surgery and on resuming anticoagulation.

SEROMA

Seroma formation is reported in up to 50% of patients after breast and axillary surgery.[9] Seromas consist of fluid accumulation in the postresection dead space and are more common after mastectomy and ALND than BCS and SLNB.[9] The exact cause of seroma formation is multifactorial, and lymph leak after the resection of axillary nodes is a known contributing factor for axillary seroma development.[10] Fluid output is highly variable between patients, although output typically declines in the first 48 hours after surgery.[11] Seromas can cause pain and discomfort, delay of subsequent treatments such as radiation therapy, impaired wound healing and dehiscence, flap ischemia, and poor cosmetic outcome. Seroma formation is associated with obesity, diabetes, increasing comorbidities, use of electrocautery, male sex, and vigorous postoperative shoulder exercise.[12–14]

Incidence of seroma after breast and axillary surgery is greatly reduced with the routine use of closed suction drains after mastectomy, large volume lumpectomies, and ALND.[15] There is no consensus criteria for optimal timing of drain removal after surgery based on duration or output; however, a recent meta-analysis found that drain removal within 24-48 hours after surgery was associated with a 50% increased risk of seroma development compared with drains removed more than 72 hours after surgery or after hospital discharge.[16] Axillary exclusion is a closure technique wherein the superior skin flap is sutured to the free edge of the pectoralis major and lateral chest wall to exclude the axillary fossa from the mastectomy cavity after MRM; small series have shown decreased overall fluid output and time to drain removal.[17] As is the case for postoperative hematoma, ancillary techniques including tissue sealants, fibrin glue, or sclerotherapy have not been shown to be effective in reducing seroma formation.[11] Seromas presenting after drain removal can be managed with percutaneous aspiration and/or drain replacement. When infection is suspected, fluid cultures should be sent before starting empiric antibiotics for accurate source determination. Ultrasound evaluation can visualize loculations, which may lead to incomplete percutaneous drainage, to assure that all fluid has been removed at the time of aspiration or that drains are located within the appropriate space. Operative drainage should be pursued in the case of multiple incomplete aspirations, concern for continued infection, or abscess.

INFECTION

Surgical site infections (SSIs) after breast and axillary surgery range in presentation from superficial cellulitis overlying the area of surgical incisions to deep abscesses accumulating in the dead-space, or implant, or tissue flap infection. Two large studies found the rate of SSI to be 3.2% to 3.3% after mastectomy and 1.3% to 1.4% after BCS.[18,19] SSIs occur in up to 10% to 15% of patients after mastectomy with immediate reconstruction, particularly when implants are placed.[20] Rates of SSI are neither different when comparing between various tissue flap techniques nor different when comparing between implant-based techniques.[21,22] The rate of uncomplicated cellulitis treated conservatively with outpatient antibiotics is often not captured in most studies and may be underreported. Risk factors for SSI after breast and axillary surgery include obesity, current smoking, diabetes, chronic obstructive pulmonary disease, and a hospital length of stay shorter than 1 day. A history of radiation treatment of previous breast cancer treatment is not associated with a significant increase in the rate of SSI in patients who undergo completion mastectomy with reconstruction for a local recurrence.[23,24] The rate of SSI is mildly increased among patients who receive ALND compared with SLNB.[25] Patients should be counseled to watch for local symptoms including spreading warmth/erythema of the skin, fullness in their resection site, incisional discharge, or a change in their drain output, as well as systemic symptoms including fever.

Management of SSIs after breast and axillary surgery depends on the severity of the infection. Superficial SSIs, including uncomplicated cellulitis, can be treated with outpatient oral antibiotics. Persistent infection or physical examination findings indicating an underlying fluid collection should prompt an ultrasound evaluation with aspiration and culture of fluid to direct antibiotic choice. Abscesses with loculations or those otherwise resistant to aspiration require operative drainage through the original incision. Suspicion of infection in the setting of a tissue expander or implant should be investigated promptly with ultrasound or cross-sectional imaging. Any fluid around the implant must be drained and cultured. Implant salvage is possible with inpatient intravenous antibiotics; however, if the infection progresses to dehiscence or fails to resolve within 48 hours, then operative exploration is necessary.[26] The presence of a biofilm makes implant salvage beyond 48 hours unlikely.

Perioperative prophylactic antibiotics have been shown in multiple clinical trials to reduce the incidence of SSIs after breast and axillary surgery.[27,28] The American Society of Breast Surgeons recommends the use of antibiotic prophylaxis before any type of mastectomy.[29] Although antibiotic prophylaxis before BCS and excisional biopsies should be considered for patients with risk factors for infection, there is no clear benefit among patients at low or average risk for SSI.[30–32] First-line antimicrobials include cefazolin or ampicillin-sulbactam. For beta-lactam allergies, clindamycin or vancomycin is appropriate. Perioperative prophylaxis should not extend beyond 24 hours, even with drains or implants in place.[33,34] The antibiotic choice must be made in the context of the local antibiogram and surgeons should consult with their institution's infectious disease service and pharmacy team to determine the most appropriate choice for antibiotic coverage at their location.

SKIN FLAP NECROSIS

The objective of performing a mastectomy is complete removal of the breast parenchyma, which inevitably leaves the overlying skin with a thin layer of subcutaneous tissue from which it receives vascular and nutritional support. The skin flaps are at risk of ischemia from overdissection that may progress to necrosis, which jeopardizes cosmesis and reconstruction. Extreme cases may require surgical debridement and skin grafting. The reported rates of skin necrosis after mastectomy with or without reconstruction vary considerably (5%–30%) owing to heterogeneity in defining necrosis, especially in minor cases.[35,36] Risk factors for skin flap necrosis after mastectomy include older age, obesity, large breasts, hypertension, active smoking, sarcopenia, prior radiation treatment, incision placement, and tissue expander volume.[36–38] Skin-sparing mastectomies are not associated with an increased risk of skin necrosis compared with conventional flat mastectomy. However, nipple-sparing mastectomies have been shown to be at increased risk of skin necrosis due the longer skin flaps that are created.[39]

Ultimately, the risk of skin flap necrosis depends on the technique of the breast surgeon to balance oncologic resection of all breast tissue while sparing appropriate subcutaneous fat. The thickness of the subcutaneous layer between the dermis and the breast parenchyma is highly variable between patients and does not correlate with age or obesity.[40] The presence of an investing fascia superficialis between breast parenchyma and subcutaneous fat is not macroscopically visible in all patients. In cases where the familiar avascular plane of dissection is not apparent, it has been shown that skin flaps with a thickness 5 mm or lesser are at increased risk of postoperative necrosis.[41] Newer technologies have emerged to aid in the evaluation of skin flap perfusion. Fluorescent angiography with indocyanine green allows the plastic surgeon to monitor tissue perfusion in real time and has been shown to decrease the incidence of postoperative necrosis.[42] Hyperspectral imaging of tissue oxygenation is a contrast-free method that allows for perfusion assessment during and after the operation to identify at risk skin before becoming clinically apparent.[43] When areas of skin do become ischemic or threatened, initial conservative management includes removing volume from tissue expanders, avoiding external pressure, and maintaining patient euthermia. Topical nitroglycerin ointment and dimethyl sulfoxide may be applied and have been shown to reduce postoperative skin necrosis when applied as part of the surgical dressing in a randomized controlled trial.[44] In the absence of superimposed infection or implant exposure, full thickness necrosis can be observed and allowed to heal and contract by secondary intention. Hyperbaric oxygen treatment may reduce the surface area threatened by ischemia and allow some patients to avoid additional operation.[45] Excisional debridement and skin grafting is reserved for large areas of necrosis and those refractory to conservative measures.

NIPPLE AND NIPPLE–AREOLAR COMPLEX NECROSIS

Nipple-sparing mastectomy with immediate reconstruction is an oncologically acceptable technique in carefully selected patients. Dissection of the glandular tissue under the nipple–areolar complex (NAC) disrupts the complex of vasculature, smooth muscle, and sensory nerves leading to denervation and ischemia.[46] Full-thickness nipple necrosis has been reported in up to 5% of patients and partial thickness necrosis in up to 24%.[47] As with skin necrosis, the true rate of nipple necrosis may be underreported.[48] Risk factors for nipple necrosis include smoking, large ptotic breasts (due to a longer distance from the NAC to intact perforators), periareolar incisions, and certain direct-to-implant techniques.[39,48] When a periareolar incision is necessary, an inferior incision results in less vascular disruption than a superior incision. Although radiation is associated with higher odds of skin necrosis, a meta-analysis found no association between a prior history of radiotherapy or receipt of adjuvant radiotherapy and nipple necrosis.[49]

Management of nipple necrosis follows the same principles as with skin flap necrosis. Most cases are treated conservatively allowing the necrotic tissue to demarcate and to salvage the cosmetic outcome later. Negative pressure wound vacuums may help increase blood flow to a threatened NAC.[50]

VENOUS THROMBOEMBOLISM

The risk of venous thromboembolism (VTE), defined as deep vein thrombosis (DVT) and/or pulmonary embolism (PE), is inherently increased in the perioperative period. Malignancy itself is a thrombophilic condition and many of the cytotoxic and hormonal therapies for breast cancer treatment further increase the risk. The incidence of VTE after breast and axillary surgery is lower compared with operations within the chest and abdomen; however, patients with breast cancer still represent 14% of all cancer-related VTE.[51,52] Previous studies report DVT occurring in 0.2% to 4% and PE in 0.12% to 2% after breast and axillary surgery.[53–55] VTE is more common after mastectomy compared with BCS, and immediate autologous reconstruction techniques are associated with the highest risk.[53,56] The addition of ALND to the operation may increase the risk of VTE.[57] Further risk factors include malignancy (as opposed to in situ lesions or benign pathologic condition), age younger than 65 years, obesity, general anesthesia, increased operating time, longer hospitalization (>3 days), and prior history of VTE.[53,55,58]

The American Society of Breast Surgeons has published consensus guidelines for the use of VTE prophylaxis for breast and axillary operations.[59] As with all major operations, early ambulation and sequential compression devices are recommended for all patients. The decision to use preoperative chemoprophylaxis is made on an individualized basis. For patients without prior risk factors for VTE, preoperative chemoprophylaxis is recommended before mastectomy with immediate reconstruction and for those under general anesthesia for less than 3 hours. For those undergoing less extensive operations, risk of VTE may be stratified with the Caprini score.[60] The use of preoperative chemoprophylaxis is not associated with a difference in bleeding complications after breast surgery.[61] For patients on chronic anticoagulation, the American College of Chest Physicians guidelines provide recommendations on the timing of anticoagulation interruption and the use of bridging anticoagulation.[62–64] In the context of these guidelines, breast and axillary surgery is normally considered low-risk for major bleeding. Certain individual factors may raise the risk among some patients receiving more extensive resections (including ALND) into the high-risk category. Postoperative chemoprophylaxis is commonly used after surgery for other solid tumors (eg, colorectal) and has been explored after surgery for breast cancer because most instances of VTE occur after discharge.[54] Perioperative and postoperative VTE prophylaxis regimens have shown inconsistent efficacy after surgery for breast cancer and some studies associate a higher bleeding risk.[54,65] The use of postoperative prophylaxis is not supported by any guidelines at this time.

NERVE INJURY AND POSTOPERATIVE PAIN

Injury to major motor and sensory nerves in the axilla during dissection and clearance of the nodal tissue may lead to pain, paresthesia, and motor deficits with variable resolution over time. The incidence of nerve injury is higher among patients who receive ALND compared with SLNB; however, SLNB still carries a risk.[66] In one prospective trial, more than 30% of patients who underwent SLNB for breast cancer reported sensory deficits 6 months after surgery.[67]

The long thoracic nerve courses from its cervical origin posterior to the brachial plexus and axillary vasculature to run along the chest wall and terminates in the lower border of the serratus anterior muscle. The long thoracic nerve provides motor innervation to the serratus anterior, where dysfunction leads to an unstable winged scapula that inhibits shoulder abduction and overhead arm movement.[68] Although complete transection of the long thoracic nerve is uncommon, the incidence of scapular asymmetry is reportedly greater than 50% immediately after ALND and most patients recover quickly.[69] A prospective series examining scapular winging after ALND for breast cancer using electromyography found 11.3% of patients had long thoracic injury at 1 month from surgery but only 2.3% had evidence at 12 months.[69] Patients with low BMI may be more likely to notice and report mild scapular asymmetry, which may not be apparent in patients with higher BMI.[70]

The thoracodorsal nerve originates from the posterior cord of the brachial plexus and courses along the posterior wall of the axilla to innervate the latissimus dorsi muscle. Injury to the thoracodorsal nerve results in weakness of shoulder adduction and internal rotation. The medial pectoral nerve arises from the medial cord of the brachial plexus and crosses the axilla to pierce the pectoralis minor muscle before continuing to innervate the pectoralis major. The lateral pectoral nerve originates from the lateral cord of the brachial plexus and crosses the axilla superiorly to the medial pectoral nerve where it terminates on the deep surface of the pectoralis major.[71] Injury to the lateral pectoral nerve during ALND results in limited shoulder mobility and atrophy of the pectoralis major and minor. Isolated injuries to the lateral pectoral nerve typically do not result in significant disability and do not affect the cosmetic outcome of subpectoral implant-based reconstructions.[72]

Injury to the intercostobrachial nerve during ALND is the most common iatrogenic nerve injury among all surgical procedures.[73] The intercostobrachial nerve originates from the lateral cutaneous branch of the second intercostal nerve, and its pathway across the axilla into the posteromedial border of the upper arm frequently varies.[74] The intercostobrachial nerve provides cutaneous sensation to the skin of the upper half of the posterior and medial arm. Injury to the nerve can cause paresthesia to this area and is associated with increased postoperative pain and reduced quality of life.[75] The nerve is susceptible to traction injury and neuroma formation on intact but injured nerves and may cause delayed symptoms that have been reported as high as 80% to 100% in patients after ALND but is significantly lower after SLNB.[75-77] Moderate-to-severe pain is seen is 50% of patients after ALND beyond the first postoperative week but many report improvement with time.[78,79]

Nerve injury is primarily avoided with technical diligence and awareness of potential anatomic variations. Many surgeons avoid paralysis during MRM or ALND. For patients with persistent pain after mastectomy or axillary surgery, conservative treatment begins with physical and cognitive therapy as well as medications such as antidepressants and neuromodulators.[80] Targeted interventions including nerve blocks, radiofrequency neurolysis, and steroid injections have been shown to provide durable relief and improve quality of life.[81] Intraoperative nerve monitoring during MRM is currently being explored to determine efficacy.[82] Operative approaches, including nerve transfers, have been described for select patients with chronic pain secondary to intercostobrachial injury or palsy related to long thoracic injury.[83] Postmastectomy pain syndrome is a form of chronic neuropathic pain caused by direct injury in the operating room, from subsequent scar tissue, or from radiation therapy. Postmastectomy pain syndrome is further discussed in the "Quality of Life" article.

BRACHIAL PLEXOPATHY

Breast and axillary operations require the patient to lie supine with the ipsilateral arm extended. Malposition of the patient or inattentive repositioning of the arm during the operation can lead to overstretch and subsequent injury to the brachial plexus. Postoperative brachial plexopathies usually present as painless weakness along the distribution of the upper cords: proximally the deltoid and biceps may be weak while the distal hand may be relatively spared. Brachial plexopathy after breast and axillary surgery is uncommon and can be avoided largely with careful padding and ensuring the arm position is abducted no more than 90°.[84,85] Brachial plexopathy can also occur secondary to direct extension of the breast tumor and can also occur in 1% to 2% of patients after radiation treatment.[86,87] The majority of operative and radiation-induced cases of brachial plexopathy is due to demyelination of intact nerves and will resolve with conservative management such as occupational or physical therapy.

LONG-TERM COMPLICATIONS
Lymphedema

Oncologic clearance of the axillary lymph nodes can lead to clinically significant lymphedema. Interstitial fluid from the skin and subcutaneous tissue of the breast and arm is collected by superficial lymphatic capillaries, which drain into the deep lymphatics and eventually into the axillary lymph nodes.[88] Lymph drains first into 1 to 2 dominant sentinel nodes in the lateral axilla before distributing into 20 to 40 regional axillary nodes. Lymphedema develops gradually with mild swelling and asymptomatic volume increase of the affected upper arm. This swelling can progress to the ipsilateral chest and distal arm and will initially resolve with arm elevation and night rest. Eventually the swelling and edema may become refractory to positioning and significant disability can develop as the arm becomes more encumbered. In later stages, the fluid edema progresses to fat deposition and tissue fibrosis.[89]

More than 20% of patients will experience symptomatic lymphedema after an extensive ALND.[90-92] The incidence of lymphedema after SLNB is still 3% to 8%

despite the comparatively limited dissection.[93,94] Although advances in axillary surgery have allowed for less aggressive treatments while maintaining disease control, surgeons and radiation oncologists may still be overtreating the axilla resulting in increased rates of lymphedema.[95–100] Patients should be educated on the risk of lymphedema development before therapy and survey data has found variability in the risk of lymphedema quoted by surgeons and radiation oncologists when discussing lymphedema.[90] The onset of lymphedema after breast and axillary surgery is typically delayed, with symptoms beginning approximately 12 to 30 months after surgery; ALND is associated with early onset (<12 months) lymphedema while delayed onset is usually seen after regional radiotherapy.[93] Early asymptomatic increases in arm volume within 3 months of surgery may predict eventual lymphedema development.[101] Risk factors for lymphedema development include ALND, mastectomy (compared with BCS), greater number of nodes harvested (after both ALND and SLNB), age older than 65 years, obesity, postoperative cellulitis, regional lymph node radiation, and prolonged adjuvant chemotherapy (particularly taxanes).[92,102,103] Secondary ALND after positive SLNB does not increase the risk of lymphedema compared with primary ALND.[104]

Early recognition and application of conservative treatments are key in minimizing the morbidity associated with lymphedema. Risk assessment tools exist to stratify the risk profile of individual patients.[102] Patients should be counseled to monitor the ipsilateral limb. Although avoidance of venipuncture and blood pressure cuffs in the ipsilateral limb is commonly recommended, there is no data supporting their association with increased risk of lymphedema development, and they are not contraindicated in patients without lymphedema.[105] Surveillance programs that include limb circumference measurements at defined intervals have been shown to reduce and maintain limb volume and prevent lymphedema progression.[106] Conservative strategies are frequently effective in treating early stage lymphedema and patients should be referred to a certified lymphedema therapist when available. Initial management aims to reduce limb volume and consists of supervised manual lymphatic drainage and multiple layer compression bandaging over several weeks.[107] Once volume and symptom reduction is achieved, the maintenance phase transitions to self-drainage and compression garments.[93] Exercise (aerobic and resistance-based), skin care, and patient education are important during all phases.[108] Patients with refractory symptoms without significant tissue changes may be candidates for operative strategies that attempt to restore drainage of the accumulated lymph. Vascularized lymph node transplants and lymphovenous bypass are operations that have been demonstrated to effectively reduce limb volume and symptoms in select patients.[109] Once fatty and fibrous deposition occurs in late stages, operative strategies shift toward reducing fibrofatty tissue in the form of direct excision and liposuction. Selective sparing of key drainage routes during ALND using the axillary reverse mapping technique has shown promising initial results and further study and physician education aim to elucidate its ability to reduce rates of lymphedema.[110,111]

AXILLARY WEB SYNDROME

Axillary web syndrome (also known as cording) is a common condition after breast and axillary surgery wherein subcutaneous cord-like scarring develops in the axilla and may extend down the arm and chest wall. The cause of these cords, which can be painful and limit shoulder movement, is thought to be related to lymphatic injury.[112] Axillary webbing of any severity occurs in up to 50% of patients and often presents within the first 2 months after surgery although cords may also develop and relapse years afterward.[113] The incidence is highest after ALND but is also seen after SLNB. Risk factors include lower BMI, younger age, greater number of lymph nodes removed, and adjuvant chemotherapy and radiation.[113,114] It is imperative that surgeons can clinically distinguish cording of the chest wall from Mondor disease of the breast. Cording in the axilla is sometimes associated with nodules, which may mimic metastasis and should be promptly evaluated. Treatment of axillary web syndrome is primarily physiotherapy with gentle manual cord manipulating, stretching, and myofascial release.[115]

SECONDARY ANGIOSARCOMA

Radiation-associated angiosarcoma of the breast is a rare but devastating sequela of a commonly delivered treatment of breast cancer. Although the receipt of radiation to the breast, chest, and axilla raises the risk of angiosarcoma 26-fold, the incidence remains less than 0.1%.[116] Therefore, for most patients, the benefits of disease control with postoperative radiation far outweigh the risk of angiosarcoma. However, patients with certain heritable mutation syndromes who are at higher risk for radiation-induced tumors (eg, retinoblastoma) should be counseled regarding this risk of radiation and tailor the patient's treatment plan accordingly.[117] Radiation-associated angiosarcomas occur at a median 10 years after breast radiation, although cases have been reported as early as 14 months and as late as 54 years.[118–120] Cases usually present as skin changes that can be confused for infection, moderate or severe radiation skin changes, or recurrence of the primary breast cancer and any suspicion should prompt biopsy to differentiate the diagnosis. Treatment involves wide local excision and often chemotherapy given the metastatic propensity of angiosarcoma. Short-course hyperfractionated reirradiation in selected patients who previously received BCS and radiation is shown to improve local disease control and is well tolerated.[121]

Lymphangiosarcoma in the setting of longstanding lymphedema of the extremity (Stewart-Treves syndrome) is a very rare entity with less than 1000 cases reported in the literature, and the majority is associated with MRM.[122] This cutaneous malignancy progresses slowly and subtly, eventually leading to purpuric macules and extensive masses with a high rate of metastasis.[123] Radical resection is required while chemotherapy and radiation are minimally effective.

DELAYED BREAST RECONSTRUCTION-RELATED COMPLICATIONS

Although the various plastic reconstructive techniques for breast surgery are associated with their own specific complications to be comanaged by the patient and the plastic surgeon, certain delayed complications may present as a remote change in the shape of the breast and prompt presentation to the oncologic surgeon. Capsular contracture may occur after implant-based reconstruction where the normally thin fibrous capsule around the implant grows to become firm and calcified. This contracture can lead to pain and distortion of the breast.[124] Capsular contracture may develop years after implant placement and the cumulative risk increases the longer it is in place.[5] Radiation therapy may increase the risk of capsular contracture and submuscular and subfascial implants are associated with decreased risk.[125] Diagnosis and grading of the contracture is typically made clinically with physical examination, although concern for alternate diagnoses should trigger appropriate imaging. Correction requires the removal of the implant along with capsulectomy or capsulotomy. Incidentally discovered recurrence or second primary breast cancer is rare but has been reported, and excised capsules should be sent for pathologic evaluation.[126]

Breast implant-associated anaplastic large cell lymphoma (ALCL) is a rare T-cell lymphoma originating specifically around textured implants.[127] More than 500 cases have been reported since 2012 along with more than 30 deaths.[128] Implant associated ALCL typically presents as a malignant effusion around the implant causing swelling, asymmetry, and pain. The median time to occurrence is 11 years after implant surgery. ALCL should be suspected if a fluid collection develops more than 1 year after implant surgery. Workup of this condition requires ultrasound evaluation and aspiration of any fluid surrounding the implant to rule out infectious cause, and fluid should be sent for cytology. Fluid analysis yields positive staining for CD30 and negative for anaplastic lymphoma kinase expression in implant-associated ALCL.[129] For patients with localized disease, complete excision of the implant, capsule, and any associated masses completes treatment. Patients with unresectable chest wall invasion or regional lymphadenopathy require adjuvant chemotherapy with lymphoma regimens.

PSYCHOSOCIAL IMPACTS OF BREAST SURGERY

Changes in physical appearance and function related to surgery are a common source of psychological distress for patients with breast cancer. Aside from the morbidity related to postoperative complications described above, operations of the breast can lead to measurable changes in quality of life, self-esteem and body image, sexual function and satisfaction, and future perspective.[130,131] Factors associated with decreased psychosocial well-being after surgery include younger age at diagnosis, more extensive surgery, lower income, history of depression, and a lack of social support.[132–134] Compared with mastectomy, BCS is associated with higher self-reported body image and sexual function.[135,136] Nonetheless, many patients who undergo BCS experience breast asymmetry (sometimes delayed due to radiation changes) and changes to nipple sensation and function, and patients should be counseled accordingly.[137] Patients who receive prophylactic mastectomy report relatively higher ratings of satisfaction and quality of life, and low rates of decisional regret.[138,139] Discussing these potential outcomes with patients can help set expectations and facilitate informed treatment decisions.

For the majority of patients who receive an operation for breast cancer, self-evaluations of psychological and emotional well-being will improve with time and often return to preoperative levels.[132,137] Cognitive-behavioral and psychoeducational therapies are effective and becoming more accessible as psychologic support is increasingly recognized as an important component of the multidisciplinary oncology team.[140] There is a growing library of information technology to empower health literacy that is shown to improve quality of life for patients with breast cancer.[140] Early involvement of a breast reconstruction surgeon informs patients of an expanding array of techniques aimed at improving postoperative satisfaction. Nipple-sparing mastectomy, when feasible, is associated with improved body image and sexual well-being compared with other types of mastectomy.[141,142] Newer techniques that aim to reinnervate the NAC after nipple-sparing mastectomy in order to improve sensation are under investigation.[143]

CLINICS CARE POINTS

- The incidence of postoperative hematoma requiring operative evacuation after breast surgery is estimated at less than 2%. Expanding hematoma, jeopardized skin flaps, or hemodynamic instability require early recognition and return to the operating room.

- Seroma formation is reported in up to 50% of patients after breast and axillary surgery. Large or symptomatic seromas presenting after drain removal can be managed with percutaneous aspiration and/or drain replacement.

- The rate of surgical site infection is 1.3% to 1.4% after lumpectomy and 3.2% to3.3% after mastectomy, although certain reconstructive techniques are associated with rates of 10% to 15%. Preoperative antibiotic prophylaxis is recommended for all types of mastectomy. For average risk patients, preoperative antibiotics show no benefit for lumpectomy or excisional biopsy.

- Venous thromboembolism occurs in up to 4% of patients after breast and axillary surgery and is more common after mastectomy than lumpectomy especially in the setting of immediate autologous reconstruction. For patients without risk factors, preoperative chemoprophylaxis is recommended before mastectomy with immediate reconstruction, for general anesthesia less than 3 hours, and for those meeting criteria based on a risk stratification assessment.

- Injury to major motor and sensory nerves in the axilla may lead to pain, paresthesia, and motor deficits with variable resolution over time. Nerve injury is primarily avoided with technical diligence and awareness of potential anatomic variations. Many surgeons avoid paralysis during formal axillary dissection.

DISCLOSURE

No relevant disclosures.

REFERENCES

1. Bernat JL, Peterson LM. Patient-Centered Informed Consent in Surgical Practice. Arch Surg 2006;141(1):86–92.
2. Browne JP, Jeevan R, Gulliver-Clarke C, et al. The association between complications and quality of life after mastectomy and breast reconstruction for breast cancer. Cancer 2017;123(18):3460–7.
3. Barton MB, West CN, Liu ILA, et al. Complications following bilateral prophylactic mastectomy. J Natl Cancer Inst Monogr 2005;35:61–6.
4. Seth AK, Hirsch EM, Kim JYS, et al. Hematoma after mastectomy with immediate reconstruction: an analysis of risk factors in 883 patients. Ann Plast Surg 2013;71(1):20–3.
5. Handel N, Cordray T, Gutierrez J, et al. A long-term study of outcomes, complications, and patient satisfaction with breast implants. Plast Reconstr Surg 2006; 117(3):757–67.
6. Almasarweh S, Sudah M, Joukainen S, et al. The Feasibility of Ultrasound-guided Vacuum-assisted Evacuation of Large Breast Hematomas. Radiol Oncol 2020;54(3):311.
7. O'Hea BJ, Ho MN, Petrek JA. External compression dressing versus standard dressing after axillary lymphadenectomy. Am J Surg 1999;177(6):450–3.
8. Bullocks J, Basu CB, Hsu P, et al. Prevention of Hematomas and Seromas. Semin Plast Surg 2006;20(4):233.
9. Srivastava V, Basu S, Shukla VK. Seroma Formation after Breast Cancer Surgery: What We Have Learned in the Last Two Decades. J Breast Cancer 2012;15(4):373.
10. Montalto E, Mangraviti S, Costa G, et al. Seroma fluid subsequent to axillary lymph node dissection for breast cancer derives from an accumulation of afferent lymph. Immunol Lett 2010;131(1):67–72.

11. Van Bemmel AJM, Van De Velde CJH, Schmitz RF, et al. Prevention of seroma formation after axillary dissection in breast cancer: a systematic review. Eur J Surg Oncol 2011;37(10):829–35.

12. Unger J, Rutkowski R, Kohlmann T, et al. Potential risk factors influencing the formation of postoperative seroma after breast surgery - a prospective study. Anticancer Res 2021;41(2):859–67.

13. Shamley DR, Barker K, Simonite V, et al. Delayed versus immediate exercises following surgery for breast cancer: a systematic review. Breast Cancer Res Treat 2005;90(3):263–71.

14. de Oliveira LL, de Aguiar SS, Bender PFM, et al. Men have a higher incidence of seroma after breast cancer surgery. Asian Pac J Cancer Prev 2017;18(5):1423–7.

15. He XD, Guo ZH, Tian JH, et al. Whether drainage should be used after surgery for breast cancer? A systematic review of randomized controlled trials. Med Oncol 2011;28(SUPPL. 1):22–30.

16. Shima H, Kutomi G, Sato K, et al. An optimal timing for removing a drain after breast surgery: a systematic review and meta-analysis. J Surg Res 2021;267:267–73.

17. Faisal M, Abu-Elela ST, Mostafa W, et al. Efficacy of axillary exclusion on seroma formation after modified radical mastectomy. World J Surg Oncol 2016;14(1):1–5.

18. De Blacam C, Ogunleye AA, Momoh AO, et al. High body mass index and smoking predict morbidity in breast cancer surgery: a multivariate analysis of 26,988 patients from the national surgical quality improvement program database. Ann Surg 2012;255(3):551–5.

19. Pastoriza J, McNelis J, Parsikia A, et al. Predictive factors for surgical site infections in patients undergoing surgery for breast carcinoma. Am Surg 2021;87(1):68–76.

20. McCullough MC, Chu CK, Duggal CS, et al. Antibiotic prophylaxis and resistance in surgical site infection after immediate tissue expander reconstruction of the breast. Ann Plast Surg 2016;77(5):501–5.

21. Chen CM, Halvorson EG, Disa JJ, et al. Immediate postoperative complications in DIEP versus free/muscle-sparing TRAM flaps. Plast Reconstr Surg 2007;120(6):1477–82.

22. Sbitany H, Serletti JM. Acellular dermis-assisted prosthetic breast reconstruction: a systematic and critical review of efficacy and associated morbidity. Plast Reconstr Surg 2011;128(6):1162–9.

23. Chang DW, Barnea Y, Robb GL. Effects of an autologous flap combined with an implant for breast reconstruction: an evaluation of 1000 consecutive reconstructions of previously irradiated breasts. Plast Reconstr Surg 2008;122(2):356–62.

24. Thiruchelvam PTR, Leff DR, Godden AR, et al. Primary radiotherapy and deep inferior epigastric perforator flap reconstruction for patients with breast cancer (PRADA): a multicentre, prospective, non-randomised, feasibility study. Lancet Oncol 2022;23(5):682–90.

25. Degnim AC, Throckmorton AD, Boostrom SY, et al. Surgical site infection (SSI) after breast surgery: impact of 2010 CDC Reporting Guidelines. Ann Surg Oncol 2012;19(13):4099.

26. Viola GM, Selber JC, Crosby M, et al. Salvaging the infected breast tissue expander: a standardized multidisciplinary approach. Plast Reconstr Surg Glob Open 2016;4(6). https://doi.org/10.1097/GOX.0000000000000676.

27. Gallagher M, Jones DJ, Bell-Syer SV. Prophylactic antibiotics to prevent surgical site infection after breast cancer surgery. Cochrane Database Syst Rev 2019; 9(9). https://doi.org/10.1002/14651858.CD005360.PUB5.

28. Bold RJ, Mansfield PF, Berger DH, et al. Prospective, randomized, double-blind study of prophylactic antibiotics in axillary lymph node dissection. Am J Surg 1998;176(3):239–43.

29. American Society of Breast Surgeons T. Consensus Guideline on Preoperative Antibiotics and Surgical Site Infection in Breast Surgery. Available from: https://www.breastsurgeons.org/docs/statements/Consensus-Guideline-on-Preoperative-Antibiotics-and-Surgical-Site-Infection-in-Breast-Surgery.pdf.

30. Giguère GB, Poirier B, Provencher L, et al. Do preoperative prophylactic antibiotics reduce surgical site infection following wire-localized lumpectomy? A single-blind randomized clinical trial. Ann Surg Oncol 2022;29(4):2202–8.

31. Petersen L, Carlson K, Kopkash K, et al. Preoperative antibiotics do not reduce postoperative infections following needle-localized lumpectomy. Breast J 2017; 23(1):49–51.

32. Kong A, Tartter PI, Zappetti D. The Significance of Risk Factors for Infection in Patients Undergoing Lumpectomy and Axillary Dissection. Breast J 1997; 3(2):81–4.

33. Alderman A, Gutowski K, Ahuja A, et al. ASPS clinical practice guideline summary on breast reconstruction with expanders and implants. Plast Reconstr Surg 2014;134(4):648e–55e.

34. Bağhaki S, Soybir GR, Soran A. Guideline for antimicrobial prophylaxis in breast surgery. J Breast Heal 2014;10(2):79.

35. Robertson SA, Jeevaratnam JA, Agrawal A, et al. Mastectomy skin flap necrosis: challenges and solutions. Breast Cancer (Dove Med Press) 2017. https://doi.org/10.2147/BCTT.S81712.

36. Matsen CB, Mehrara B, Eaton A, et al. Skin flap necrosis after mastectomy with reconstruction: a prospective study. Ann Surg Oncol 2016;23(1):257–64.

37. Yabe S, Nakagawa T, Oda G, et al. Association between skin flap necrosis and sarcopenia in patients who underwent total mastectomy. Asian J Surg 2021; 44(2):465–70.

38. Chun YS, Verma K, Rosen H, et al. Use of tumescent mastectomy technique as a risk factor for native breast skin flap necrosis following immediate breast reconstruction. Am J Surg 2011;201(2):160–5.

39. Galimberti V, Vicini E, Corso G, et al. Nipple-sparing and skin-sparing mastectomy: Review of aims, oncological safety and contraindications. The Breast 2017;34:S82–4.

40. Robertson SA, Rusby JE, Cutress RI. Determinants of optimal mastectomy skin flap thickness. Br J Surg 2014;101(8):899–911.

41. Wiberg R, Andersson MN, Svensson J, et al. Prophylactic mastectomy: postoperative skin flap thickness evaluated by MRT, ultrasound and clinical examination. Ann Surg Oncol 2020;27(7):2221–8.

42. Ogawa A, Nakagawa T, Oda G, et al. Study of the protocol used to evaluate skin-flap perfusion in mastectomy based on the characteristics of indocyanine green. Photodiagnosis Photodyn Ther 2021;35:102401, 1.

43. Pruimboom T, Lindelauf AAMA, Felli E, et al. Perioperative hyperspectral imaging to assess mastectomy skin flap and DIEP flap perfusion in immediate autologous breast reconstruction: a pilot study. Diagnostics (Basel, Switzerland) 2022;12(1). https://doi.org/10.3390/DIAGNOSTICS12010184.

44. Gdalevitch P, Van Laeken N, Bahng S, et al. Effects of nitroglycerin ointment on mastectomy flap necrosis in immediate breast reconstruction: a randomized controlled trial. Plast Reconstr Surg 2015;135(6):1530–9.

45. Spruijt NE, Hoekstra LT, Wilmink J, et al. Hyperbaric oxygen treatment for mastectomy flap ischaemia: a case series of 50 breasts. Diving Hyperb Med 2021; 51(1):2.

46. Nicholson BT, Harvey JA, Cohen MA. Nipple-areolar complex: normal anatomy and benign and malignant processes. Radiographics 2009;29(2):509–23.

47. Mallon P, Feron JG, Couturaud B, et al. The role of nipple-sparing mastectomy in breast cancer: a comprehensive review of the literature. Plast Reconstr Surg 2013;131(5):969–84.

48. Ahn SJ, Woo TY, Lee DW, et al. Nipple-areolar complex ischemia and necrosis in nipple-sparing mastectomy. Eur J Surg Oncol 2018;44(8):1170–6.

49. Zheng Y, Zhong M, Ni C, et al. Radiotherapy and nipple–areolar complex necrosis after nipple-sparing mastectomy: a systematic review and meta-analysis. Radiol Med 2017;122(3):171–8.

50. Chicco M, Huang TCT, Cheng HT. Negative-pressure wound therapy in the prevention and management of complications from prosthetic breast reconstruction: a systematic review and meta-analysis. Ann Plast Surg 2021;87(4):478–83.

51. De Martino RR, Goodney PP, Spangler EL, et al. Variation in thromboembolic complications among patients undergoing commonly performed cancer operations. J Vasc Surg 2012;55(4):1035–40.e4.

52. Tafur A, Fuentes H, Caprini J, et al. Predictors of early mortality in cancer-associated thrombosis: analysis of the RIETE database. TH Open Companion J Thromb Haemost 2018;2(2):e158–66.

53. Castaldi M, George G, Stoller C, et al. Independent predictors of venous thromboembolism in patients undergoing reconstructive breast cancer surgery. Plast Surg (Oakville, Ont) 2021;29(3):160–8.

54. Rochlin DH, Sheckter CC, Pannucci C, et al. Venous thromboembolism following microsurgical breast reconstruction: a longitudinal analysis of 12,778 patients. Plast Reconstr Surg 2020;146(3):465–73.

55. Londero AP, Bertozzi S, Cedolini C, et al. Incidence and risk factors for venous thromboembolism in female patients undergoing breast surgery. Cancers (Basel) 2022;14(4). https://doi.org/10.3390/CANCERS14040988/S1.

56. Konoeda H, Yamaki T, Hamahata A, et al. Incidence of deep vein thrombosis in patients undergoing breast reconstruction with autologous tissue transfer. Phlebology 2017;32(4):282–8.

57. Lovely JK, Nehring SA, Boughey JC, et al. Balancing venous thromboembolism and hematoma after breast surgery. Ann Surg Oncol 2012;19(10):3230–5.

58. Nwaogu I, Yan Y, Margenthaler JA, et al. Venous thromboembolism after breast reconstruction in patients undergoing breast surgery: an american college of surgeons NSQIP analysis. J Am Coll Surg 2015;220(5):886–93.

59. American Society of Breast Surgeons T. Consensus Guideline on Venous Thromboembolism (VTE) Prophylaxis for Patients Undergoing Breast Operations. Available from: https://www.breastsurgeons.org/docs/statements/Consensus-Guideline-on-Venous-Thromboembolism-VTE-Prophylaxis-for-Patients-Undergoing-Breast-Operations.pdf.

60. Pannucci CJ, Swistun L, MacDonald JK, et al. Individualized venous thromboembolism risk stratification using the 2005 caprini score to identify the benefits and harms of chemoprophylaxis in surgical patients: a meta-analysis. Ann Surg 2017;265(6):1094–103.

61. Keith JN, Chong TW, Davar D, et al. The timing of preoperative prophylactic low-molecular-weight heparin administration in breast reconstruction. Plast Reconstr Surg 2013;132(2):279–84.

62. Stevens SM, Woller SC, Baumann Kreuziger L, et al. Executive summary: antithrombotic therapy for VTE disease: second update of the CHEST guideline and expert panel report. Chest 2021;160(6):2247–59.

63. Kearon C, Akl EA, Ornelas J, et al. Antithrombotic therapy for VTE disease: CHEST guideline and expert panel report. Chest 2016;149(2):315–52.

64. Douketis JD, Spyropoulos AC, Spencer FA, et al. Perioperative management of antithrombotic therapy: antithrombotic therapy and prevention of thrombosis, 9th ed: american college of chest physicians evidence-based clinical practice guidelines. Chest 2012;141(2):e326S–50S.

65. Klifto KM, Gurno CF, Major M, et al. Pre-, intra-, and/or postoperative arterial and venous thromboembolism prophylaxis for breast surgery: Systematic review and meta-analysis. J Plast Reconstr Aesthet Surg 2020;73(1):1–18.

66. Lucci A, McCall LM, Beitsch PD, et al. Surgical complications associated with sentinel lymph node dissection (SLND) plus axillary lymph node dissection compared with SLND alone in the American College of Surgeons Oncology Group trial Z0011. J Clin Oncol 2007;25(24):3657–63.

67. Kozak D, Głowacka-Mrotek I, Nowikiewicz T, et al. Analysis of undesirable sequelae of sentinel node surgery in breast cancer patients – a prospective cohort study. Pathol Oncol Res 2018;24(4):891.

68. Meininger AK, Figuerres BF, Goldberg BA. Scapular winging: an update. J Am Acad Orthop Surg 2011;19(8):453–62.

69. Flávia De Oliveira J, Bezerra T, Carolina A, et al. Incidence and risk factors of winged scapula after axillary lymph node dissection in breast cancer surgery. Appl Cancer Res 2009;29(2):69–73.

70. Adriaenssens N, De Ridder M, Lievens P, et al. Scapula alata in early breast cancer patients enrolled in a randomized clinical trial of post-surgery short-course image-guided radiotherapy. World J Surg Oncol 2012;10. https://doi.org/10.1186/1477-7819-10-86.

71. Macchi V, Tiengo C, Porzionato A, et al. Medial and lateral pectoral nerves: course and branches. Clin Anat 2007;20(2):157–62.

72. Prakash KG, Saniya K. Anatomical study of pectoral nerves and its implications in surgery. J Clin Diagn Res 2014;8(7). https://doi.org/10.7860/JCDR/2014/8631.4545.

73. Sharp E, Roberts M, Żurada-Zielińska A, et al. The most commonly injured nerves at surgery: a comprehensive review. Clin Anat 2021;34(2):244–62.

74. Zhu JJ, Liu XF, Zhang PL, et al. Anatomical information for intercostobrachial nerve preservation in axillary lymph node dissection for breast cancer. Genet Mol Res 2014;13(4):9315–23.

75. Henry BM, Graves MJ, Pękala JR, et al. Origin, Branching, and Communications of the Intercostobrachial Nerve: a Meta-Analysis with Implications for Mastectomy and Axillary Lymph Node Dissection in Breast Cancer. Cureus 2017;9(3). https://doi.org/10.7759/CUREUS.1101.

76. Vadivelu N, Schreck M, Lopez J, et al. Pain after mastectomy and breast reconstruction. Am Surg 2008;74(4):285–96.

77. Mansel RE, Fallowfield L, Kissin M, et al. Randomized multicenter trial of sentinel node biopsy versus standard axillary treatment in operable breast cancer: the ALMANAC Trial. J Natl Cancer Inst 2006;98(9):599–609.

78. Andersen KG, Aasvang EK, Kroman N, et al. Intercostobrachial nerve handling and pain after axillary lymph node dissection for breast cancer. Acta Anaesthesiol Scand 2014;58(10):1240–8.

79. Gärtner R, Jensen MB, Nielsen J, et al. Prevalence of and factors associated with persistent pain following breast cancer surgery. JAMA 2009;302(18): 1985–92.

80. Chappell AG, Yuksel S, Sasson DC, et al. Post-mastectomy pain syndrome: an up-to-date review of treatment outcomes. JPRAS Open 2021;30:97–109.

81. Yang A, Nadav D, Legler A, et al. An interventional pain algorithm for the treatment of postmastectomy pain syndrome: a single-center retrospective review. Pain Med 2021;22(3):677–86.

82. Tokgöz S, Karaca Umay E, Yilmaz KB, et al. Role of intraoperative nerve monitoring in postoperative muscle and nerve function of patients undergoing modified radical mastectomy. J Investig Surg 2021;34(7):703–10.

83. Noland SS, Krauss EM, Felder JM, et al. Surgical and clinical decision making in isolated long thoracic nerve palsy. Hand (N Y) 2018;13(6):689.

84. Warner MA, Blitt CD, Butterworth JF, et al. Practice advisory for the prevention of perioperative peripheral neuropathies: a report by the American Society of Anesthesiologists Task Force on Prevention of Perioperative Peripheral Neuropathies. Anesthesiology 2000;92(4):1168–82.

85. Zhang J, Moore AE, Stringer MD, et al. Iatrogenic upper limb nerve injuries: a systematic review. ANZ J Surg 2011;81(4):227–36.

86. Rudra S, Roy A, Brenneman R, et al. Radiation-Induced Brachial Plexopathy in Patients With Breast Cancer Treated With Comprehensive Adjuvant Radiation Therapy. Adv Radiat Oncol 2020;6(1). https://doi.org/10.1016/J.ADRO.2020. 10.015.

87. Jack MM, Smith BW, Capek S, et al. The spectrum of brachial plexopathy from perineural spread of breast cancer. J Neurosurg 2022;1–10. https://doi.org/10. 3171/2021.12.JNS211882.

88. Suami H, Scaglioni MF. Lymphedema Management: Anatomy of the Lymphatic System and the Lymphosome Concept with Reference to Lymphedema. Semin Plast Surg 2018;32(1):5.

89. Campisi CC, Molinari L, Campisi CS, et al. Surgical research, staging-guided technical procedures and long-term clinical outcomes for the treatment of peripheral lymphedema: the Genoa Protocol. J Surg Surg Res 2020;6(1):041–50.

90. Cortina CS, Yen TWF, Bergom C, et al. Breast cancer-related lymphedema rates after modern axillary treatments: How accurate are our estimates? Surgery 2022;171(3):682–6.

91. Naoum GE, Roberts S, Brunelle CL, et al. Quantifying the impact of axillary surgery and nodal irradiation on breast cancer-related lymphedema and local tumor control: Long-term results from a prospective screening trial. J Clin Oncol 2020;38(29):3430–8.

92. DiSipio T, Rye S, Newman B, et al. Incidence of unilateral arm lymphoedema after breast cancer: a systematic review and meta-analysis. Lancet Oncol 2013; 14(6):500–15.

93. McLaughlin SA, Brunelle CL, Taghian A. Breast cancer–related lymphedema: risk factors, screening, management, and the impact of locoregional treatment. J Clin Oncol 2020;38(20):2341.

94. Galimberti V, Cole BF, Zurrida S, et al. Axillary dissection versus no axillary dissection in patients with sentinel-node micrometastases (IBCSG 23-01): a phase 3 randomised controlled trial. Lancet Oncol 2013;14(4):297–305.

95. Cortina CS, Kong AL. ASO author reflections: the evolving multidisciplinary management of the axilla in mastectomy patients. Ann Surg Oncol 2021;1–2. https://doi.org/10.1245/S10434-021-10585-Y.
96. Cortina CS, Bergom C, Craft MA, et al. A national survey of breast surgeons and radiation oncologists on contemporary axillary management in mastectomy patients. Ann Surg Oncol 2021;28(10):5568–79.
97. Cortina CS, Kong AL. Comment on "women could avoid axillary lymph node dissection by choosing breast-conserving therapy instead of mastectomy. Ann Surg Oncol 2021;28(3):772–3.
98. Morrow M, Jagsi R, Chandler M, et al. Surgeon attitudes toward the omission of axillary dissection in early breast cancer. JAMA Oncol 2018;4(11):1511–6.
99. Donker M, van Tienhoven G, Straver ME, et al. Radiotherapy or surgery of the axilla after a positive sentinel node in breast cancer (EORTC 10981-22023 AMAROS): a randomised, multicentre, open-label, phase 3 non-inferiority trial. Lancet Oncol 2014;15(12):1303–10.
100. Giuliano AE, Ballman KV, McCall L, et al. Effect of axillary dissection vs no axillary dissection on 10-year overall survival among women with invasive breast cancer and sentinel node metastasis: the ACOSOG Z0011 (Alliance) randomized clinical trial. JAMA 2017;318(10):918–26.
101. McDuff SGR, Mina AI, Brunelle CL, et al. Timing of lymphedema after treatment for breast cancer: when are patients most at risk? Int J Radiat Oncol 2019; 103(1):62–70.
102. Basta MN, Wu LC, Kanchwala SK, et al. Reliable prediction of postmastectomy lymphedema: the risk assessment tool evaluating lymphedema. Am J Surg 2017;213(6):1125–33.e1.
103. Armer JM, Ballman KV, McCall L, et al. Factors associated with lymphedema in women with node-positive breast cancer treated with neoadjuvant chemotherapy and axillary dissection. JAMA Surg 2019;154(9):800–9.
104. Husted Madsen A, Haugaard K, Soerensen J, et al. Arm morbidity following sentinel lymph node biopsy or axillary lymph node dissection: a study from the Danish Breast Cancer Cooperative Group. Breast 2008;17(2):138–47.
105. McLaughlin SA, DeSnyder SM, Klimberg S, et al. Considerations for clinicians in the diagnosis, prevention, and treatment of breast cancer-related lymphedema, recommendations from an expert panel: part 2: preventive and therapeutic options. Ann Surg Oncol 2017;24(10):2827–35.
106. Stout Gergich NL, Pfalzer LA, McGarvey C, et al. Preoperative assessment enables the early diagnosis and successful treatment of lymphedema. Cancer 2008;112(12):2809–19.
107. McNeely ML, Magee DJ, Lees AW, et al. The addition of manual lymph drainage to compression therapy for breast cancer related lymphedema: a randomized controlled trial. Breast Cancer Res Treat 2004;86(2):95–106.
108. Schmitz KH, Ahmed RL, Troxel A, et al. Weight lifting in women with breast-cancer-related lymphedema. N Engl J Med 2009;361(7):664–73.
109. Schaverien MV, Asaad M, Selber JC, et al. Outcomes of vascularized lymph node transplantation for treatment of lymphedema. J Am Coll Surg 2021; 232(6):982–94.
110. Tummel E, Ochoa D, Korourian S, et al. Does axillary reverse mapping prevent lymphedema after lymphadenectomy? Ann Surg 2017;265(5):987–92.
111. DeSnyder SM, Yi M, Boccardo F, et al. American society of breast surgeons' practice patterns for patients at risk and affected by breast cancer-related lymphedema. Ann Surg Oncol 2021;28(10):5742–51.

112. YANG E, LI X, LONG X. Diagnosis and treatment of axillary web syndrome: an overview. Chin J Plast Reconstr Surg 2020;2(2):128–36.

113. Koehler LA, Haddad TC, Hunter DW, et al. Axillary web syndrome following breast cancer surgery: symptoms, complications, and management strategies. Breast Cancer (London) 2019;11:13.

114. O'Toole J, Miller CL, Specht MC, et al. Cording following treatment for breast cancer. Breast Cancer Res Treat 2013;140(1):105–11.

115. Fourie WJ, Robb KA. Physiotherapy management of axillary web syndrome following breast cancer treatment: discussing the use of soft tissue techniques. Physiotherapy 2009;95(4):314–20.

116. Cohen-Hallaleh RB, Smith HG, Smith RC, et al. Radiation induced angiosarcoma of the breast: outcomes from a retrospective case series. Clin Sarcoma Res 2017;7(1):15.

117. Kleinerman RA, Tucker MA, Tarone RE, et al. Risk of new cancers after radiotherapy in long-term survivors of retinoblastoma: an extended follow-up. J Clin Oncol 2005;23(10):2272–9.

118. Mito JK, Mitra D, Barysauskas CM, et al. A Comparison of outcomes and prognostic features for radiation-associated angiosarcoma of the breast and other radiation-associated sarcomas. Int J Radiat Oncol Biol Phys 2019;104(2):425–35.

119. Deutsch M, Safyan E. Angiosarcoma of the breast occurring soon after lumpectomy and breast irradiation for infiltrating ductal carcinoma: a case report. Am J Clin Oncol 2003;26(5):471–2.

120. De Smet S, Vandermeeren L, Christiaens MR, et al. Radiation-induced sarcoma: analysis of 46 cases. Acta Chir Belg 2008;108(5):574–9.

121. Smith TL, Morris CG, Mendenhall NP. Angiosarcoma after breast-conserving therapy: Long-term disease control and late effects with hyperfractionated accelerated re-irradiation (HART) 2014;53(2):235–41. https://doi.org/10.3109/0284186X.2013.819117.

122. Sharma A, Schwartz RA. Stewart-treves syndrome: pathogenesis and management. J Am Acad Dermatol 2012;67(6):1342–8.

123. Bernia E, Rios-Viñuela E, Requena C. Stewart-treves syndrome. JAMA Dermatol 2021;157(6):721.

124. Araco A, Caruso R, Araco F, et al. Capsular contractures: a systematic review. Plast Reconstr Surg 2009;124(6):1808–19.

125. Namnoum JD, Largent J, Kaplan HM, et al. Primary breast augmentation clinical trial outcomes stratified by surgical incision, anatomical placement and implant device type. J Plast Reconstr Aesthet Surg 2013;66(9):1165–72.

126. Lapid O., Noels E.C., Meijer S.L., et al., Pathologic findings in primary capsulectomy specimens: analysis of 2531 patients, Aesthet Surg J, 34 (5), 2014, 714-718.

127. Doren EL, Miranda RN, Selber JC, et al. U.S. epidemiology of breast implant-associated anaplastic large cell lymphoma. Plast Reconstr Surg 2017;139(5):1042–50.

128. McCarthy CM, Loyo-Berríos N, Qureshi AA, et al. Patient registry and outcomes for breast implants and anaplastic large cell lymphoma etiology and epidemiology (PROFILE): initial report of findings, 2012-2018. Plast Reconstr Surg 2019;143:65S–73S (3S A Review of Breast Implant-Associated Anaplastic Large Cell Lymphoma).

129. Clemens MW, Jacobsen ED, Horwitz SM. 2019 NCCN Consensus guidelines on the diagnosis and treatment of breast implant-associated anaplastic large cell lymphoma (BIA-ALCL). Aesthet Surg J 2019;39(Supplement_1):S3–13.
130. Helms RL, O'Hea EL, Corso M. Body image issues in women with breast cancer 2008;13(3):313–25. https://doi.org/10.1080/13548500701405509.
131. Cornell LF, Mussallem DM, Gibson TC, et al. Trends in sexual function after breast cancer surgery. Ann Surg Oncol 2017;24(9):2526–38.
132. Rosenberg SM, Dominici LS, Gelber S, et al. Association of breast cancer surgery with quality of life and psychosocial well-being in young breast cancer survivors. JAMA Surg 2020;155(11):1035–42.
133. Campbell-Enns H, Woodgate R. The psychosocial experiences of women with breast cancer across the lifespan: a systematic review protocol. JBI Database Syst Rev Implement Reports 2015;13(1):112–21.
134. Janowski K, Tatala M, Jedynak T, et al. Social support and psychosocial functioning in women after mastectomy. Palliat Support Care 2020;18(3):314–21.
135. Ng ET, Ang RZ, Tran BX, et al. Comparing quality of life in breast cancer patients who underwent mastectomy versus breast-conserving surgery: a meta-analysis. Int J Environ Res Public Health 2019;16(24):4970.
136. Aerts L, Christiaens MR, Enzlin P, et al. Sexual functioning in women after mastectomy versus breast conserving therapy for early-stage breast cancer: a prospective controlled study. Breast 2014;23(5):629–36.
137. Parker PA, Youssef A, Walker S, et al. Short-term and long-term psychosocial adjustment and quality of life in women undergoing different surgical procedures for breast cancer. Ann Surg Oncol 2007;14(11):3078–89.
138. Anderson C, Islam JY, Elizabeth Hodgson M, et al. Long-term satisfaction and body image after contralateral prophylactic mastectomy. Ann Surg Oncol 2017;24(6):1499–506.
139. Parker PA, Peterson SK, Shen Y, et al. Prospective study of psychosocial outcomes of having contralateral prophylactic mastectomy among women with nonhereditary breast cancer. J Clin Oncol 2018;36(25):2630–8.
140. Guarino A, Polini C, Forte G, et al. The Effectiveness of Psychological Treatments in Women with Breast Cancer: A Systematic Review and Meta-Analysis. J Clin Med 2020;9(1). https://doi.org/10.3390/JCM9010209.
141. Didier F, Radice D, Gandini S, et al. Does nipple preservation in mastectomy improve satisfaction with cosmetic results, psychological adjustment, body image and sexuality? Breast Cancer Res Treat 2009;118(3):623–33.
142. Wei CH, Scott AM, Price AN, et al. Psychosocial and sexual well-being following nipple-sparing mastectomy and reconstruction. Breast J 2016;22(1):10–7.
143. Tevlin R, Brazio P, Tran N, et al. Immediate targeted nipple-areolar complex re-innervation: Improving outcomes in immediate autologous breast reconstruction. J Plast Reconstr Aesthet Surg 2021;74(7):1503–7.

Novel Approaches to Breast Reconstruction

Anne Warren Peled, MD[a],*, Nicholas W. Clavin, MD[b]

KEYWORDS

- Mastectomy • Oncoplastic surgery • Autologous reconstruction
- Breast neurotization

KEY POINTS

- Option of nipple-sparing mastectomy can be offered to patients with macromastia or significant ptosis through a staged approach.
- Advanced oncoplastic reconstruction techniques can expand possibilities for breast conservation even with larger tumors.
- Newer reconstructive options allow for preserving and restoring sensation after mastectomy.

INTRODUCTION

As breast oncologic surgical procedures and approaches have evolved in recent years, so have breast reconstruction techniques. Newer advances focus on expanding the options of reconstructive approaches and patient selection, optimizing quality of life, and helping improve postsurgical survivorship. These advances span from techniques to expand criteria for nipple-sparing mastectomies, optimizing and enhancing oncoplastic surgery, evolving autologous reconstruction options, and preserving and restoring sensation after mastectomy.

Expanding the Option of Nipple-Sparing Mastectomy

During the past 2 decades as nipple-sparing mastectomy (NSM) has become more widely adopted, oncologic indications have expanded to now include nearly all patients from an oncologic standpoint other than those with gross involvement of the nipple–areolar complex or other contraindications to preserving the breast skin envelope. However, many people are still not considered good candidates for NSM because of large or ptotic breasts, which can significantly increase the chance of

a Sutter Health California Pacific Medical Center Breast Cancer Program, 2100 Webster Street, Suite 222, San Francisco, CA 94115, USA; b Department of Plastic Surgery, Atrium Health, 1025 Morehead Medical Drive, #200; Charlotte, NC 28204, USA
* Corresponding author.
E-mail address: Drpeled@apeledmd.com

Surg Clin N Am 103 (2023) 141–153
https://doi.org/10.1016/j.suc.2022.08.008
0039-6109/23/© 2022 Elsevier Inc. All rights reserved.

surgical complications and be challenging from a reconstructive standpoint.[1,2] These patients are typically recommended to have skin-sparing mastectomies as an alternative,[3] which prevents them from getting the known esthetic and psychological benefits of preservation of the entire breast skin envelope.[4]

Multiple alternatives to skin-sparing mastectomies in patients with large or ptotic breasts have been described, including simultaneous mastopexy/reduction of the skin envelope using a dermal pedicle at the time of NSM[5,6] or the use of free nipple grafting.[7,8] One of the most popular approaches is a staged NSM, with an initial breast reduction/mastopexy to act as a vascular delay before subsequent NSM. This approach was pioneered by Spear and colleagues,[9] who reported performing staged NSM through the mastopexy incisions a minimum of 4 weeks following mastopexy/reduction, with low rates of ischemic complications. Other authors have published subsequent large case series using this approach for both therapeutic and prophylactic indications in combination with implant-based and autologous reconstructions, showing excellent outcomes concerning nipple–areolar complex viability and reconstructive success.[10–12]

We offer a staged approach to NSM for any patient with larger than D/DD-cup sized-breasts or moderate Grade II ptosis or greater, both in prophylactic and therapeutic settings. For patients with diagnosed cancer, the initial procedure involves lumpectomy with/without axillary surgery as indicated and bilateral oncoplastic reduction mastopexy/mammoplasty. The staged NSM is then done approximately 2.5 to 3 months after the lumpectomy, or earlier if thought to be necessary from an oncology perspective. Immediate reconstruction with either direct-to-implant, immediate autologous, or 2-stage reconstruction with initial tissue expander placement is performed at the time of mastectomy (**Fig. 1**). If adjuvant chemotherapy is recommended, this is

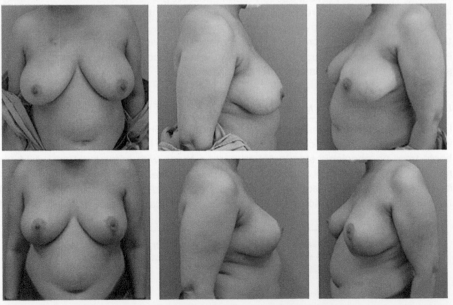

Fig. 1. A 39-year-old woman with BRCA1 mutation and left Stage I breast cancer before (*above*) and after (*below*) initial lumpectomy and bilateral oncoplastic reduction mammoplasty followed by staged NSM and prepectoral implant reconstruction.

done before mastectomy. Additionally, if surgical pathologic condition from the lumpectomy/axillary surgery leads to a recommendation for postmastectomy radiation therapy, further discussion regarding the true "need" for the mastectomy is had as part of a shared decision-making conversation with the patient. Given the increased risk of complications following postmastectomy radiation therapy in patients having implant-based (and to a lesser extent, autologous) reconstruction and the improved safety profile with lumpectomy and oncoplastic reconstruction,[13,14] these patients are encouraged to consider going on to postlumpectomy radiation rather than proceeding with the staged mastectomy if mastectomy is not truly medically indicated.

For prophylactic mastectomies, staged NSM is typically done a minimum of 3 months following initial reduction mastopexy/mammoplasty to optimize healing and minimize the chance of complications. Reconstructive options at the staged mastectomy are similar to those for therapeutic cases. Our preference is to do a superior/superior-medial pedicle for the initial reduction mastopexy/mammoplasty and then do the staged NSM through the inferior vertical portion of the reduction incision, thus completely avoiding the dermal pedicle created during the reduction and ideally optimizing the vascularity to the rest of the mastectomy skin flap (**Fig. 2**).

Optimizing and Enhancing Oncoplastic Surgery

The term oncoplastic surgery typically describes reconstruction of lumpectomy defects, usually involving immediate reconstruction done at the time of lumpectomy. The spectrum of oncoplastic surgery includes everything from esthetic scar placement for lumpectomy with limited local tissue rearrangement to more complex reconstruction involving oncoplastic mastopexies or reduction mammoplasties. Several classification systems based on the volume of resection and anticipated reconstructive technique have been developed to help guide clinical management.[15-17]

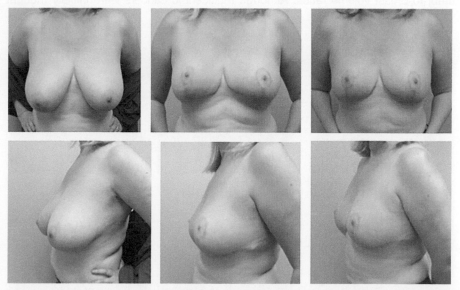

Fig. 2. A 55-year-old woman with BRCA2 mutation before (*left*) and after (*center*) initial reduction mammoplasty followed by staged NSM and prepectoral implant reconstruction (*right*).

More advanced oncoplastic techniques can be especially helpful for patients with large breasts or macromastia, particularly given the potential challenges of performing postmastectomy reconstruction in this patient population. Studies have shown numerous benefits from oncoplastic reduction mammoplasty for these patients. First, many patients with macromastia have significant baseline functional symptoms from their large breasts, which are known to be well relieved through reduction mammoplasty.[18] Offering large-breasted patients newly diagnosed with breast cancer a simultaneous breast reduction at the time of lumpectomy has been shown to provide a number of quality-of-life benefits and high levels of patient satisfaction.[19–21] We have found in our practices that these patients are some of our happiest patients who undergo breast reconstruction, with many patients feeling and looking much better than they did before their diagnosis (**Fig. 3**). Of note, oncoplastic reduction mammoplasty can be offered to any patient who can safely undergo the procedure from a medical standpoint and would like to reduce the size of their breasts, whether they truly require it from a reconstructive standpoint based on tumor size/extent of lumpectomy reconstruction or not.[22] In addition to the quality-of-life and functional benefits, oncoplastic reduction mastopexy/mammoplasty is thought to improve radiation delivery given the known increase in dose inhomogeneity seen in patients with larger, more ptotic breasts.[23,24] It has also been shown to improve margin control as compared with standard lumpectomy due to the ability to take more generous resection specimens, leading to lower rates of unplanned return to the OR for re-excision or completion mastectomy.[25,26] Finally, for patients with large breasts who might otherwise consider mastectomy, oncoplastic reduction has been shown to significantly lower the risk of complications as compared with mastectomy and reconstruction, including the need for additional operative procedures and complications leading to delays in adjuvant therapy.[13,27,28]

Other indications for more advanced oncoplastic reconstruction techniques include reconstruction of multifocal/multicentric lumpectomy defects and patients with large tumor-to-breast volume ratios. Although multicentric cancers were initially thought

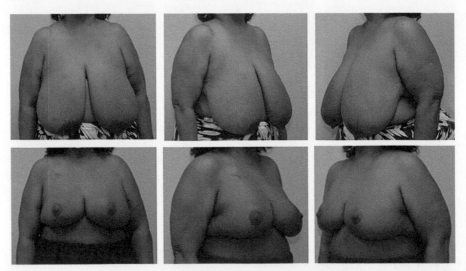

Fig. 3. A 52-year-old woman with Stage II left breast cancer before (*above*) and after (*below*) lumpectomy and bilateral oncoplastic reduction mammoplasty.

of as a contraindication to breast conservation,[29] more recent studies have reconsidered this recommendation and shown it to be oncologically equivalent if clear margins can be achieved.[30–32] Reconstruction, however, can be more challenging, particularly with multicentric disease where resection is required from multiple quadrants. In these cases, more advanced approaches such as round block, circumvertical, or Wise pattern reduction/mastopexy can be helpful both to allow for access to all of the area of resection and to allow for more extensive soft tissue reconstruction. Using extended pedicles or secondary pedicles for additional reconstructive volume may be necessary if reconstruction of multiple defects is required.[33,34] Additionally, patients with smaller breasts and larger tumor-to-breast volume ratios as well as patients of any breast size requiring extensive resection may be able to avoid mastectomy if more advanced oncoplastic approaches are offered. The concept of "extreme oncoplasty" was coined by Dr Mel Silverstein and colleagues in 2015,[35] which describes approaches to breast conservation through oncoplastic reconstruction in these more complex scenarios. Their workhorses for reconstruction of larger lumpectomy defects include Wise pattern reductions and split reduction procedures, which entail reconfiguring the Wise pattern design to allow for skin removal over the tumor.[36] Other surgeons have taken these principles and expanded indications for breast conservation and oncoplastic reconstruction in their practices as well, demonstrating good oncologic outcomes even in scenarios traditionally managed with mastectomy.[37,38]

Advancements in Autologous Reconstruction

Breast reconstruction using autologous flaps was first described in 1906 by Tanzini,[39] who reported using a myocutaneous latissimus dorsi flap to reconstruct a mastectomy defect. Earlier approaches such as this and flap reconstruction options throughout much of the twentieth century required complete muscle sacrifice harvest typically with either latissimus dorsi or transverse rectus abdominis myocutaneous (TRAM) flap reconstruction. As the concept of perforator flaps was introduced and techniques were optimized,[40] flap reconstruction evolved to allow for muscle-sparing options, with the deep inferior epigastric perforator flap being the most commonly described and utilized perforator flap option.[41] At many centers, deep inferior epigastric perforator (DIEP) flaps are the workhorse of their flap reconstruction programs, allowing patients the benefits of decreased abdominal donor site morbidity including lower rates of abdominal wall hernias as well as lower rates of fat necrosis.[42,43]

Although the abdomen is usually the preferred donor site for autologous reconstruction, some patients may not be candidates due to insufficient tissue or prior abdominal surgery affecting the vascular supply to the flaps.[44] In these cases, other perforator flaps can be considered, typically either the superior or inferior gluteal artery perforator (SGAP/IGAP) or profunda artery perforator (PAP) flaps. Some centers routinely use gluteal artery perforator flaps when abdominal flaps are not available or even as a first choice for reconstruction, describing the benefits of safe and reliable harvest with low rates of complications.[45] Limitations of the flap include the need for harvest in the prone position, which can add significant time to the procedure and precludes simultaneous flap harvest during the mastectomy in immediate reconstruction cases, as well as some concerns for donor site morbidity, particularly with IGAP flaps.[46,47] PAP flaps have been described more frequently in the literature recently, likely due to the reliable vascular anatomy,[48] minimal donor site morbidity and low complication rates,[49,50] and the ability to harvest the flap in the supine position potentially concurrently with the mastectomy, as well as the ability to shape the flap to achieve good esthetic outcomes (**Fig. 4**).[51]

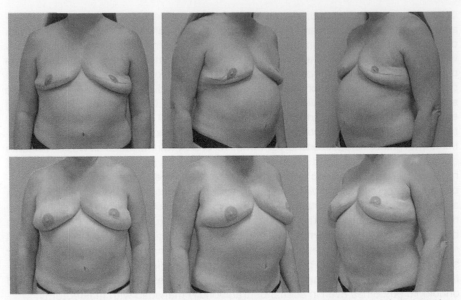

Fig. 4. A 47-year-old woman with a history of bilateral mastectomies and failed implant reconstruction as well as abdominoplasty before (*above*) and after (*below*) bilateral PAP flap reconstruction.

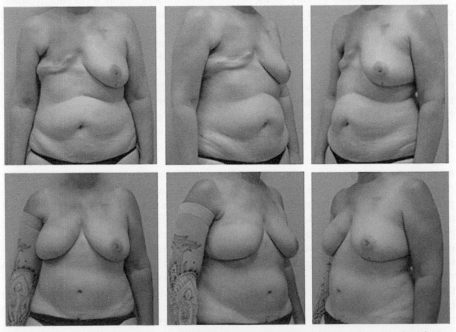

Fig. 5. A 43-year-old woman with a history of Stage II right breast cancer treated with simple mastectomy before (*above*) and after (*below*) stacked DIEP flap reconstruction.

Other options for flap reconstruction when there is insufficient donor site tissue are stacked flaps, where more than one flap is used to reconstruct the breast, or hybrid flap reconstruction, where an implant is placed deep to the flap to add more volume. For stacked flaps, typical combinations included stacked combination DIEP/PAP flaps, stacked PAP flaps,[44] and stacked DIEP flaps for unilateral reconstruction.[52-54] These combinations allow for more volume than a single flap could provide, although still allowing patients a fully autologous reconstruction (**Fig. 5**). Although operative times are significantly longer with stacked flaps, studies comparing complication profiles following stacked flap reconstruction to single flap reconstruction have not shown increased risk of complications including flap loss or donor site complications.[55]

Another option for patients who need more volume than a single flap can provide is hybrid reconstruction, which combines autologous and implant-based reconstruction.[56] The technique has been described as either delayed or simultaneous placement of a prepectoral implant at the time of flap (typically DIEP flap or latissimus dorsi) reconstruction in order to achieve patients' desired size goals.[57] This approach has shown a favorable safety profile[58,59] and high rates of patient satisfaction.[60]

Preserving and Restoring Sensation After Mastectomy

Although so many advances have been made over time to improve the esthetics of postmastectomy reconstruction, one of the major limitations of mastectomy has been the loss of sensation following surgery. Prior studies have shown the loss of sensation to be very common in people undergoing mastectomy, with rates of return of breast skin and nipple sensation reported in the range of 2% to 26% following NSM,[61-63] indicating the vast majority of patients do not have meaningful sensation following mastectomy. The loss of sensation not only affects erogenous sensation and intimacy following mastectomy[64] but the loss of protective sensation can also lead to burns and other injuries, which can have devastating reconstructive consequences.[65,66] For some patients the loss of sensation can be very distressing and can significantly affect patient satisfaction as well as quality of life.[63,67]

Although there has been a more recent focus on preserving and restoring sensation after mastectomy, sensation restoration has actually been described with autologous reconstruction since the early 1990s. Early reports by Slezak and colleagues in 1992[68] involved intercostal nerve reconstruction at the time of delayed TRAM flap reconstruction for patients who had undergone prior mastectomy, with improved sensation seen in reinnervated reconstructed breasts compared with controls. Subsequent studies describing nerve reconstruction using either nerve conduits or nerve autografts at the time of flap reconstruction have shown improved objective return of sensation as well as better patient-reported overall and erogenous sensation with reinnervated flaps.[69-71] More recent data have come out of the Sensation-NOW trial, which is a multisite prospective case-control registry study assessing outcomes following autologous reconstruction and flap neurotization.[72] Momeni and colleagues[73] described outcomes from 22 patients who had abdominally based autologous reconstruction with or without neurotization at a minimum of 1-year follow-up. Patients who underwent neurotization were significantly more likely to have return of protective sensation on cutaneous pressure threshold evaluation compared to controls.

Although the majority of studies describing neurotization and autologous reconstruction are focused on restoring sensation after mastectomy has already been completed, more recent advances have focused on trying to preserve sensation at the time of mastectomy. This is done through a combination of nerve preservation (when oncologically feasible) and nerve reconstruction with either autografts or allografts. Ducic[74] and Djohan[75] have significantly contributed to our understanding of

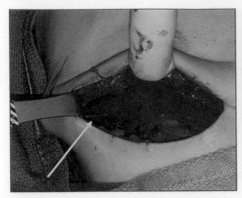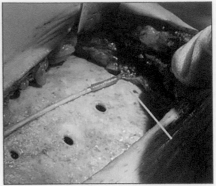

Fig. 6. Example of nerve preservation during NSM (*left*) and intercostal nerve reconstruction using a nerve allograft coapted to a subareolar nerve (*right*).

breast nerve anatomy to allow for nerve preservation and immediate reconstruction through cadaver studies of dissections of mastectomies and abdominal flaps with nerve harvest. Based on their dissections, they have recommended consideration for use of nerve allograft for reconstruction to ensure complete sensory nerve repair as well as delineated anticipated nerve anatomy to assist with identification during mastectomy. Peled and Peled described their approach to preserving sensation at the time of mastectomy in 2019,[76] reporting that they carefully identify the lateral thoracic intercostal nerves at the time of mastectomy (typically T4 and T5, although sometimes T3) and preserve them if oncologically safe, wherein the nerves run in the subcutaneous tissue rather than the breast parenchyma itself. In their study, they combine nerve preservation with nipple–areolar complex neurotization at the time of NSM (**Fig. 6**).

With the technological advancements of nerve allografts, nerve reconstruction can be done not only with flap reconstruction, where donor site nerves can be used but also with implant-based reconstruction. A small number of studies have been published to date describing nerve reconstruction at the time of mastectomy and implant-based reconstruction but more data are anticipated with the growing interest in the procedure from both surgeons and patients.[77] Djohan and colleagues[78] first described their experience with nipple–areolar complex neurotization at the time of NSM and immediate implant reconstruction in 2020. They performed nerve reconstruction with allografts from the lateral fourth intercostal nerves to carefully identified subareolar nerves and reported on the improvement in objective sensation over time. Peled and Peled[76] described a similar approach to nerve reconstruction in their initial study, with 91% of patients achieving return to baseline sensation of their nipple–areolar complex by a mean follow-up of 13 months. Neurotization at the time of immediate autologous reconstruction has also been described, with a similar approach concerning preservation of as much length of the native intercostal nerve as possible at coaptation to a subareolar nerve. Tevlin and colleagues[79] reported sensory outcomes in their case-control study of nipple reinnervation during immediate autologous reconstruction, demonstrating full return to baseline sensation in the group undergoing neurotization.

Outcomes research around sensation preservation and restoration after mastectomy continues to evolve as well, with an increased focus on determining the optimal patient-reported outcomes tools and metrics to assess sensation,[67,80] as well as more objective sensory outcomes assessment.[81,82] Advances in outcomes measures as well as more outcomes data from these procedures will be essential in helping determine best practices and selection criteria, as well as ensuring insurance coverage for patients.

CLINICS CARE POINTS

- Nerve preservation and reconstruction at the time of mastectomy can safely and effectively provide patients with sensation after mastectomy.
- Use of initial reduction mammoplasty or mastopexy can extend the option of nipple-sparing mastectomy in therapeutic and prophylactic situations.

DISCLOSURE

Dr A.W. Peled is a consultant/speaker for Axogen, Allergan, Sientra, and Stryker. Dr N.W. Clavin is a consultant/speaker for Allergan and Stryker.

REFERENCES

1. Stolier AJ, Levine EA. Reducing the risk of nipple necrosis: technical observations in 340 nipple-sparing mastectomies. Breast J 2013;19:173–9.
2. McCarthy CM, Mehrara BJ, Riedel E, al at. Predicting complications following expander/implant breast reconstruction: an outcomes analysis based on preoperative clinical risk. Plast Reconstr Surg 2008;121:1886–92.
3. Nava MB, Cortinovis U, Ottolenghi J, et al. Skin-reducing mastectomy. Plast Reconstr Surg 2006;118:603–10.
4. Howard MA, Sisco M, Yao K, et al. Patient satisfaction with nipple-sparing mastectomy: a prospective study of patient reported outcomes using the BREAST-Q. J Surg Oncol 2016;114:416–22.
5. Salibian AH, Harness JK, Mowlds DS. Primary buttonhole mastopexy and nipple-sparing mastectomy: a preliminary report. Ann Plast Surg 2016;77:388–95.
6. Aliotta RE, Scomacao I, Duraes EFR, et al. Pushing the envelope: skin-only mastopexy in single-stage nipple-sparing mastectomy with direct-to-implant breast reconstruction. Plast Reconstr Surg 2021;147:38–45.
7. Doren EL, Kuykendall LVE, Lopez JJ, et al. Free nipple grafting: an alternative for patients ineligible for nipple-sparing mastectomy? Ann Plast Surg 2014;72:S112–5.
8. Kim EK, Cho JM, Lee JW. Skin-sparing mastectomy and immediate nipple graft for large, ptotic breast. J Breast Cancer 2019;22:641–6.
9. Spear SL, Rottman SJ, Seiboth LA, et al. Breast reconstruction using a staged nipple-sparing mastectomy following mastopexy or reduction. Plast Reconstr Surg 2012;129:572–81.
10. Momeni A, Kanchwala S, Sbitany H. Oncoplastic procedures in preparation for nipple-sparing mastectomy and autologous breast reconstruction: controlling the breast envelope. Plast Reconstr Surg 2020;145:914–20.
11. Salibian AA, Frey JD, Karp NS, et al. Does staged breast reduction before nipple-sparing mastectomy decrease complications? A matched cohort study between staged and nonstaged techniques. Plast Reconstr Surg 2019;144:1023–32.
12. Economides JM, Graziano F, Tousimis E, et al. Expanded algorithm and updated experience with breast reconstruction using a staged nipple-sparing mastectomy

following mastopexy or reduction mammaplasty in the large or ptotic breast. Plast Reconstr Surg 2019;143:688e, 97e.

13. Peled AW, Sbitany H, Foster RD, et al. Oncoplastic mammoplasty as a strategy for reducing reconstructive complications associated with postmastectomy radiation therapy. Breast J 2014;20:302–7.

14. Stein MJ, Karir A, Arnaout A, et al. Quality-of-life and surgical outcomes for breast cancer patients treated with therapeutic reduction mammoplasty versus mastectomy with immediate reconstruction. Ann Surg Oncol 2020;27:4502–12.

15. Clough KB, Kaufman GJ, Nos C, et al. Improving breast cancer surgery: a classification and quadrant per quadrant atlas for oncoplastic surgery. Ann Surg Oncol 2010;17:1375–91.

16. Chatterjee A, Gass J, Patel K, et al. A consensus definition and classification system of oncoplastic surgery developed by the American Society of Breast Surgeons. Ann Surg Oncol 2019;26:3436–44.

17. Patel K, Bloom J, Nardello S, et al. An oncoplastic surgery primer: common indications, techniques, and complications in Level I and 2 volume displacement oncoplastic surgery. Ann Surg Oncol 2019;26:3063–70.

18. Strong B, Hall-Findlay EJ. How does volume of resection relate to symptom relief for reduction mammaplasty patients? Ann Plast Surg 2015;75:376–82.

19. Acea-Nebril B, Cereijo-Garea C, Garcia-Novoa A, et al. The role of oncoplastic breast reduction in the conservative management of breast cancer: complications, survival, and quality of life. J Surg Oncol 2017;115:679–86.

20. Denis-Katz HS, Ghaedi BB, Fitzpatrick A, et al. Oncological safety, surgical outcome, and patient satisfaction of oncoplastic breast-conserving surgery with contralateral balancing reduction mammoplasty. Plast Surg (Oakv) 2021;29:235–42.

21. Patel K, Hannah CM, Gatti ME, et al. A head-to-head comparison of quality of life and aesthetic outcomes following immediate, staged-immediate, and delayed oncoplastic reduction mammaplasty. Plast Reconstr Surg 2011;127:2167–75.

22. Di Micco R, O'Connell RL, Barry PA, et al. Standard wide local excision or bilateral reduction mammoplasty in large-breasted women with small tumours: surgical and patient-reported outcomes. Eur J Surg Oncol 2017;43:636–41.

23. Prabhakar R, Rath GK, Julka PK, et al. Breast dose heterogeneity in CT-based radiotherapy treatment planning. J Med Phys 2008;33:43–8.

24. Fernando IN, Ford HT, Powles TJ, et al. Factors affecting acute skin toxicity in patients having breast irradiation after conservative surgery: a prospective study of treatment practice at the Royal Marsden Hospital. Clin Oncol (R Coll Radiol) 1996;8:226–33.

25. Losken A, Pinell-White X, Hart AM, et al. The oncoplastic reduction approach to breast conservation therapy: benefits for margin control. Aesthet Surg J 2014;34:1185–91.

26. Piper ML, Esserman LJ, Sbitany H, et al. Outcomes following oncoplastic reduction mammoplasty: a systematic review. Ann Plast Surg 2016;76:S222–6.

27. Losken A, Pinell XA, Eskenazi BR. The benefits of partial versus total breast reconstruction for women with macromastia. Plast Reconstr Surg 2010;125:1051–6.

28. Tong WMY, Baumann DP, Villa MT, et al. Obese women experience fewer complications after oncoplastic breast repair following partial mastectomy than after immediate total breast reconstruction. Plast Reconstr Surg 2016;137:777–91.

29. Morrow M, Strom EA, Bassett LW, et al. Standard for breast conservation therapy in the management of invasive breast carcinoma. CA Cancer J Clin 2002;52: 277–300.

30. Masannat YA, Agrawal A, Maraqa L, et al. Multifocal and multicentric breast cancer, is it time to think again? Ann R Coll Surg Engl 2020;102:62–6.

31. Tan MP, Sitoh NY, Sim AS. Breast conservation treatment for multifocal and multicentric breast cancers in women with small-volume breast tissue. ANZ J Surg 2017;87:E5–10.

32. Kadioglu H, Yucel S, Yildiz S, et al. Feasibility of breast conserving surgery in multifocal breast cancers. Am J Surg 2014;208:457–64.

33. Losken A, Hart AM, Dutton JW, et al. The expanded use of autoaugmentation techniques in oncoplastic breast surgery. Plast Reconstr Surg 2018;141:10–9.

34. Bellizzi A, Vella Baldacchino R, Kazzazi F, et al. The successful use of disparate pedicle types for bilateral therapeutic mammaplasties during breast conservation surgery. J Surg Case Rep 2021;3:rjab064.

35. Silverstein MJ, Savalia N, Khan S, et al. Extreme oncoplasty: breast conservation for patients who need mastectomy. Breast J 2015;21:52–9.

36. Silverstein MJ, Savalia NB, Khan S, et al. Oncoplastic split reduction with intraoperative radiation therapy. Ann Surg Oncol 2015;22:3405–6.

37. Savioli F, Seth S, Morrow E, et al. Extreme oncoplasty: breast conservation in patients with large, multifocal, and multicentric breast cancer. Breast Cancer 2021; 13:353–9. Dove Med Press.

38. Koppiker CB, Noor AU, Dixit S, et al. Extreme oncoplastic surgery for multifocal/multicentric and locally advanced breast cancer. Int J Breast Cancer 2019;4262589.

39. Tanzini I. Spora il mio nuova processo di amputazione della mammella. Riforma Med 1906;22:757.

40. Koshima I, Soeda S. Inferior epigastric artery skin flap without rectus abdominis muscle. Br J Plast Surg 1989;42:645.

41. Healy C, Allen RJ Sr. The evolution of perforator flap breast reconstruction: twenty years after the first DIEP flap. J Reconstr Microsurg 2014;30:121–5.

42. Garvey PB, Buchel EW, Pockaj BA, et al. DIEP and pedicled TRAM flaps: a comparison of outcomes. Plast Reconstr Surg 2006;117:1711–9.

43. Knox ADC, Ho AL, Leung L, et al. Comparison of outcomes following autologous breast reconstruction using the DIEP and pedicled TRAM flaps: a 12-year clinical retrospective study and literature review. Plast Reconstr Surg 2016;138:16–28.

44. Haddock NT, Cho MJ, Gassman A, et al. Stacked profunda artery perforator flap for breast reconstruction in failed or unavailable deep inferior epigastric perforator flap. Plast Reconstr Surg 2019;143:488e, 94e.

45. Granzow JW, Levine JL, Chiu ES, et al. Breast reconstruction with gluteal artery perforator flaps. J Plast Reconstr Aesthet Surg 2006;59:614–21.

46. Godbout E, Farmer L, Bortoluzzi P, et al. Donor-site morbidity of the inferior gluteal artery perforator flap for breast reconstruction in teenagers. Can J Plast Surg 2013;21:19–22.

47. Mirzabeigi M, Au A, Jandali S, et al. Trials and tribulations with the inferior gluteal artery perforator flap in autologous breast reconstruction. Plast Reconstr Surg 2011;128:614e, 24e.

48. Largo RD, Chu CK, Chang EI, et al. Perforator mapping of the profunda artery perforator flap: anatomy and clinical experience. Plast Reconstr Surg 2020; 146:1135–45.

49. Qian B, Xiong L, Li J, et al. A systematic review and meta-analysis on microsurgical safety and efficacy of profunda artery perforator flap in breast reconstruction. J Oncol 2019;29:9506720.
50. Allen RJ Jr, Lee Z, Mayo JL, et al. The profunda artery perforator flap experience for breast reconstruction. Plast Reconstr Surg 2016;138:968–75.
51. Atzeni M, Salzillo R, Haywood R, et al. Breast reconstruction using the profunda artery perforator (PAP) flap: technical refinements and evolution, outcomes, and patient satisfaction based on 116 consecutive flaps. J Plast Reconstr Aesthet Surg 2022;75:1617–24.
52. Martinez CA, Fairchild B, Secchi-Del Rio R, et al. Bilateral outpatient breast reconstruction with stacked DIEP and vertical PAP flaps. Plast Reconstr Surg Glob Open 2021;9:e3878.
53. Haddock NT, Suszynski TM, Teotia SS. Consecutive bilateral breast reconstruction using stacked abdominally based and posterior thigh free flaps. Plast Reconstr Surg 2021;147:294–303.
54. DellaCroce FJ, Sullivan SK, Trahan C. Stacked deep inferior epigastric perforator flap breast reconstruction: a review of 110 flaps in 55 cases over 3 years. Plast Reconstr Surg 2011;127:1093–9.
55. Haddock NT, Cho MJ, Teotia SS. Comparative analysis of single versus stacked free flap breast reconstruction: a single center experience. Plast Reconstr Surg 2019;144:369e, 77e.
56. Kanchwala S, Momeni A. Hybrid breast reconstruction- the best of both worlds. Gland Surg 2019;8:82–9.
57. Scafati ST, Cavaliere A, Aceto B, et al. Combining autologous and prosthetic techniques: the breast reconstruction scale principle. Plast Reconstr Surg Glob Open 2017;5:e1602.
58. Momeni A, Kanchwala S. Hybrid prepectoral breast reconstruction: a surgical approach that combines the benefits of autologous and implant-based reconstruction. Plast Reconstr Surg 2018;142:1109–15.
59. Lee HC, Lee J, Park SH, et al. The hybrid latissimus dorsi flap in immediate breast reconstruction: a comparative study with the abdominal-based flap. Ann Plast Surg 2021;86:394–9.
60. Bach AD, Morgenstern IH, Horch RE. Secondary "hybrid reconstruction" concept with silicone implants after autologous breast reconstruction: is it safe and reasonable? Med Sci Monit 2020;26:e921329.
61. Chirappapha P, Srichan P, Lertsithichai P, et al. Nipple-areola complex sensation after nipple-sparing mastectomy. Plast Reconstr Surg Glob Open 2018;6:e1716.
62. Dossett LA, Lowe J, Sun W, et al. Prospective evaluation of skin and nipple-areola sensation and patient satisfaction after nipple-sparing mastectomy. J Surg Oncol 2016;114:11–6.
63. Djohan R, Gage E, Gatherwright J, et al. Patient satisfaction following nipple-sparing mastectomy and immediate breast reconstruction: an 8-year outcome study. Plast Reconstr Surg 2010;125:818–29.
64. Boswell EN, Dizon DS. Breast cancer and sexual function. Transl Androl Urol 2015;4:160–8.
65. Faulkner HR, Colwell AS, Liao EC, et al. Thermal injury to reconstructed breasts from commonly used warming devices: a risk for reconstructive failure. Plast Reconstr Surg Glob Open 2016;4:e1033.
66. Seth R, Lamyman MJ, Athanassopoulos A, et al. Too close for comfort: accidental burn following subcutaneous mastectomy and immediate implant reconstruction. J R Soc Med 2008;101:39–40.

67. Peled AW, Amara D, Piper ML, et al. Development and validation of a nipple-specific scale for the BREAST-Q to assess patient-reported outcomes following nipple-sparing mastectomy. Plast Reconstr Surg 2019;143:1010–7.
68. Slezak S, McGibbon B, Dellon AL. The sensational transverse rectus abdominis musculocutaneous (TRAM) flap: return of sensibility after TRAM breast reconstruction. Ann Plast Surg 1992;28:210–7.
69. Blondeel PN, Demuynck M, Mete D, et al. Sensory nerve repair in perforator flaps for autologous breast reconstruction: sensational or senseless? Br J Plast Surg 1999;52:37–44.
70. Spiegel AJ, Menn ZK, Eldor L, et al. Breast reinnervation: DIEP neurotization using the third anterior intercostal nerve. Plast Reconstr Surg Glob Open 2013; 1:e72.
71. Beugels J, Bijkerk E, Lataster A, et al. Nerve coaptation improves the sensory recovery of the breast in DIEP flap breast reconstruction. Plast Reconstr Surg 2021; 148:273–84.
72. Available at: https://clinicaltrials.gov/ct2/show/NCT01526681 -. Accessed 6.1.22.
73. Momeni A, Meyer S, Shefren K, et al. Flap neurotization in breast reconstruction with nerve allografts: 1-year clinical outcomes. Plast Reconstr Surg Glob Open 2021;9:e3328.
74. Ducic I, Yoon J, Momeni A, et al. Anatomical considerations to optimize sensory recovery in breast neurotization with allograft. Plast Reconstr Surg Glob Open 2018;6:e1985.
75. Gatherwright J, Knackstedt R, Djohan R. Anatomic targets for breast reconstruction neurotization: past results and future possibilities. Ann Plast Surg 2019;82: 207–12.
76. Peled AW, Peled ZM. Nerve preservation and allografting for sensory innervation following immediate implant breast reconstruction. Plast Reconstr Surg Glob Open 2019;7:e2332.
77. Peled AW, Peled ZM. Sensory reinnervation after mastectomy with implant-based reconstruction. Ann Breast Surg. Submitted for publication.
78. Djohan R, Scomacao I, Knackstedt R, et al. Neurotization of the nipple-areola complex during implant-based reconstruction: evaluation of early sensation recovery. Plast Reconstr Surg 2020;146:250–4.
79. Tevlin R, Brazio P, Tran N, et al. Immediate targeted nipple-areolar complex reinnervation: improving outcomes in immediate autologous breast reconstruction. J Plast Reconstr Aesthet Surg 2021;74:1503–7.
80. Tsangaris E, Klassen AF, Kaur MN, et al. Development and psychometric validation of the BREAST-Q sensation module for women undergoing post-mastectomy breast reconstruction. Ann Surg Oncol 2021;28:7842–53.
81. Vartanian ED, Lo AY, Hershenhouse KS, et al. The role of neurotization in autologous breast reconstruction: can reconstruction restore breast sensation? J Surg Oncol 2021;123:1215–31.
82. Weissler JM, Koltz PF, Carney MJ, et al. Sifting through the evidence: a comprehensive review and analysis of neurotization in breast reconstruction. Plast Reconstr Surg 2018;141:550–65.

Quality of Life Issues Following Breast Cancer Treatment

James Abdo, MD*, Holly Ortman, MD, Natalia Rodriguez, MD,
Rachel Tillman, MD, Elizabeth O. Riordan, MD, Anna Seydel, MD

KEYWORDS

- Breast cancer • Survivorship • Lymphedema • Side effects • Quality of life
- Cancer-related cognitive deficit • Hormone therapy • Radiation therapy

KEY POINTS

- As more women develop and survive breast cancer with the increasing length of survival, we review the effects of therapy on their quality of life.
- Provide a patient viewpoint of life with breast cancer and side effects of treatment as well as common topics not often discussed.
- Identify common side effects of therapy, the risk factors leading to side effects, as well as their management.
- Understanding that as breast cancer survival continues to improve, survivorship and quality of life become increasingly important, and may influence cancer treatment, or guide care of common side effects.

INTRODUCTION

With an estimated 5 million breast cancer survivors in 2030,[1] it is important for the breast specialist to understand the impact recommended treatments have on patients to lessen the unwanted effects and improve the overall quality of life. This article explores what patients need beyond good outcomes to maintain a satisfactory quality of life. Quality of Life scoring systems cannot fully describe the subjective effects of cancer and its treatment. These metrics instead reflect the degree of patients' social support and lend evidence to patients' resilience. Subjective scores are minimally affected by measurable morbidities as patients adjust to their new baseline tolerating the side effects of treatment and minimizing the impact on their daily life. Instead of discussing the quality of life scores, this article aims to review the intangible effects

No authors have financial disclosures.
Marshfield Medical Center, 1000 North Oak Street, Marshfield, WI 54449, USA
* Corresponding author.
E-mail address: abdo.james@marshfieldclinic.org

Surg Clin N Am 103 (2023) 155–167
https://doi.org/10.1016/j.suc.2022.08.014
0039-6109/23/© 2022 Elsevier Inc. All rights reserved.

of breast cancer treatment, the more concrete side effects of systemic and local therapy, and offer strategies to mitigate them.

Dr O'Riordan, a breast cancer surgeon who is also a breast cancer survivor, offers her insights from the patient's perspective, discussing those aspects of patient care that aren't easily measured or often discussed—that is, sex, intimacy, and fear of recurrence. This is followed by a more didactic review of the commonly investigated side effects of systemic and local treatment. We hope to arm the clinician with the tools necessary to discuss strategies that support behavior modifications and interventions to improve the quality of life for our patients with breast cancer.

Intangible Effects of Treatment

Social media

Patients with breast cancer are talking among themselves on multiple forums about the topics of self-esteem, diet, exercise, sex, intimacy, and anxiety regarding recurrence. Surgeons and oncologists should be potential participants in these conversations. Once a patient with a new diagnosis of breast cancer leaves the office, one of the first things s/he may do is scour the internet for information. It is worth spending a couple of hours walking in your patients' shoes to see what is available to them via social media and the internet. Are you familiar with any breast cancer patient forums, apps, or websites? Have you read any books or blogs written by a patient? Do you know what questions your patients are asking each other and what they really need? Questions they are too scared to ask their breast cancer specialist such as "Is it safe to have sex during chemo? I'm afraid my husband's hair will fall out." These are the issues beyond our evidence-based treatment that affect their everyday lives. Tell your patients that you know they are going to open their phones and computers and give them safe and useful resources to start their journey. This small gesture will make a huge difference to the quality of care you provide for your patients.

Diet

Wellness and nutrition experts on social media claim that various diets and supplements can cure or reduce the risk of getting cancer. Our patients are vulnerable, possibly scared, and quite willing to do anything to stop their cancer from coming back. It is imperative that the clinician talks to them about what they should be eating and drinking as they move forward with their life. The WHO recommends that patients with cancer simply eat a healthy, balanced diet including 6 servings of fruit and vegetables daily. That's it. There is no robust evidence at the moment to prove that any food group can increase or decrease its their risk of recurrence.

Obesity increases the risk of breast cancer recurrence and even death by 35% to 40%.[2] Despite eating normally, many women gain more weight during breast cancer treatment, especially once hormonal manipulation begins. For many women, this information is empowering—getting to and maintaining normal body weight is something patients can do to take control of their future. This is also true for patients who do not have an existing diagnosis of breast cancer. Postmenopausal weight loss reduces the risk of developing breast cancer—a 5% weight reduction lowers the risk of postmenopausal breast cancer by 12%. Conversely, greater than 5% weight gain in the postmenopausal period is associated with a 54% higher incidence of triple-negative disease.[3]

Patients may ask whether it is safe to take supplements they have read about online. Patients with cancer are a captive market, and many are spending hundreds of dollars each month on things they believe they need. All they need is a general multivitamin on top of any bone health supplement. For less common supplements, you can direct patients to a website[4] run by the Memorial Sloan Kettering Cancer Center which will provide current information on the supplement and data regarding its relationship to cancer.

Another important piece of advice to provide patients regarding behavior modifications is to reduce alcohol intake to less than five units per week. According to the National Institutes of Health, one "standard" drink contains roughly 14 g of pure alcohol, which is found in one of the following: 12 fL oz of regular beer, 9 oz of malt liquor, 5 ox of table wine, and 1.5 oz of hard liquor. In addition to postmenopausal weight gain, regular alcohol consumption can also increase the risk of breast cancer recurrence.[5]

Exercise

Exercise should be one of the first treatments you prescribe to every patient. It is effective at reducing side effects[6] such as fatigue, anxiety, and depression, as well as improving quality of life, sleep, and bone health. Exercise can be associated with a decrease in overall mortality for patients with breast cancer and is specifically recommended for patients with bony metastases as it improves physical function and reduces psychosocial morbidity.[7] Every patient should be "prescribed" 75 to 150 weekly minutes of vigorous aerobic activity and twice-weekly progressive resistance exercise targeting all major muscle groups.[7] A good starting place to educate yourself and your patients is the website and book created by Dr Kathryn Schmitz[8] https://www.movingthroughcancer.com. It explains why exercise is so important for patients and gives clear instructions for a resistance program that patients can do at home using simple equipment.

Sex and intimacy

Breast cancer treatment will affect a patient's sex life and it is important to ensure that someone on the treatment team opens the door to these conversations and is available to discuss patient concerns and review options. Challenges with sex and intimacy following treatment of breast cancer start with body image and how patients see themselves after surgery. Some patients grieve for their femininity and sexuality— taken away at a moment's notice following an operation for breast cancer. Breast reconstructions can look realistic, but many women don't realize until they have undergone the initial operation that their reconstructed breast mound is nothing more than that—a mound of tissue or silicone, often under numb skin, without sensation. Postoperative pain and scarring can make patients avoid physical contact with their partners. The added hair loss associated with chemotherapy and burned skin from radiotherapy take their toll on any woman's body image. Additionally, the side effects of hormonal manipulation push women into menopause overnight. Night sweats can cause unbroken sleep and separate bed covers. Vaginal dryness can make intercourse painful, cause bleeding and tearing, and lack of lubrication. Providing patients with information about vaginal dryness and lubricants (used during intercourse) and moisturizers (daily use) is an important component of a patient's cancer care. It is recommended that individuals use a natural lubricant with no parabens or preservatives. Start the conversation by asking patients what lubricant they use, so it seems like a normal part of sex. Have an "intimacy bag" in your clinic with samples of items that women could explore after talking to you and plan follow-up discussions as part of the routine cancer surveillance office visit.

The loss of libido can be damaging to relationships. Some women never feel the urge to have sex after their diagnosis of cancer. Two medications, Vyleesi and Addyi, have been approved by the Food & Drug Administration (FDA) for low sexual drive in premenopausal women, along with one over-the-counter supplement, Ristela, that benefit women of any age.[9,10] These medications have been shown to improve arousal, orgasm, satisfaction, and desire and can be considered for patients undergoing breast cancer treatment.[11]

Also important when counseling patients about sexual intercourse after breast cancer treatment is to remember to talk about the importance of contraception for any premenopausal woman having chemotherapy, HER2 treatment, or tamoxifen as these treatments are all teratogenic.

Vaginal estrogen does not increase the risk of recurrence for women taking Tamoxifen and aromatase inhibitors and should be offered to patients who need more help with lubrication. Vaginal estrogen may need to be used daily for severe symptoms. Dilators may also need to be used with a lubricant to gently stretch the vaginal walls and make intercourse less painful. Advocate for a sexual psychotherapist or advanced practice provider who has been trained in sexual health to be a part of the cancer treatment team and can see your patients in consultation from the time of diagnosis and throughout treatment into survivorship.

Mental health

The fear of recurrence is real for many patients with breast cancer. It can cause extreme anxiety, or "scanxiety" and "labxiety," whenever a patient has a routine mammogram, scan, or laboratories. Alternatively, some women do not realize that their cancer can come back, either locally or as a Stage IV disease. Indeed, a large number of women don't know what symptoms to look for, and more importantly, what to do if they're worried. It is important to provide clear instructions at surveillance visits about the signs and symptoms of a recurrence and who to call should symptoms develop or questions arise.

While nearly all patients with cancer exhibit depressive symptoms at the time of a new breast cancer diagnosis, approximately 25% of patients suffer from a major depressive episode following initial diagnosis.[12] Major depression is not uncommon after breast cancer[13] and can occur months or even years after treatment, often when patients need the most support. It is important that clinicians involved in breast cancer care have a mental health team or referral source to provide patients with options for both situational as well as prolonged depression.

Effects of Systemic Treatment

Cancer-related cognitive impairment

One of the most significant side effects of breast cancer and its treatment is the associated cognitive impairment, often referred to as "chemo-brain." Cancer-related cognitive impairment (CRCI) is a well-identified pattern of cognitive deficits reflecting the CNS toxic effects of not only chemotherapy, but of a systemic malignancy.[1] While most commonly the acquired cognitive deficits are found in verbal memory, sustained attention, executive function, and processing speed, additional domains can be affected such as visual memory, verbal fluency, and upper extremity fine motor dexterity. Even though these effects are well studied, the reported prevalence varies greatly, ranging from 12% to 82% of women with breast cancer.[1] Patients are very aware of these symptoms and discuss them routinely within patient support groups. Living with these cognitive deficits and developing coping strategies is a frequent topic in Facebook groups and other social media outlets. It is the connectivity of patients that have advanced the awareness of the systemic effects of cancer and its treatments among physicians and investigators and helped push the research into these fields.

Despite the frequent occurrence of these symptoms, obtaining objective evidence of cognitive dysfunction has been difficult.[14] Initial cross-sectional studies showed patients performed lower than expected on the neuropsychological testing for cognitive impairment. Subsequent prospective studies challenged the concept of "chemo brain" with some reporting no cognitive impairment and others limiting their effects to a few cognitive domains which are discordant with the patient's experience. Additionally, studies showed that CRCI was independent of chemotherapy, with deficits seen before receiving chemotherapy and in patients that did not receive chemotherapy.[14-16] Additional studies have added objective evidence with neuroimaging showing structural and functional changes in those patients who underwent chemotherapy raising further questions about the impact of cognitive decline on patients.[14,15] Several possibilities could explain these discrepancies—patient's abilities to compensate for the cognitive impairment in the affected domains, inability of testing to accurately capture the cognitive deficits, overlap of effects of depression and anxiety on cognitive function, or the possibility of small deficits having a large effect on patient's perception.

One suggested model for the conceptualization of the interaction between cancer, treatment, and cognitive function is the "soil, seed, and pesticides model," referring to the patient's predisposing factors, the disease-related factors of cancer, and the systemic treatments used to eradicate the cancer. While chemotherapy has been an obvious culprit, there is evidence that hormonal treatments and radiation therapy can also affect cognition.[1] While early age-related cognitive decline may put patients at risk of CRCI, cancer-related cognitive impairment does not seem to increase the risk of dementia.[17,18]

While patient risk factors such as age, diabetes, and hypertension may have an important role in determining chemotherapy regimens in the future,[16] the best predictor of the effects of CRCI is a patient's cognitive reserve (CR). Defined as innate and developed cognitive capacity, the cognitive reserve may be one of our most reliable predictors of severity. CR, which is influenced by education, occupational attainment, and lifestyle has been used as a measurement in studies evaluating brain pathology in disease states such as Alzheimer's, Parkinson's, traumatic brain injury, and multiple sclerosis. CR is influenced by both mentally or physically stimulating activities and it may be of use to identify those at risk of CRCI to guide resources available to attenuate the functional decline. Cognitive rehab training, meditation, and exercise are lifestyle modifications that have been shown to improve recovery from CRCI. In addition to comprehensive therapy, medications can also be used to mitigate the development and severity of cognitive impairment for our patients, including modafinil, antidepressants, cotinine, donepezil, and antioxidants.[18]

Peripheral neuropathy

Patients with breast cancer have some of the highest rates of chemotherapy-induced peripheral neuropathy (CIPN), with effects so severe it may affect oncologic outcomes by forcing dose modifications. The mechanism is through the demyelination of the dorsal root ganglion and peripheral nerves, causing numbness, paresthesias, or pain.[19,20] Common complaints include tingling, cold sensitivity, a feeling of wearing gloves or stockings, burning, freezing, shock-like, or electric pain.[21,22] While sensory and not motor nerves are often affected, patients have loss of proprioception and touch which lead to decreased dexterity and mobility impairing the patient's ability to perform activities of daily living. While neuropathy itself is distressing, these effects are compounded by worsening mental health for patients as they experience frustration, loss of purpose, and depression because they can no longer participate in activities of daily living.[23] Patients adjust to their degree of impairment due to CIPN and the impact of peripheral neuropathy on their daily life is not accurately reflected in the routine quality of life scores.[20] Introduction of more standardized scales such as the total neuropathy score, CIPN 20, and the FACT/GOG-NTX may help generalize findings amongst future studies to adequately measure the impact on quality of life.

Recognition of CIPN's effect on the quality of life has led to the search for treatments and prevention. Strategies to prevent peripheral neuropathy, which are being developed and include nutritional supplements and cryotherapy, have yet to show definitive benefits.[24] Pharmacologic treatment of neuropathy is limited, with duloxetine and pregabalin being the few medications shown to have an effect. Exercise has been shown to have some benefits as well. Presently, the only proven practice to manage peripheral neuropathy is to implement dose reductions to reduce the risk of developing permanent disabling neuropathy.

Hormone therapy

Approximately 75% of all patients with breast cancer are eligible to receive adjuvant endocrine therapy, such as a selective estrogen receptor modulator (SERM) like tamoxifen or an aromatase inhibitor like anastrozole.[25] When these medications are taken as directed, these therapies can reduce the risk of recurrence by 40% and reduce mortality by 33%.[26] However, side effects can be so severe that often patients choose to discontinue this essential therapy. Side effects of endocrine therapy include alopecia, anxiety, cognitive dysfunction, fatigue, hot flashes, sleep disturbances, loss of sexual interest, musculoskeletal pain, nausea, osteoporosis, dyspareunia, vaginal dryness, weight gain, and many more. In younger patients, the effects can be amplified due to the abrupt suppression of estrogen which pushes patients into menopause.[27]

Some studies have looked into the patient quality of life and how the medication's side effects correlate to medication adherence.[26] Multiple factors were assessed, most notably the daily impact of hormone therapy side effects. Patients report side effects as "excruciating," and many states that these side effects have limited their ability to do household maintenance, perform their work duties, or even do things as simple as getting out of bed. Effects can also exacerbate others; for example, hot flashes can cause sleep disturbances which then lead to fatigue, and can then result in cognitive decline or "brain fog."

Management strategies to combat hot flashes include pharmacologic options, such as gabapentin, venlafaxine, clonidine, oxybutynin, and progesterone analogs.[27] Offering support and recommending patients wear layers have a fan at their desk and air conditioning nearby, can help patients navigate their inevitable symptoms of hormonal treatment and improve compliance. Other side effects that play a key role in the quality of life for many patients taking hormone therapy are sexual dysfunction due to associated vulvovaginal changes, decreased libido, and psychosocial effects which can contribute to poor communication between partners. It has been shown that 79% of patients on an aromatase inhibitor report sexual dysfunction, and 24% of patients have stopped having sex with their partners.[28] As previously discussed, it is important to review vaginal lubricants and moisturizers with your patients as they embark on hormone therapy.

During follow-up appointments the focus is often on disease recurrence and side effects are downplayed or overlooked.[27] However, with the emergence of therapies to counteract these potentially debilitating side effects inclusive exercise; improved diet, additional medications, it is important to discuss these interventions as well as signs of recurrence in order to improve the patient's quality of life.

Effects of Local Treatment

Breast/chest wall pain

Postmastectomy pain syndrome (PMPS) is localized to the axilla, medial upper arm, breast, and chest wall, is described as neuropathic in nature, and persists more than 3 to 18 months after surgery.[29] Pain can be severe enough to not only interfere with sleep and daily activities but also lead to decreased use of the arm and the development of a frozen shoulder or complex regional pain syndrome. PMPS is caused by direct nerve injury or subsequent formation of a traumatic neuroma or scar tissue and presents with tingling, burning, and numbness. Often the anterior and lateral cutaneous branches are injured. Treatment often starts with pharmacotherapy with drugs targeting neuropathic pain such as gabapentin, carbamazepine, venlafaxine, and duloxetine which have been shown to be effective. If this is ineffective, surgical treatment such as axillary scar release or autologous fat grafting may be appropriate, along with physical therapy, to improve symptoms.[30]

Chronic breast/chest wall pain after surgery affects 25% to 60% of patients.[29] The prevalence of chronic pain varies by treatment and has been found to be 25% for patients treated with mastectomy without adjuvant therapy, and 60% for patients treated with breast-conserving therapy, axillary lymph node dissection, and radiation.[31] As in lymphedema, obesity is an independent risk factor for the development of breast pain. Age is also a significant risk factor with several studies showing young age to be a predictive factor for the development of chronic breast pain. In fact, increasing age is associated with a decrease in postoperative pain.[29] High-quality evidence and review of the literature—30 studies involving 19,813 patients—showed a significant association between persistent pain after breast cancer surgery and 2 nonmodifiable factors: younger age and radiotherapy.[32] The most significant associated modifiable factor is ALND, regardless of whether lumpectomy or mastectomy was performed. Women who underwent ALND experienced a 21% increase in the absolute risk of chronic postoperative pain. In addition to modifying the risk of lymphedema, efforts to omit ALND will also have a favorable impact on reducing the incidence of chronic postoperative pain. Other potentially modifiable associated risk factors for persistent pain are the degree of acute postoperative pain and presence of preoperative pain. Despite this, the use of regional anesthesia has not shown any improvement in reducing chronic pain or improving the overall quality of life.[32]

Lymphedema

Lymphedema is one of the most common and yet underestimated complications of breast cancer treatment. It is caused by the disruption of the lymphatics of the axillary system by cancer and its treatment. It is one of the most significant complications of breast cancer treatment and additionally can add a significant financial burden to patients affected. Lymphedema is progressive and debilitating and requires proactive diagnosis, surveillance, and therapy to reverse early stages and prevent progressing to later stages. Management has been modernized, and new techniques in limiting risk as well as managing lymphedema have been developed.

The risk of developing lymphedema is dependent on the extent of surgery or radiation performed in the axilla. As each additional therapy seems to have synergistic effects that increase the risk of lymphedema, limiting therapies to either one adjuvant therapy or no adjuvant therapy will be essential in limiting the incidence of lymphedema in breast cancer survivors.

Treatment of lymphedema should start at diagnosis as it is a progressive disease and in later stages is irreversible. Classically lymphedema was identified by symptoms such as swelling of the affected limb, pain, weakness, fatigue, impaired mobility, skin changes with "brawny edema," and recurrent infections.[33] But, waiting for patients to become symptomatic leads to later presentations with irreversible changes. Early diagnosis requires proactive surveillance with adequate follow-up. Developing a protocol for determining limb measurement and standardizing this within a practice is essential. Multiple studies have shown that objectively measured lymphedema may have little to no effect on patients' quality of life (QoL), while self-reported or symptomatic lymphedema has a severe effect on QoL. Factors affecting QoL include increased financial burden, restricted lifestyles and activities, and potential negative career impact with missed days at work and hospitalizations.[34–37] It is important to note that most reported incidences of lymphedema are likely to be low as many studies have inadequate follow-up periods of only 1 to 2 years.[34] Even though approximately 75% of lymphedema patients will present within 3 years of their operation,[38] a recent meta-analysis has shown the cumulative incidence of lymphedema increases to 40% at 10 years after treatment.[34,39]

In a review by Eaton and colleagues, upper extremity pain and decreased limb function were found to be the 2 primary physical health factors affecting the quality of life; while the psychological health factors included body image disturbance and psychological stress in the form of anxiety, depression, emotional distress, fatigue, self-care, relationship issues, impaired mobility, and ability to participate in social activities.[40] Recent reviews have challenged the lifestyle-limiting "risk-reducing factors" such as IV placement, blood pressure monitoring, and blood draws in the affected arm. This recent data suggests no increased risk of lymphedema with these common procedures.[41]

Obesity—specifically a BMI $\geq$ 30 kg/m2 at breast cancer diagnosis—is the only independent risk factor for the development of lymphedema.[34,42] Emerging data support that monitored, low-impact exercise is actually beneficial in reducing the risk and symptoms of lymphedema. Additionally exercise improves the quality of life and can help with weight loss goals which decrease the risk and severity of lymphedema.[34,43,44]

Lymphedema treatment has expanded in recent years and includes a patient-specific regimen that is in line with their goals. The mainstay of lymphedema treatment is Complete Decongestive Therapy. This includes lymphatic massage, physical therapy, and compression stockings with surgical intervention being limited to those who fail medical management. The two microsurgical techniques that are most widely used are vascularized lymph node transfer and lymphaticovenous anastomosis. The indication for vascularized lymph node transfer is complete blockage and loss of lymph nodes in a patient who has failed conservative treatment.[45] Lymphaticovenous anastomosis, initially described in 1969, is indicated when patients still have a functional lymphatic system with an underlying blockage and a venous system with intact valves (Brahma and colleagues). A meta-analysis by Basta and colleagues, compared LVA and VLN, demonstrating that both interventions are efficient in short-term outcomes; however, patients with VLN showed better long-term improvement with an increased likelihood of not needing to wear compression stockings.[33,46] In patients who are plagued by recurrent infection or failure of medical management, surgical interventions can be considered, although not widely used due to the morbidities and inability to show generalizable results.[47]

Preventative surgical options are being evaluated such as arm lymph node mapping at the time of surgery to try to find lymph nodes or sentinel lymph nodes away from those that drain the arm. Studied techniques include primary lymphovenous bypass performed at the time of axillary treatment. Again, initial findings are hopeful, but are not strong enough to make these operations commonplace.

Radiation
Radiation has evolved into a refined and precise process that is pivotal in breast cancer care. Radiotherapy techniques have continued to improve to minimize adverse

effects such as cardiomyopathy and lung damage which occurred when radiation fields of early breast cancer protocols were much larger. This is especially significant now as the indications for radiation in breast cancer continue to expand.

Overall, radiotherapy is initially tolerated fairly well, but early toxicities and late complications greatly impact the quality of life of our patients. Often, the hyperacute side effects are immediately noticeable and include fatigue, skin changes (dermatitis), and breast edema. These effects are often limited to the duration of the treatment and resolve completely within 2 weeks of completion of radiation.

The indications for radiotherapy for local control continue to increase as the treatment of the axilla moves away from axillary dissection due to the morbid complication of lymphedema. However, while the morbidity is lower, there are still long-term effects of radiation that may become more significant as the treated population continues to grow.

Early and late pulmonary complications may occur following radiation therapy as portions of the lung lie within the radiation portals: anterolateral peripheral in the setting of breast and chest wall irradiation and the lung apex in the setting of supraclavicular irradiation. One early occurring syndrome of note is bronchiolitis obliterans organizing pneumonia or bilateral lymphocytic alveolitis. This is a rare entity with symptoms including cough, dyspnea, asthenia, and weight loss that responds well to corticosteroids, has a high recurrence rate, and an excellent prognosis, virtually never progressing or developing into chronic fibrosis.[48,49] More commonly, radiation pneumonitis can occur and is seen typically in 4 to 12 weeks following the completion of radiotherapy. Symptoms can include dry cough, dyspnea, and low-grade fever. Corticosteroids are the treatment of choice and maximal improvement can be expected within 48 months. Symptoms that persist beyond 48 months will not typically improve.[48,50] Lung fibrosis can be seen as early as 6 months, peaks at 2 years, and remains stable thereafter. This is associated with limited changes in pulmonary function tests, and when occurs is irreversible.[48,50]

Cardiac toxicity is associated with the radiation of the internal mammary chain which is increasingly included in the clinical target volume as it increases overall survival.[51,52] Cardiac toxicities as a result of breast cancer treatment include left ventricular dysfunction, congestive heart failure, pericarditis, myocardial ischemia, arterial hypertension, conduction abnormalities, atrial and ventricular arrhythmias, and thromboembolic disease with the major cardiovascular toxicity of radiation therapy being coronary artery disease.[52] Techniques of radiation including proton therapy, breath-holding, optimization of the beam angles, intensity-modulated radiotherapy, and prone positioning among others are being used to attempt to decrease the cardiac effects of radiation therapy.[51]

Advances in radiation therapy have led to more favorable outcomes and radiotherapy can be routinely used in those who choose implant-based or autologous reconstruction with high satisfaction. The longer the time interval between surgery and radiation, the less likely patients are to encounter wound healing complications following reconstruction surgery (wound dehiscence).[53] Capsular contraction is seen more commonly in those patients that have radiation directly to the permanent implant as opposed to the tissue expander, but this disparity is attributed to the capsulotomy performed at the time of exchanging the tissue expander for the permanent implant. Anecdotal evidence supports the use of acellular dermal matrices for breast reconstruction as well as fat grafting to correct contour deformities, but the benefits have not been studied in a controlled manner.[54] Skin fibrosis is seen in approximately 11% of patients and is associated with ptosis (grade $^2/_3$) or pseudoptosis, bra size >/ = cup C, and a decreased time interval from surgery to radiotherapy.[53]

Telangiectasias and impaired cosmetic outcomes are also seen in late radiation toxicity and may significantly impact the quality of life of the patient.

Radiation fibrosis results in other side effects including the relatively rare complication of brachial plexus neuropathy, which is motor or sensory symptoms or physical signs with or without pain in a nerve-root distribution and may include paresthesias, hypoesthesia, hypoalgesia, dysesthesia, paresis, hyporeflexia, and muscle atrophy; this plexopathy is irreversible.[48] Fibrosis may also lead to shoulder stiffness requiring physical therapy to alleviate this fibrosis, but again, is also irreversible.

Hyperbaric therapy (HBOT) has been studied in the Netherlands as a means to alleviate late radiation toxicity and is approved by insurance in the Netherlands for different tumor sites. Late radiation toxicity is primarily characterized by breast/chest wall pain, breast and/or arm edema, fibrosis, impaired arm movement, telangiectasia, and impaired cosmetic outcome following breast cancer treated with radiotherapy.[55] Batenburg and colleagues describe the reduced pain, breast and arm symptoms, and improved quality of life following hyperbaric treatment of late radiation toxicity.[55] In 1005 patients, pain scores improved from 43.4 to 29.7 at 3 months post-HBOT; breast symptoms decreased from 44.6 to 28.9 and arm symptoms decreased from 38.2 to 27.4; all of these being significant ($P < .05$). There were minimal side effects with the most prevalent being myopia and mild barotrauma.[55]

SUMMARY

To improve the quality of life for our patients, it is essential to recognize the side effects of breast cancer treatment, identify root causes of nonspecific symptoms, and understand cancer survivorship and the anxiety, self-image, and interpersonal relationship issues that patients experience. Comprehensive counseling begins at diagnosis and includes knowing available resources and appropriate treatment at each step along our patients' breast cancer journey. The number of breast cancer survivors will continue to grow and our understanding of life after breast cancer treatment must keep pace to maximize the quality of life in survivorship.

REFERENCES

1. Cristian A. Breast cancer and gynecologic cancer rehabilitation. 2021 [Online]. Available: https://www.clinicalkey.com.au/dura/browse/bookChapter/3-s2.0-C20180032375. Accessed date May 25, 2022.
2. Jiralerspong S, Goodwin PJ. Obesity and Breast Cancer Prognosis: Evidence, Challenges, and Opportunities. J Clin Oncol 2016;34(35):4203–16. https://doi.org/10.1200/JCO.2016.68.4480.
3. Chlebowski RT, et al. Weight loss and breast cancer incidence in postmenopausal women. Cancer 2019;125(2):205–12.
4. Integrative Medicine: Search About Herbs | Memorial Sloan Kettering Cancer Center. Available at: https://www.mskcc.org/cancer-care/diagnosis-treatment/symptom-management/integrative-medicine/herbs/search. Accessed May 26, 2022.
5. Simapivapan P, Boltong A, Hodge A. To what extent is alcohol consumption associated with breast cancer recurrence and second primary breast cancer?: a systematic review. Cancer Treat. Rev 2016;50:155–67.
6. Coletta AM, Basen-Engquist KM, Schmitz KH. Exercise Across the Cancer Care Continuum: Why It Matters, How to Implement It, and Motivating Patients to Move. Am Soc Clin Oncol Educ Book 2022;42:1–7.

7. Campbell KL, et al. Exercise Recommendation for People With Bone Metastases: Expert Consensus for Health Care Providers and Exercise Professionals. JCO Oncol Pract 2022;18(5):e697–709.

8. Moving Through Cancer," Moving Through Cancer. Available at: https://www.movingthroughcancer.com. Accessed May 26, 2022.

9. Kingsberg SA, Simon JA. Female Hypoactive Sexual Desire Disorder: A Practical Guide to Causes, Clinical Diagnosis, and Treatment. J Womens Health 2020; 29(8):1101–12.

10. Kim L. Hypoactive sexual desire disorder: How do you identify it and treat it? Women's Healthc 2019. Available at: https://www.npwomenshealthcare.com/hypoactive-sexual-desire-disorder-how-do-you-identify-it-and-treat-it/. Accessed July 16, 2022.

11. Dupree B. The American Society of Breast Surgeons | ASBrS," The American Society of Breast Surgeons Fellows Webinars, Surveillance and Survivorship. 2021. https://www.breastsurgeons.org/resources/videos?v=214. Accessed May 25, 2022.

12. Gass J, et al. Breast Cancer Survivorship: Why, What and When? Ann Surg Oncol 2016;23(10):3162–7.

13. Fann JR, et al. Major depression after breast cancer: a review of epidemiology and treatment. Gen Hosp Psychiatry 2008;30(2):112–26.

14. Hermelink K. Chemotherapy and Cognitive Function in Breast Cancer Patients: The So-Called Chemo Brain. JNCI Monogr 2015;51:67–9.

15. McDonald BC, Conroy SK, Ahles TA, et al. Alterations in Brain Activation During Working Memory Processing Associated With Breast Cancer and Treatment: A Prospective Functional Magnetic Resonance Imaging Study. J Clin Oncol 2012; 30(20):2500–8.

16. Pomykala KL, de Ruiter MB, Deprez S, et al. Integrating imaging findings in evaluating the post-chemotherapy brain. Brain Imaging Behav 2013;7(4):436–52.

17. Raji MA, et al. Risk of subsequent dementia diagnoses does not vary by types of adjuvant chemotherapy in older women with breast cancer. Med Oncol Northwood Lond Engl 2009;26(4):452–9.

18. Bai L, Yu E. A narrative review of risk factors and interventions for cancer-related cognitive impairment. Ann Transl Med 2021;9(1):72.

19. Bhatnagar B, et al. Chemotherapy dose reduction due to chemotherapy induced peripheral neuropathy in breast cancer patients receiving chemotherapy in the neoadjuvant or adjuvant settings: a single-center experience. SpringerPlus 2014;3(1):366.

20. Mols F, Beijers T, Vreugdenhil G, et al. Chemotherapy-induced peripheral neuropathy and its association with quality of life: a systematic review. Support Care Cancer 2014;22(8):2261–9.

21. Stubblefield MD, et al. NCCN Task Force Report: Management of Neuropathy in Cancer. J Natl Compr Cancer Netw J Natl Compr Canc Netw 2009;7(Suppl_5). https://doi.org/10.6004/jnccn.2009.0078. S-1-S-26.

22. Stubblefield MD, McNeely ML, Alfano CM, et al. A prospective surveillance model for physical rehabilitation of women with breast cancer. Cancer 2012;118(S8): 2250–60.

23. Tofthagen C. Patient Perceptions Associated With Chemotherapy-Induced Peripheral Neuropathy. Clin J Oncol Nurs 2010;14(3). E22–E28.

24. Gutiérrez-Gutiérrez G, Sereno M, Miralles A, et al. Chemotherapy-induced peripheral neuropathy: clinical features, diagnosis, prevention and treatment strategies. Clin Transl Oncol 2010;12(2):81–91.

25. Zwart W, Terra H, Linn SC, et al. Cognitive effects of endocrine therapy for breast cancer: keep calm and carry on? Nat Rev Clin Oncol 2015;12(10). https://doi.org/10.1038/nrclinonc.2015.124. Art. no. 10.

26. Peddie N, Agnew S, Crawford M, et al. The impact of medication side effects on adherence and persistence to hormone therapy in breast cancer survivors: A qualitative systematic review and thematic synthesis. The Breast 2021;58:147–59.

27. Franzoi MA, et al. Evidence-based approaches for the management of side-effects of adjuvant endocrine therapy in patients with breast cancer. Lancet Oncol 2021;22(7). https://doi.org/10.1016/S1470-2045(20)30666-5. e303–e313.

28. Kagan R, Kellogg-Spadt S, Parish SJ. Practical Treatment Considerations in the Management of Genitourinary Syndrome of Menopause. Drugs Aging 2019;36(10):897–908.

29. Andersen KG, Kehlet H. Persistent Pain After Breast Cancer Treatment: A Critical Review of Risk Factors and Strategies for Prevention. J Pain 2011;12(7):725–46.

30. Larsson IM, Ahm Sørensen J, Bille C. The Post-mastectomy Pain Syndrome—A Systematic Review of the Treatment Modalities. Breast J 2017;23(3):338–43.

31. Gärtner R, Jensen M-B, Nielsen J, et al. Prevalence of and Factors Associated With Persistent Pain Following Breast Cancer Surgery. JAMA 2009;302(18):1985–92.

32. Chhabra A, Roy Chowdhury A, Prabhakar H, et al. Paravertebral anaesthesia with or without sedation versus general anaesthesia for women undergoing breast cancer surgery. Cochrane Database Syst Rev 2021;2. https://doi.org/10.1002/14651858.CD012968.pub2.

33. Pappalardo M, Starnoni M, Franceschini G, et al. Breast Cancer-Related Lymphedema: Recent Updates on Diagnosis, Severity and Available Treatments. J Pers Med 2021;11(5):402. https://doi.org/10.3390/jpm11050402.

34. McLaughlin S. The Valuable Ounce: Surgical and Radiation Oncology Considerations for Lymphedema Prevention," Lymphedema- Diagnosis and management. 2021. Available at: https://www.breastsurgeons.org/resources/videos?v=211. Accessed May 30, 2022.

35. Fleissig A, et al. Post-operative arm morbidity and quality of life. Results of the ALMANAC randomised trial comparing sentinel node biopsy with standard axillary treatment in the management of patients with early breast cancer. Breast Cancer Res Treat 2006;95(3):279–93.

36. Grada AA, Phillips TJ. Lymphedema: Pathophysiology and clinical manifestations. J Am Acad Dermatol 2017;77(6):1009–20.

37. Armer JM, et al. Lymphedema symptoms and limb measurement changes in breast cancer survivors treated with neoadjuvant chemotherapy and axillary dissection: results of American College of Surgeons Oncology Group (ACOSOG) Z1071 (Alliance) substudy. Support Care Cancer 2019;27(2):495–503.

38. McDuff SGR, et al. Timing of Lymphedema After Treatment for Breast Cancer: When Are Patients Most At Risk? Int J Radiat Oncol Biol Phys 2019;103(1):62–70.

39. Gillespie TC, Sayegh HE, Brunelle CL, et al. Breast cancer-related lymphedema: risk factors, precautionary measures, and treatments. Gland Surg 2018;7(4):379–403.

40. Eaton LH, Narkthong N, Hulett JM. Psychosocial Issues Associated with Breast Cancer-Related Lymphedema: a Literature Review. Curr Breast Cancer Rep 2020;12(4):216–24.

41. Asdourian MS, et al. Association Between Precautionary Behaviors and Breast Cancer–Related Lymphedema in Patients Undergoing Bilateral Surgery. J Clin Oncol 2017;35(35):3934–41.

42. McLaughlin SA, et al. Trends in Risk Reduction Practices for the Prevention of Lymphedema in the First 12 Months after Breast Cancer Surgery. J Am Coll Surg 2013;216(3):380–9.

43. Kwan ML, Cohn JC, Armer JM, et al. Exercise in patients with lymphedema: a systematic review of the contemporary literature. J Cancer Surviv 2011;5(4): 320–36.

44. Schmitz KH, et al. Effect of Home-Based Exercise and Weight Loss Programs on Breast Cancer–Related Lymphedema Outcomes Among Overweight Breast Cancer Survivors: The WISER Survivor Randomized Clinical Trial. JAMA Oncol 2019; 5(11):1605–13.

45. Gasteratos K, Morsi-Yeroyannis A, Vlachopoulos NC, et al. Microsurgical techniques in the treatment of breast cancer-related lymphedema: a systematic review of efficacy and patient outcomes. Breast Cancer Tokyo Jpn 2021;28(5): 1002–15.

46. Basta MN, et al. Complicated breast cancer–related lymphedema: evaluating health care resource utilization and associated costs of management. Am J Surg 2016;211(1):133–41.

47. Brahma B, Yamamoto T. Breast cancer treatment-related lymphedema (BCRL): An overview of the literature and updates in microsurgery reconstructions. Eur J Surg Oncol 2019;45(7):1138–45.

48. Senkus-Konefka E, Jassem J. Complications of breast-cancer radiotherapy. Clin Oncol R Coll Radiol G B 2006;18(3):229–35.

49. Ducray J, et al. [Radiation-induced bronchiolitis obliterans with organizing pneumonia]. Cancer Radiother J Soc Francaise Radiother Oncol 2017;21(2):148–54.

50. Hanania AN, Mainwaring W, Ghebre YT, et al. Radiation-Induced Lung Injury: Assessment and Management. Chest 2019;156(1):150–62.

51. Taylor CW, Kirby AM. Cardiac Side-effects From Breast Cancer Radiotherapy. Clin Oncol R Coll Radiol G B 2015;27(11):621–9.

52. Caron J, Nohria A. Cardiac Toxicity from Breast Cancer Treatment: Can We Avoid This? Curr Oncol Rep 2018;20(8):61.

53. Hille-Betz U, et al. Late radiation side effects, cosmetic outcomes and pain in breast cancer patients after breast-conserving surgery and three-dimensional conformal radiotherapy : Risk-modifying factors. Strahlenther Onkol Organ Dtsch Rontgengesellschaft Al 2016;192(1):8–16.

54. Ho AY, Hu ZI, Mehrara BJ, et al. Radiotherapy in the setting of breast reconstruction: types, techniques, and timing. Lancet Oncol 2017;18(12):e742–53.

55. Batenburg MCT, et al. The impact of hyperbaric oxygen therapy on late radiation toxicity and quality of life in breast cancer patients. Breast Cancer Res Treat 2021;189(2):425–33.

Follow-up and Cancer Survivorship

Heather B. Neuman, MD, MS[a,b,*], Jessica R. Schumacher, PhD[a,b,1]

KEYWORDS

• Breast cancer • Survivorship • Follow-up • Recurrence

KEY POINTS

• High-quality survivorship care focuses on individual's health and well-being, including disease recurrence, physical sequelae of treatment, psychosocial concerns, quality of life, and healthy behaviors.

• Breast cancer survivors have the potential to experience long-term sequelae of having a cancer diagnosis and their completed therapy, ranging from cardiotoxicity to lymphedema to sexual functioning to psychological distress.

• As most breast cancer survivors will ultimately die of non–cancer-related causes, survivors should be encouraged to have ongoing visits with their primary care provider to screening for other health conditions and cancers.

• Alternative models of survivorship care, such as transitioning survivors to a distinct survivorship clinic, sharing care with primary care, or transferring the responsibility of survivorship care to primary care, are likely all equally effective at delivering survivorship care.

Currently, more than 3.5 million breast cancer survivors live in the United States.[1] With 5-year survival for local-regional cancer exceeding 90%,[1] that number will continue to grow. Survivorship is a continuum that starts at the time of diagnosis and continues until death.[2] Survivorship focuses on individual's health and well-being, considering disease recurrence, physical symptoms associated with treatment, psychosocial concerns, quality of life, and the economic impact of cancer. In addition, survivorship includes an emphasis on healthy behaviors (**Fig. 1**). This article reviews the recommendations for survivors in the post-treatment phase of the cancer continuum and the level of evidence supporting each aspect of high-quality survivorship care.

CANCER RECURRENCE

Both providers and survivors consider evaluating for cancer recurrence as the priority for follow-up care.[3,4] In fact, in our work with survivor stakeholders, survivors describe

[a] Wisconsin Surgical Outcomes Research Program, Department of Surgery, Madison, WI, USA;
[b] University of Wisconsin Carbone Cancer Center, Madison, WI, USA
[1] Present address: K6/144 CSC, 600 Highland Avenue, Madison, WI 53792-1690.
* Corresponding author. K6/142 CSC, 600 Highland Avenue, Madison, WI.
E-mail address: neuman@surgery.wisc.edu

Surg Clin N Am 103 (2023) 169–185
https://doi.org/10.1016/j.suc.2022.08.009
0039-6109/23/© 2022 Elsevier Inc. All rights reserved.

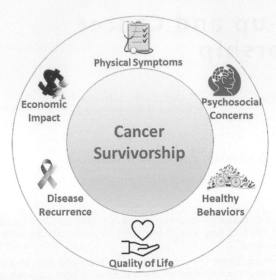

Fig. 1. Key survivorship domains.

the reassurance they received from a visit where no evidence of cancer was found to be the most valued aspect of follow-up.[4] However, survivors commonly experience anticipatory anxiety before follow-up clinic visits or breast imaging.[5,6] In addition, follow-up can be associated with both financial and emotional costs for survivors due to visit co-pays and travel, and time away from work or family. Providing follow-up care for the growing number of survivors can also be burdensome for the health care system. Given the workforce shortages facing both primary care and oncology,[7,8] provision of survivorship care could impede access for newly diagnosed patients or even delay care. It is critical that follow-up care be delivered deliberately in order to optimize access to high-quality care while reducing the burden for both survivors and providers.

Current clinical practice guidelines exist for follow-up care, published by the American Society for Clinical Oncology (ASCO) and the National Comprehensive Cancer Network (NCCN).[9–11] Both recommend frequent history and physical examinations (**Fig. 2**). The NCCN recommended 1 to 4 visits per year for the first 5 years, as "clinically appropriate." The ASCO recommends a follow-up visit every 3 to 6 months for the first 3 years, then every 6 to 12 months until year 5. Both guidelines recommend annual visits after year 5. No systemic surveillance imaging or laboratory testing is recommended for survivors who are asymptomatic.

	NCCN	ASCO
History & Physical Exam	• 1–4 times per year for 5 y • Annual after 5 y	• Every 3–6 mo for 3 y • Every 6–12 mo for 2 y • Annual after 5 y
Mammogram	Annual[a]	Annual[a]
Gynecologic exam	Age-appropriate screening[b]	Annual[b]
Bone mineral density[c]	Baseline and periodically	Baseline and every 2 y

Fig. 2. Overview of clinical practice guidelines follow-up recommendations. ASCO, American Society for Clinical Oncology; NCCN, National Comprehensive Cancer Network. [a]For women with at-risk breast tissue. [b]For women on tamoxifen. [c]For women on AI or premenopausal with chemotheraphy-induced ovarian failure.

It is worth emphasizing that follow-up recommendations from the NCCN and ASCO are one-size-fits-all, regardless of cancer stage or receptor subtype.[9-11] Current recommendations for frequent follow-up visits within the first 5 years are largely based on older data, such as that published by Saphner and colleagues.[12] In this study published in 1996, researchers evaluated patients who were enrolled in 7 Eastern Cooperative Oncology Group trials and estimated the annual hazard of breast cancer recurrence. The researchers demonstrated that the peak hazard of recurrence occurred during the first 5 years. In addition, the researchers observed a difference in the hazard of recurrence based on estrogen receptor (ER) status, with patients with ER-negative cancer having a higher hazard in years 0 to 5 compared to patients with ER-positive cancer. Of note, the trials included in this analysis were all conducted before routine HER2 testing and HER2-targeted therapy, which is a significant limitation.

With modern era targeted therapy toward ER, progesterone receptors (PR), and HER2, the absolute rates of both local and distant recurrence for breast cancer survivors have declined. There is also clear variability in outcomes based on receptor subtype. The current 8th edition AJCC prognostic staging system reflects the importance of receptor subtype by incorporating ER, PR, and HER2 into the staging.[13,14] This has led to shifts in staging when comparing the prognostic staging system with the traditional anatomic staging (Table 1).[15] For example, many triple-negative cancers are staged higher relative to similar ER- and PR-positive and/or HER2-positive cancers, in recognition of the differences in survival outcomes based on receptor subtype.[13,14] Importantly, evidence demonstrates that the timing of recurrence also varies based on the receptor subtype. For example, several studies have reported that some patients with ER-positive cancers have delayed recurrence as late as 15 to 20 years after diagnosis.[16,17] This data supports that the common conceptualization of focused cancer follow-up within the first 5 years after diagnosis might be outdated for some patients.

In current clinical practice, there is significant variation observed in how frequently follow-up visits occur.[18,19] This suggests that providers may be personalizing their follow-up recommendations to the given patient. Although practice guidelines do not give specific guidance as to how to personalize follow-up, these guidelines do encourage personalization in that they delineate a range of follow-up frequency that is acceptable.[9-11] Based on the available evidence, providers should consider both the likelihood and the timing of recurrence based on tumor size, lymph nodes status, and receptor subtype when making recommendations for frequency of follow-up visits

Table 1			
Examples of stage migration within the 8th edition AJCC staging			
Tumor Size and Lymph Node Status	Receptor Subtype and Grade	Anatomic Stage	Prognostic Stage
T3N0	ER- PR- Her2-Grade 3	Stage IIB	Stage IIIA
T2N1	ER + PR + Her2+Grade 1	Stage IIB	Stage IA
T1N0	ER- PR- Her2-Grade 2	Stage IA	Stage IB
T1N1	ER + PR + Her2-Grade 3	Stage IIA	Stage IB

Abbreviations: ER, estrogen receptor; PR progesterone receptor.

for a given survivor. It is likely that genomic testing could also contribute to follow-up recommendations, although that data are still evolving.

Current practice guidelines recommend against systemic imaging or laboratory testing when assessing for distant recurrence, relying solely on a thorough review of symptoms.[9–11] These practice guidelines are based on randomized controlled trials from the 1980s that evaluated whether "more" versus "less" intensive follow-up regimens impact survival (**Table 2**).[20,21] None of these trials, or a subsequent 2005 Cochrane review, reported a benefit to a "more" intensive regimen.[20–22] Although these trials provide level I evidence to inform practice guidelines, they have several limitations. First, the imaging modalities within the "more" intensive arm of the trials were liver ultrasounds and chest x-rays. More advanced imaging modalities, such as computed tomography (CT) scans or PET/CTs, are substantially more sensitive, with the potential to identify smaller volume diseases at an earlier time point. Furthermore, the randomized controlled trials were conducted before receptor subtyping of cancer and the availability of targeted therapy. It is possible that survivors with certain receptor subtypes may benefit relatively more or less from earlier identification of metastatic disease. A recent cohort study evaluated this hypothesis by comparing survival for women who developed distant metastatic disease based on whether the metastasis was identified on asymptomatic surveillance imaging versus based on patient's symptoms.[23] The authors evaluated whether the association between reasons for detection and survival differed by receptor subtype. In this study, detection of metastatic disease through asymptomatic surveillance imaging was associated with improved survival for women with triple-negative cancer. This datum is intriguing and suggests that a future clinical trial may be warranted to test whether surveillance imaging for survivors with high-risk triple-negative cancer improves survival. Importantly, this study also demonstrated no difference in survival based on the method of detection of metastasis for women with ER, PR, and/or HER2-positive cancer. This observation provides important confirmatory evidence in support of current recommendations against asymptomatic surveillance imaging for these receptor subtypes. Observational studies have reported that breast cancer survivors are receiving surveillance imaging to evaluate for asymptomatic metastases despite the lack of proven benefits.[24–27] However, a more recent study suggests that most women undergoing systemic imaging actually have symptoms, with only a minority undergoing sequential asymptomatic imaging.[28] In this retrospective study based on the National Cancer Database, registrars were asked to abstract all follow-up imaging received, including the indication. The low rate of asymptomatic imaging observed may represent a successful outcome for the Choosing Wisely campaign, which recommended asymptomatic surveillance testing for breast cancer surveillance be considered low-value care.[29]

Assessing for local recurrence and new primary cancer are additional key aspects of follow-up. In general, guidelines recommend annual surveillance mammography for any remaining at-risk tissue. This should start at least 6 months following radiation. Prior studies have not demonstrated a benefit to more frequent mammograms,[9–11,30] unless driven by patient-reported symptoms.

MRI screening may play a complementary role to screening mammography for some cancer survivors. In general, the utility of MRI screening in women with a personal history of breast cancer is poorly defined.[31,32] MRI screening for breast cancer survivors can be considered for survivors who meet American Cancer Society Guidelines for Breast Cancer Screening with MRI,[33] or for women whose lifetime risk of breast cancer exceeded 20% before their cancer diagnosis.[10] However, women with a personal history of breast cancer are at higher risk of developing a future breast

Table 2
Overview of randomized controlled trials evaluating systemic imaging as a component of breast cancer follow-up

Publication Year	Intensive Follow-Up	Control Follow-Up	
Roselli, et al.1994[101]	Chest x-ray and bone scan every 6 mo	Physical examination alone	No difference in 5-y mortality (18.6% vs 19.5%)
GIVIO Investigators,[20] 1994	Chest x-ray every 6 mo; bone scan annually; liver ultrasound annually	Physical examination alone	No difference in 5-y mortality (20% vs 18%)

cancer based solely on their own personal history.[34–36] At our institution, we noted substantial variation in the use of MRI screening for women with a personal history of cancer.[37] We created a multidisciplinary stakeholder group composed of UW Breast Center members to review available data and develop an algorithm to inform the use of MRI screening within our own institution (**Fig. 3**). In the developed algorithm, survivors with a lifetime risk of breast cancer >20% before their cancer would be eligible to consider MRI, consistent with prior recommendations.[10,33] However, the algorithm also considers women's own personal history of cancer in the risk estimation. In calculating their lifetime risk, we allowed a generous annual new cancer incidence of 0.25% to 0.5% per year, making all women less than 50 years of age eligible based on their personal history alone. The algorithm also considers women with occult primary cancer or extremely dense breasts to be eligible.[37–39] This algorithm can be a framework to guide clinician and survivor discussions about the role of MRI screening for women with a personal history of cancer, until more robust data are available.

One final topic worth commenting on is the use of imaging to evaluate for local recurrence in women treated with mastectomy. Physical examination is the primary means of assessing for local recurrence in this setting, with no routine imaging recommended even for women who underwent postmastectomy reconstruction.[40] For women with subpectoral implants, the physical examination is sensitive, as the at-risk tissue is projected anteriorly. There has been debate around the merits of imaging for women with either prepectoral implants or autologous reconstruction, given that the pectoralis margin cannot be examined. However, if the pectoralis fascia is removed, which should be the standard for an oncologic mastectomy, the risk of recurrent disease under the reconstruction should be very uncommon.

EVALUATION OF ADHERENCE TO ONGOING ENDOCRINE THERAPY

Although survivors cite reassurance about recurrence as their priority for follow-up, oncology providers additionally prioritize assessing for adherence to ongoing therapy.[41] This is most relevant for women with ER+ and/or PR+ cancers being treated with endocrine therapy. Endocrine therapy is an important component of cancer treatment and contributes to the good prognosis observed for women with ER- and PR-positive cancer. However, adherence to endocrine therapy is mixed, with as many as 50% of women not completing their prescribed course of endocrine therapy.[42–45] Side effects are commonly cited as the reason for discontinuation, specifically hot flashes and musculoskeletal concerns. These symptoms can have a significant impact on women's quality of life and impact adherence to treatment. For women with

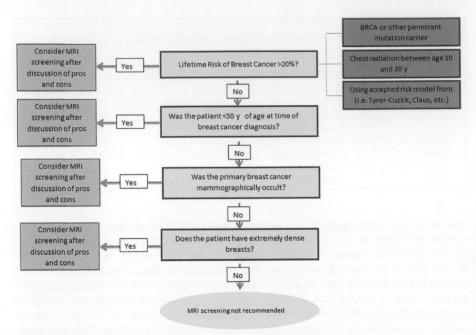

Fig. 3. University of Wisconsin health system algorithm to inform the use of MRI screening in women with a personal history of breast cancer.

significant vasomotor symptoms, medications such as selective serotonin reuptake inhibitors have been reported to decrease the intensity of hot flashes.[11] Some studies have also demonstrated that complementary therapies such as acupuncture may reduce the burden of symptoms. Finally, lifestyle modifications, including avoiding food or alcohol triggers, may be beneficial for some women. Musculoskeletal concerns such as arthralgias are common for women taking aromatase inhibitors, and in some cases severe enough to lead to treatment discontinuation. Changing from one endocrine therapy to another can sometimes be beneficial (either to another aromatase inhibitor or to tamoxifen). Long-term sequelae of aromatase inhibitors can be osteopenia. Ensuring that ongoing assessment of bone health for women who are treated with aromatase inhibitors occurs is another important component of follow-up for women on these endocrine therapies.[9–11] The existing literature suggests that in addition to managing side effects, provider encouragement and reinforcement of the importance of adhering to endocrine therapy to optimize cancer outcomes are critical to improving adherence.[46–48] Discussing adherence to endocrine therapy should therefore be a priority during all follow-up visits.

SEQUELAE OF COMPLETED TREATMENT

As we described at the start of the article, breast cancer survival is excellent because of the success of mammogram screening and improvements in modern-era targeted therapy.[1] However, more women surviving their breast cancer also means more women have the potential to experience long-term sequelae of having a cancer diagnosis and their completed therapy. These sequelae include a wide range of potential concerns ranging from cardiotoxicity to lymphedema to sexual functioning to psychological distress. The prevalence of symptoms or concerns in breast cancer survivors is high.[49,50] The American Cancer Society/American Society of Clinical Oncology Breast Cancer Survivorship Care Guidelines include a very detailed list of the domains that should be considered when caring for breast cancer survivors (**Table 3**). We will highlight some of the areas in the section that follows.

Sequelae of Chemotherapy and HER2-Targeted Therapy

Chemotherapy and other systemic therapy, such as HER2-targeted therapy, can be associated with long-term sequelae. Symptoms or concerns most common for breast cancer survivors after chemotherapy include cardiotoxicity, changes in cognition, fatigue, and neuropathy. These symptoms are especially challenging as they may overlap with symptoms nonsurvivors experience over the course of aging. Fortunately, the proportion of breast cancer survivors who have received chemotherapy has decreased over the past decade.[51,52] For survivors who still require systemic therapy, monitoring for further evaluation of intervention is warranted and should be considered during both primary care and oncology visits.

Sequelae of Local-Regional Therapy

The vast majority of breast cancer survivors undergo some type of local regional treatment, either surgery alone or combined with radiation. Body image is a significant concern for most breast cancer survivors. Current guidelines on acceptable margin width have decreased the volume of breast tissue that must be removed and oncoplastic surgical techniques have helped to improve the cosmetic outcome after breast-conserving surgery. Postmastectomy breast reconstruction is increasingly available, and as many as 50% of women undergoing mastectomy receive breast reconstruction.[53,54] Despite these improvements, breast surgery can have an impact on body image. The changes in body image can impact survivors differently, with some survivors experiencing a negative impact on quality of life. Assessing for satisfaction with cosmetic outcome to identify opportunities to intervene, either through referrals to plastic surgery or to cancer psychologists, is important.

Breast surgery can also frequently lead to chest/breast pain and limitations to range of motion, as high as 40% in our own institutional experience. For many survivors, the presence of pain is distressing in part because it raises concerns about cancer recurrence and is a constant reminder of their cancer. Reassurance is sometimes all that is required. For other women, nonsteroidal anti-inflammatory drugs, gabapentin, or referral to occupational therapists or pain service may be necessary.

Finally, routine assessment for lymphedema is critical. Lymphedema related to breast cancer is common after axillary interventions to control disease. Lymphedema is most commonly observed after axillary lymph node dissection, occurring in 13% to 60% of patients.[55-57] However, lymphedema can also develop after a sentinel lymph node biopsy alone, albeit at lower rates. The ACOSOG Z0010 trial prospectively tracked rates of lymphedema (defined as a change in baseline arm circumference of >2 cm) for patients undergoing sentinel lymph node biopsy and reported a rate of 6.9% at 6 months postoperative.[58] Increasingly, axillary radiation is being used as a component of breast cancer treatment, which when combined with axillary surgery increases lymphedema rates.[59] However, axillary radiation used instead of axillary surgery to obtain local-regional control is associated with lower overall rates.[60]

Early identification and intervention is important to provide durable control of symptoms. Current practice guidelines endorse routine screening for lymphedema using both clinical symptoms and objective measures. The American Society of Breast Surgeons[61] and the NCCN[10] encourage preoperative baseline arm measurements to account for baseline asymmetry in arm circumference. Numerous means of objectively

Table 3
Overview of treatment modality and potential sequelae

Treatment Type	Potential Sequelae
Endocrine therapy	• Hot flashes •Bone health •Musculoskeletal symptoms/pain •Increased risk of stroke •Increased risk of endometrial cancer
Chemotherapy and Her2-targeted therapy	•Cognitive impairment •Fatigue •Infertility •Weight gain •Neuropathy •Cardiac toxicity
Local-regional therapy	•Body image •Sexual function •Breast/Chest wall pain •Limited range of motion •Poor cosmetic outcome •Lymphedema •Neuropathy
Other	•Sexual health •Infertility •Mental health concerns (depressions, anxiety) •Financial hardship

assessing for lymphedema exist. However, limb circumference is most commonly used given the ease of integrating into clinical practice. Patients with signs or symptoms of lymphedema should be referred to a certified lymphedema therapist. Early interventions are composed of manual lymphatic drainage and compression. For more advanced lymphedema, surgical intervention may have merit.[62]

A variety of precautionary recommendations have historically been considered with the goal of minimizing the risk of lymphedema. These include things like avoiding blood draws, intravenous catheters or blood pressure cuffs in the "at-risk" arm, avoiding use of hot tubs, and wearing compression sleeves when flying. These guidelines were largely developed based on consensus opinion. However, more recent data demonstrate that these precautionary measures may have limited effect at either preventing or decreasing the risk of lymphedema.[63,64] Although it is likely still reasonable to preferentially avoid the "at-risk" arm for medical procedures, survivors should be reassured that the actual risk of developing lymphedema as a consequence of this mild trauma is likely quite low.

On a final note, there has been much discussion over the years about the role of exercise, specifically upper body weight lifting, for breast cancer survivors at risk of lymphedema. Randomized clinical trials have demonstrated that slow progressive weight lifting program does not increase the risk of lymphedema.[65,66] Exercise should be encouraged for breast cancer survivors.

Other Sequelae of Breast Cancer

Although there are several other sequelae that can result from a cancer diagnosis, 3 are especially relevant for breast cancer survivors. First, sexual function is frequently impacted by a breast cancer diagnosis.[67,68] This is multifactorial and can stem from changes in body image due to surgery, changes in sensitivity of the breast, and general side effects of systemic treatment (vaginal dryness, dyspareunia, loss of desire). These symptoms are common in breast cancer survivors. However, sexual function is not routinely discussed as a part of follow-up visits, due to the sensitive nature of the topic and the number of competing priorities that must be addressed during a visit.[69] It is important to assess for sexual health in order to identify opportunities to improve symptoms through recommendation for lubricants, counseling, and in severe cases, vaginal estrogens. At our institution, we are fortunate to have a Women's Integrated Sexual Health clinic to which we can refer cancer survivors experiencing symptoms.

Assessing for mental health is another significant aspect of breast cancer follow-up. Many survivors struggle with anxiety and fear of recurrence,[70–72] especially early in the transition from active treatment to surveillance. For some women, discussion of these fears with their oncology and primary care providers is enough to provide reassurance. However, for others, treatment with medication and/or psychotherapy is necessary. Routine screening for mental health using validated tools such as the Patient Health Questionnaire-9[73] and the Generalized Anxiety Disorder 7-item scale[74] may be beneficial as a way of identifying survivors who may benefit from further intervention.

Finally, diagnosis of breast cancer impacts survivors and their families financially, often long after diagnosis and treatment.[75,76] A recent study of breast cancer survivors up to 12 years following their diagnosis suggests survivors have annual adjusted health-related out-of-pocket costs of $2792, with higher costs ($3325) if the survivor has lymphedema.[77] These higher out-of-pocket costs are an important driver of quality of life for survivors.

HEALTH PROMOTION

Because of the high survival rate associated with an early-stage breast cancer diagnosis, most breast cancer survivors will ultimately die of other causes.[78–80] However, cancer survivors often prioritize their cancer care over care, including wellness visits or management of other chronic conditions.[81–83] Survivors should be encouraged to have ongoing visits with their primary care provider (and establish care if they do not have one) to ensure screening for other health conditions (hypertension, hypercholesterolemia, diabetes) and cancers (colon cancer, cervical cancer, lung cancer). This likely will have as high of an impact on their longevity as will their cancer follow-up care.

Weight Loss and Maintaining a Healthy Weight

The majority of women (~60%) newly diagnosed with breast cancer are overweight or obese.[11] Obesity has been associated with both an increased rate of breast cancer recurrence and cancer-related death, as high as 35% increase.[84] In addition, obesity is associated with numerous other chronic conditions that can decrease longevity, such as diabetes and heart disease. Providers of survivorship care can play a key role in motivating survivors to prioritize weight loss by emphasizing the importance of obesity on cancer outcomes.

Physical Activity

Current guidelines recommend that survivors engage in regular physical activity, aiming for at least 150 minutes of moderate or 75 minutes of vigorous aerobic exercise per week; strength training is recommended at least 2 days per week.[85] Existing data suggest that physical activity improves not only physical functioning but also mental health and quality of life. Physical activity has also been associated with reductions in cancer recurrence and improvements in breast cancer-specific survival, making it another modifiable risk factor.[86]

Alcohol Intake

Alcohol intake is a known carcinogen associated with the development of a variety of cancers, including breast cancer.[87] However, a growing body of evidence also suggests that alcohol intake is associated with the risk of cancer recurrence. A 2016 systematic review demonstrated that alcohol levels as low as 6 g per day may increase the risk of a breast cancer recurrence; these effects may be stronger in women who are postmenopausal or overweight.[88] Although there is significant heterogeneity in the available data, it is reasonable to counsel survivors about the potential relationship between alcohol intake and recurrence, and encourage moderation in alcohol consumption.

MODELS OF DELIVERING SURVIVORSHIP CARE

Providing comprehensive survivorship care to breast cancer survivors is challenging. Traditionally, ongoing survivorship care occurred within the setting of oncology clinics. However, alternative models of survivorship care have been described such as transitioning survivors to a distinct survivorship clinic, sharing care with primary care, or even transferring the responsibility of survivorship care entirely to primary care.[89–91] It is likely that any model is equally able to provide high-quality care, assuming key components of care as outlined in this article are being addressed. Models may be differentially able to be implemented in different care settings, as they require different levels of resources. For example, a distinct survivorship clinic may be less feasible in a lower resource setting, although it may be highly successful in a higher volume setting with the resources to support it. Shared care requires a significant coordination between oncology and primary care to delineate each of their responsibilities and articulate this to survivors, which can be quite burdensome. Furthermore, though randomized controlled trial data demonstrate that survivorship care provided by primary care can be equivalent to oncology-based care, the primary care workforce shortage in the United States presents challenges to this model of care.[8,92] It is likely that different models of care matched to the resources of the health care delivery setting are necessary. Given that needs of survivors also vary based on their risk of recurrence and treatment received, risk-stratification of survivorship care is likely also needed.

IMPACT OF SURVIVORSHIP CARE PLANS ON SURVIVORSHIP CARE

Survivorship care plans have held a prominent position in any discussion about survivorship care over the past several years. They were recommended by the Institute of Medicine in 2005 as a way to improve the quality of survivorship care[93] and included as a quality metric by the American College of Surgeons Commission on Cancer in 2016 (Standard 3.3).[94] However, numerous clinical trials have failed to demonstrate an improvement in patient outcomes in association with the delivery of survivorship care plans.[95–98] This may be due in part to limitations in trial designs. However, integrating survivorship care plans into clinical practice has been shown to be challenging and highly resource intensive.[99,100] Because of evolving experiences with survivorship care plan implementation and the negative results of clinical trials testing their effectiveness, the CoC standard 4.8 removed the quality guideline for survivorship care plans, instead focusing on a team-based strategy for implementing high-quality survivorship care.

CLINICS CARE POINTS

- Survivforship care should include evaluation for recurrence, sequelae of treatment, and overall health and well-being.Providers should evaluate for long-term sequelae of cancer treatment, including surgical sequelae (e.g. cosmetic outcome, lymphedema), radiation (e.g. range of motion), chemotherapy (e.g. cardiotoxicity) and endocrine therapy (e.g. hot flashes).

- Survivors should be encouraged to pursue wellness care with their primary care providers

SUMMARY

Provision of high-quality survivorship care to the more than 3.5 million (and growing) breast cancer survivors is critical. As treatment for breast cancer becomes increasingly personalized, so must our approach to survivorship. Risk-stratifying survivorship care to address survivors' risk of recurrence, risk of treatment side effects, and quality of life is necessary to ensure we meet survivors' needs. No one model of survivorship care delivery has been shown to be superior. Considering available resources within the center, including which individuals have capacity, expertise, and interest in providing survivorship care, is a critical first step.

DISCLOSURE

The authors have nothing to disclose.

REFERENCES

1. DeSantis CE, Ma J, Gaudet MM, et al. Breast cancer statistics, 2019. CA: a Cancer J clinicians 2019;69(6):438–51.
2. Committee on Cancer Survivorship: improving care and quality of life, Institute of medicine and national research council. From cancer patient to cancer survivor: lost in transition. Washington, DC: National Academy of Sciences; 2006.
3. Neuman HB, Steffens NM, Jacobson N, et al. Oncologists' Perspectives of Their Roles and Responsibilities During Multi-disciplinary Breast Cancer Follow-Up. Ann Surg Oncol 2016;23(3):708–14.
4. Tucholka JL, Jacobson N, Steffens NM, et al. Breast cancer survivor's perspectives on the role different providers play in follow-up care. Support Care Cancer 2018;26(6):2015–22.
5. McGinty HL, Small BJ, Laronga C, et al. Predictors and patterns of fear of cancer recurrence in breast cancer survivors. Health Psychol 2016;35(1):1–9.
6. Stark D, Kiely M, Smith A, et al. Reassurance and the anxious cancer patient. Br J Cancer 2004;91(5):893–9.
7. Yang W, Williams JH, Hogan PF, et al. Projected supply of and demand for oncologists and radiation oncologists through 2025: an aging, better-insured population will result in shortage. J Oncol Pract/Am Soc Clin Oncol 2014;10(1):39–45.
8. The complexities of physician supply and demand: projections from 2018-2033. Washington, DC: Association of American Medical Colleges; 2020.
9. Khatcheressian JL, Hurley P, Bantug E, et al. Breast cancer follow-up and management after primary treatment: American Society of Clinical Oncology clinical practice guideline update. J Clin Oncol 2013;31(7):961–5.

10. National Comprehensive Cancer Network. National comprehensive cancer Network clinical practice guidelines in oncology: breast cancer 2022. Available at: http://www.nccn.org/professionals/physician_gls/pdf/breast.pdf. Accessed January 14, 2022.

11. Runowicz CD, Leach CR, Henry NL, et al. American Cancer Society/American Society of Clinical Oncology Breast Cancer Survivorship Care Guideline. J Clin Oncol 2016;34(6):611–35.

12. Saphner T, Tormey DC, Gray R. Annual hazard rates of recurrence for breast cancer after primary therapy. J Clin Oncol 1996;14(10):2738–46.

13. Giuliano AE, Edge SB, Hortobagyi GN. Eighth Edition of the AJCC Cancer Staging Manual: Breast Cancer. Ann Surg Oncol 2018;25(7):1783–5.

14. Weiss A, Chavez-MacGregor M, Lichtensztajn DY, et al. Validation Study of the American Joint Committee on Cancer Eighth Edition Prognostic Stage Compared With the Anatomic Stage in Breast Cancer. JAMA Oncol 2018;4(2): 203–9.

15. Plichta JK, Ren Y, Thomas SM, et al. Implications for Breast Cancer Restaging Based on the 8th Edition AJCC Staging Manual. Ann Surg 2020;271(1):169–76.

16. Colleoni M, Sun Z, Price KN, et al. Annual Hazard Rates of Recurrence for Breast Cancer During 24 Years of Follow-Up: Results From the International Breast Cancer Study Group Trials I to V. J Clin Oncol 2016;34(9):927–35.

17. Pan H, Gray R, Braybrooke J, et al. 20-Year Risks of Breast-Cancer Recurrence after Stopping Endocrine Therapy at 5 Years. N Engl J Med 2017;377(19): 1836–46.

18. Neuman HB, Weiss JM, Schrag D, et al. Patient demographic and tumor characteristics influencing oncologist follow-up frequency in older breast cancer survivors. Ann Surg Oncol 2013;20(13):4128–36.

19. Ganz PA, Hahn EE, Petersen L, et al. Quality of Posttreatment Care Among Breast Cancer Survivors in the University of California Athena Breast Health Network (Athena). Clin Breast Cancer 2016;16(5):356–63.

20. GIVIO Investigators. Impact of follow-up testing on survival and health-related quality of life in breast cancer patients. A multicenter randomized controlled trial. JAMA 1994;271(20):1587–92.

21. Rosselli Del Turco M, Palli D, Cariddi A, et al. Intensive diagnostic follow-up after treatment of primary breast cancer. A randomized trial. National Research Council Project on Breast Cancer Follow-Up. JAMA 1994;271(20):1593–7.

22. Rojas MP, Telaro E, Russo A, et al. Follow-up strategies for women treated for early breast cancer. Cochrane Database Syst Rev 2005;(1):CD001768.

23. Schumacher JR, Neuman HB, Yu M, et al. Surveillance imaging vs symptomatic recurrence detection and survival in stage II-III breast cancer (AFT-01). J Natl Cancer Inst 2022. https://doi.org/10.1093/jnci/djac131.

24. Grunfeld E, Hodgson DC, Del Giudice ME, et al. Population-based longitudinal study of follow-up care for breast cancer survivors. J Oncol Pract/Am Soc Clin Oncol 2010;6(4):174–81.

25. Panageas KS, Sima CS, Liberman L, et al. Use of high technology imaging for surveillance of early stage breast cancer. Breast Cancer Res Treat 2012;131(2): 663–70.

26. Hahn EE, Hays RD, Kahn KL, et al. Use of Imaging and Biomarker Tests for Posttreatment Care of Early-Stage Breast Cancer Survivors. Cancer-am Cancer Soc 2013;119(24):4316–24.

27. Geurts SM, de Vegt F, Siesling S, et al. Pattern of follow-up care and early relapse detection in breast cancer patients. Breast Cancer Research Treat 2012;136(3):859–68.

28. Schumacher JR, Neuman HB, Chang GJ, et al. A National Study of the Use of Asymptomatic Systemic Imaging for Surveillance Following Breast Cancer Treatment (AFT-01). Ann Surg Oncol 2018;25(9):2587–95.

29. American Board of Internal Medicine Foundation. Choosing wisely clinician lists. Available at: http://www.choosingwisely.org/clinician-lists. Accessed April 11, 2016.

30. McNaul D, Darke M, Garg M, et al. An evaluation of post-lumpectomy recurrence rates: is follow-up every 6 months for 2 years needed? J Surg Oncol 2013;107(6):597–601.

31. Haas CB, Nekhlyudov L, Lee JM, et al. Surveillance for second breast cancer events in women with a personal history of breast cancer using breast MRI: a systematic review and meta-analysis. Breast Cancer Res Treat 2020;181(2):255–68.

32. Wernli K, Brandzel S, Buist D, et al. In: Is Breast MRI Better at Finding Second Breast Cancers than Mammograms Alone for Breast Cancer Survivors? Washington (DC)2019.

33. Saslow D, Boetes C, Burke W, et al. American Cancer Society guidelines for breast screening with MRI as an adjunct to mammography. CA: a Cancer J Clinicians 2007;57(2):75–89.

34. Bouchardy C, Benhamou S, Fioretta G, et al. Risk of second breast cancer according to estrogen receptor status and family history. Breast Cancer Res Treat 2011;127(1):233–41.

35. Kurian AW, McClure LA, John EM, et al. Second primary breast cancer occurrence according to hormone receptor status. J Natl Cancer Inst 2009;101(15):1058–65.

36. Fowble B, Hanlon A, Freedman G, et al. Second cancers after conservative surgery and radiation for stages I-II breast cancer: identifying a subset of women at increased risk. Int J Radiat Oncol Biol Phys 2001;51(3):679–90.

37. Strigel RM, Bravo E, Tevaarwerk AJ, et al. Development and Implementation of an Algorithm to Guide MRI Screening in Patients With a Personal History of Treated Breast Cancer. Clin Breast Cancer 2021;21(1):26–30.

38. Yang TJ, Yang Q, Haffty BG, et al. Prognosis for mammographically occult, early-stage breast cancer patients treated with breast-conservation therapy. Int J Radiat Oncol Biol Phys 2010;76(1):79–84.

39. Boyd NF, Guo H, Martin LJ, et al. Mammographic density and the risk and detection of breast cancer. N Engl J Med 2007;356(3):227–36.

40. Zakhireh J, Fowble B, Esserman LJ. Application of screening principles to the reconstructed breast. J Clin Oncol 2010;28(1):173–80.

41. Neuman HB, Steffens N, Tevaarwerk AJ, et al. Oncologists' priorities for breast cancer follow-up. Am Soc Clin Oncol 2014.

42. Partridge AH, LaFountain A, Mayer E, et al. Adherence to initial adjuvant anastrozole therapy among women with early-stage breast cancer. J Clin Oncol 2008;26(4):556–62.

43. Nekhlyudov L, Li L, Ross-Degnan D, et al. Five-year patterns of adjuvant hormonal therapy use, persistence, and adherence among insured women with early-stage breast cancer. Breast Cancer Res Treat 2011;130(2):681–9.

44. Hershman DL, Kushi LH, Shao T, et al. Early discontinuation and nonadherence to adjuvant hormonal therapy in a cohort of 8,769 early-stage breast cancer patients. J Clin Oncol 2010;28(27):4120–8.

45. Ruddy K, Mayer E, Partridge A. Patient adherence and persistence with oral anticancer treatment. CA Cancer J Clin 2009;59(1):56–66.

46. Hershman DL. Sticking to It: Improving Outcomes by Increasing Adherence. J Clin Oncol 2016;34(21):2440–2.

47. Henry NL, Azzouz F, Desta Z, et al. Predictors of aromatase inhibitor discontinuation as a result of treatment-emergent symptoms in early-stage breast cancer. J Clin Oncol 2012;30(9):936–42.

48. Chim K, Xie SX, Stricker CT, et al. Joint pain severity predicts premature discontinuation of aromatase inhibitors in breast cancer survivors. BMC Cancer 2013; 13:401.

49. Mustafa Ali M, Moeller M, Rybicki L, et al. Prevalence and correlates of patient-reported symptoms and comorbidities in breast cancer survivors at a tertiary center. J Cancer Survivorship : Res Pract 2017;11(6):743–50.

50. de Ligt KM, Heins M, Verloop J, et al. Patient-reported health problems and healthcare use after treatment for early-stage breast cancer. Breast 2019; 46:4–11.

51. Kurian AW, Bondarenko I, Jagsi R, et al. Recent Trends in Chemotherapy Use and Oncologists' Treatment Recommendations for Early-Stage Breast Cancer. J Natl Cancer Inst 2018;110(5):493–500.

52. Dinan MA, Mi X, Reed SD, et al. Association Between Use of the 21-Gene Recurrence Score Assay and Receipt of Chemotherapy Among Medicare Beneficiaries With Early-Stage Breast Cancer, 2005-2009. JAMA Oncol 2015;1(8): 1098–109.

53. Schumacher JR, Taylor LJ, Tucholka JL, et al. Socioeconomic Factors Associated with Post-Mastectomy Immediate Reconstruction in a Contemporary Cohort of Breast Cancer Survivors. Ann Surg Oncol 2017;24(10):3017–23.

54. Jonczyk MM, Jean J, Graham R, et al. Surgical trends in breast cancer: a rise in novel operative treatment options over a 12 year analysis. Breast Cancer Res Treat 2019;173(2):267–74.

55. Boughey JC, Suman VJ, Mittendorf EA, et al. Sentinel lymph node surgery after neoadjuvant chemotherapy in patients with node-positive breast cancer: the ACOSOG Z1071 (Alliance) clinical trial. JAMA 2013;310(14):1455–61.

56. Krag DN, Anderson SJ, Julian TB, et al. Sentinel-lymph-node resection compared with conventional axillary-lymph-node dissection in clinically node-negative patients with breast cancer: overall survival findings from the NSABP B-32 randomised phase 3 trial. Lancet Oncol 2010;11(10):927–33.

57. Lucci A, McCall LM, Beitsch PD, et al. Surgical complications associated with sentinel lymph node dissection (SLND) plus axillary lymph node dissection compared with SLND alone in the American College of Surgeons Oncology Group Trial Z0011. J Clin Oncol 2007;25(24):3657–63.

58. Wilke LG, McCall LM, Posther KE, et al. Surgical complications associated with sentinel lymph node biopsy: results from a prospective international cooperative group trial. Ann Surg Oncol 2006;13(4):491–500.

59. Whelan TJ, Olivotto IA, Parulekar WR, et al. Regional Nodal Irradiation in Early-Stage Breast Cancer. N Engl J Med 2015;373(4):307–16.

60. Donker M, van Tienhoven G, Straver ME, et al. Radiotherapy or surgery of the axilla after a positive sentinel node in breast cancer (EORTC 10981-22023

AMAROS): a randomised, multicentre, open-label, phase 3 non-inferiority trial. Lancet Oncol 2014;15(12):1303–10.

61. McLaughlin SA, Staley AC, Vicini F, et al. Considerations for Clinicians in the Diagnosis, Prevention, and Treatment of Breast Cancer-Related Lymphedema: Recommendations from a Multidisciplinary Expert ASBrS Panel : Part 1: Definitions, Assessments, Education, and Future Directions. Ann Surg Oncol 2017; 24(10):2818–26.

62. Chang DW, Dayan J, Greene AK, et al. Surgical Treatment of Lymphedema: A Systematic Review and Meta-Analysis of Controlled Trials. Results of a Consensus Conference. Plast Reconstr Surg 2021;147(4):975–93.

63. Ferguson CM, Swaroop MN, Horick N, et al. Impact of Ipsilateral Blood Draws, Injections, Blood Pressure Measurements, and Air Travel on the Risk of Lymphedema for Patients Treated for Breast Cancer. J Clin Oncol 2016;34(7):691–8.

64. Asdourian MS, Skolny MN, Brunelle C, et al. Precautions for breast cancer-related lymphoedema: risk from air travel, ipsilateral arm blood pressure measurements, skin puncture, extreme temperatures, and cellulitis. Lancet Oncol 2016;17(9):e392–405.

65. Schmitz KH, Troxel AB, Dean LT, et al. Effect of Home-Based Exercise and Weight Loss Programs on Breast Cancer-Related Lymphedema Outcomes Among Overweight Breast Cancer Survivors: The WISER Survivor Randomized Clinical Trial. JAMA Oncol 2019;5(11):1605–13.

66. Schmitz KH, Ahmed RL, Troxel AB, et al. Weight lifting for women at risk for breast cancer-related lymphedema: a randomized trial. JAMA 2010;304(24): 2699–705.

67. Soldera SV, Ennis M, Lohmann AE, et al. Sexual health in long-term breast cancer survivors. Breast Cancer Res Treat 2018;172(1):159–66.

68. Gass JS, Onstad M, Pesek S, et al. Breast-Specific Sensuality and Sexual Function in Cancer Survivorship: Does Surgical Modality Matter? Ann Surg Oncol 2017;24(11):3133–40.

69. Flynn KE, Reese JB, Jeffery DD, et al. Patient experiences with communication about sex during and after treatment for cancer. Psychooncology 2012;21(6): 594–601.

70. Simard S, Thewes B, Humphris G, et al. Fear of cancer recurrence in adult cancer survivors: a systematic review of quantitative studies. J Cancer Survivorship : Res Pract 2013;7(3):300–22.

71. Harris J, Cornelius V, Ream E, et al. Anxiety after completion of treatment for early-stage breast cancer: a systematic review to identify candidate predictors and evaluate multivariable model development. Support Care Cancer 2017; 25(7):2321–33.

72. Zainal NZ, Nik-Jaafar NR, Baharudin A, et al. Prevalence of depression in breast cancer survivors: a systematic review of observational studies. Asian Pac J Cancer Prev 2013;14(4):2649–56.

73. Kroenke K, Spitzer RL, Williams JB. The Patient Health Questionnaire-2: validity of a two-item depression screener. Med Care 2003;41(11):1284–92.

74. Spitzer RL, Kroenke K, Williams JB, et al. A brief measure for assessing generalized anxiety disorder: the GAD-7. Arch Intern Med 2006;166(10):1092–7.

75. Coughlin SS, Ayyala DN, Tingen MS, et al. Financial distress among breast cancer survivors. Curr Cancer Rep 2020;2(1):48–53.

76. Jagsi R, Pottow JA, Griffith KA, et al. Long-term financial burden of breast cancer: experiences of a diverse cohort of survivors identified through population-based registries. J Clin Oncol 2014;32(12):1269–76.

77. Dean LT, Moss SL, Ransome Y, et al. It still affects our economic situation": long-term economic burden of breast cancer and lymphedema. Support Care Cancer 2019;27(5):1697–708.

78. Colzani E, Liljegren A, Johansson AL, et al. Prognosis of patients with breast cancer: causes of death and effects of time since diagnosis, age, and tumor characteristics. J Clin Oncol 2011;29(30):4014–21.

79. Patnaik JL, Byers T, Diguiseppi C, et al. The influence of comorbidities on overall survival among older women diagnosed with breast cancer. J Natl Cancer Inst 2011;103(14):1101–11.

80. Ramin C, Schaeffer ML, Zheng Z, et al. All-Cause and Cardiovascular Disease Mortality Among Breast Cancer Survivors in CLUE II, a Long-Standing Community-Based Cohort. J Natl Cancer Inst 2021;113(2):137–45.

81. Arora NK, Reeve BB, Hays RD, et al. Assessment of quality of cancer-related follow-up care from the cancer survivor's perspective. J Clin Oncol 2011; 29(10):1280–9.

82. Siembida EJ, Kent EE, Bellizzi KM, et al. Healthcare providers' discussions of physical activity with older survivors of cancer: Potential missed opportunities for health promotion. J Geriatr Oncol 2020;11(3):437–43.

83. Rai A, Chawla N, Han X, et al. Has the Quality of Patient-Provider Communication About Survivorship Care Improved? J Oncol Pract/Am Soc Clin Oncol 2019; 15(11):e916–24.

84. Jiralerspong S, Goodwin PJ. Obesity and Breast Cancer Prognosis: Evidence, Challenges, and Opportunities. J Clin Oncol 2016;34(35):4203–16.

85. Rock CL, Thomson C, Gansler T, et al. American Cancer Society guideline for diet and physical activity for cancer prevention. CA: a Cancer J Clinicians 2020;70(4):245–71.

86. Schmid D, Leitzmann MF. Association between physical activity and mortality among breast cancer and colorectal cancer survivors: a systematic review and meta-analysis. Ann Oncol 2014;25(7):1293–311.

87. LoConte NK, Brewster AM, Kaur JS, et al. Alcohol and Cancer: A Statement of the American Society of Clinical Oncology. J Clin Oncol 2018;36(1):83–93.

88. Simapivapan P, Boltong A, Hodge A. To what extent is alcohol consumption associated with breast cancer recurrence and second primary breast cancer?: A systematic review. Cancer Treat Rev 2016;50:155–67.

89. Halpern MT, Viswanathan M, Evans TS, et al. Models of Cancer Survivorship Care: Overview and Summary of Current Evidence. J Oncol Pract/Am Soc Clin Oncol 2015;11(1):e19–27.

90. Oeffinger KC, McCabe MS. Models for delivering survivorship care. J Clin Oncol 2006;24(32):5117–24.

91. Miller KD, Pandey M, Jain R, et al. Cancer Survivorship and Models of Survivorship Care: A Review. Am J Clin Oncol 2015;38(6):627–33.

92. Grunfeld E, Levine MN, Julian JA, et al. Randomized trial of long-term follow-up for early-stage breast cancer: a comparison of family physician versus specialist care. J Clin Oncol 2006;24(6):848–55.

93. Institute of Medicine. From cancer patient to cancer survivor: lost in transition. Washington, DC: National Academy Press; 2005.

94. American College of Surgeons Commission on Cancer. Available at: https://www.facs.org/quality-programs/cancer-programs/commission-on-cancer/. Accessed May 31, 2022.

95. Grunfeld E, Julian JA, Pond G, et al. Evaluating survivorship care plans: results of a randomized, clinical trial of patients with breast cancer. J Clin Oncol 2011; 29(36):4755–62.

96. Hershman DL, Greenlee H, Awad D, et al. Randomized controlled trial of a clinic-based survivorship intervention following adjuvant therapy in breast cancer survivors. Breast Cancer Res Treat 2013;138(3):795–806.

97. Joshi A, Larkins S, Evans R, et al. Use and impact of breast cancer survivorship care plans: a systematic review. Breast Cancer 2021;28(6):1292–317.

98. Jacobsen PB, DeRosa AP, Henderson TO, et al. Systematic Review of the Impact of Cancer Survivorship Care Plans on Health Outcomes and Health Care Delivery. J Clin Oncol 2018;36(20):2088–100.

99. Birken SA, Raskin S, Zhang Y, et al. Survivorship Care Plan Implementation in US Cancer Programs: a National Survey of Cancer Care Providers. J Cancer Educ 2019;34(3):614–22.

100. Klemanski DL, Browning KK, Kue J. Survivorship care plan preferences of cancer survivors and health care providers: a systematic review and quality appraisal of the evidence. J Cancer Survivorship : Res Pract 2016;10(1):71–86.

101.. Rosselli Del Turco M, Palli D, Cariddi A, et al. Intensive diagnostic follow-up after treatment of primary breast cancer. A randomized trial. National Research Council Project on Breast Cancer follow-up. JAMA 1994;271(20):1593–7.

Radiation Treatment for Breast Cancer

Anderson Bauer, MD

KEYWORDS

- Radiation • Breast conservation • Whole breast radiation
- Accelerated partial breast radiation • Postmastectomy • Regional nodes
- Hypofractionation

KEY POINTS

- Knowledge of the fundamentals of radiation allows for a better understanding of breast cancer treatment.
- There are a variety of acceptable treatment techniques and dose-fractionation schedules for adjuvant breast radiation.
- Radiation treatment plays an important adjuvant role in breast conservation and also in the postmastectomy setting.
- Careful assessment of individual patient risk factors and treatment goals is essential in identifying the appropriate radiation treatment.

INTRODUCTION

Radiation is a well-established component of breast cancer treatment. This is primarily in the adjuvant setting in both breast conservation and also for many patients who have had mastectomy. The objective of radiation is to eradicate any microscopic tumor deposits remaining after surgery. It is important to understand the various techniques that are utilized in breast radiation. A multitude of factors can help to determine an ideal combination and sequence of surgery, radiation treatment, and systemic therapy for each patient. In addition to the curative setting, radiation can also have an important palliative role.

RADIATION TREATMENT OVERVIEW AND TECHNIQUES
Radiation Treatment Overview

The first radiation treatment of cancer is claimed to have occurred in 1896.[1] The technology of radiation treatment has changed dramatically since this time. Radiation is energy deposited in tissue that kills dividing cancer cells while preferentially allowing

Radiation Oncology Department, Marshfield Clinic Health System, 1001 North Oak Avenue, Marshfield, WI 54449, USA
E-mail address: bauer.anderson@marshfieldclinic.org

Surg Clin N Am 103 (2023) 187–199
https://doi.org/10.1016/j.suc.2022.08.015
0039-6109/23/© 2022 Elsevier Inc. All rights reserved.

normal tissue cells to survive. In general, lower doses of radiation are required to treat postoperative microscopic disease compared to doses for macroscopic deposits of cancer.

The modern era of radiation began in the 1990s, when radiation oncologists began to regularly use CT-based planning. CT imaging is performed on the patient in the treatment position. Customized immobilization devices are used. Certain techniques can be used to minimize doses to specific normal tissues. For individuals with breast cancer, a deep inspiratory breath hold (DIBH) technique increases the distance between the heart and the breast/chest wall to minimize cardiac radiation dose.[2] A prone setup technique can be conducted for patients with larger, pendulous breasts to limit skin reactions while also potentially minimizing dose to the lung and heart.[3]

The CT image sets are sent to the treatment planning system computer. The radiation oncologist delineates the target volumes, which may include the whole breast, lumpectomy cavity, chest wall, and/or at-risk regional lymphatics for breast cancer. Avoidance structures anticipated to be in the treatment field are also drawn, including the heart, lungs, contralateral breast, brachial plexus, and/or thyroid gland. The computer planning software allows for the creation of a virtual treatment plan. **Fig. 1** shows a whole breast radiation treatment plan with tangent fields.

The radiation oncologist determines the treatment technique and prescribes a dose of radiation to be delivered to a specific target in a specified number of treatments. The dose is prescribed in Gray (Gy), and treatments are called fractions. Standard fractionation is typically recognized as 1.8–2.0 Gy per day to a total dose of 50–60 Gy. Hypofractionation schedules include doses of greater than 2.0 Gy per fraction to radiobiologically equivalent total doses (ie, 16 fractions of 2.66 Gy per day to a total of 42.56 Gy). The virtual plan is approved once appropriate target dose coverage and normal tissue sparing are achieved. The plan is transferred to the radiation treatment machine. Appropriate quality assurance is done on treatment plans to ensure accuracy and safety.

Techniques

A vast array of radiation techniques have been developed for cancer treatment, including for individuals with breast cancer. Different types of radiation used in these

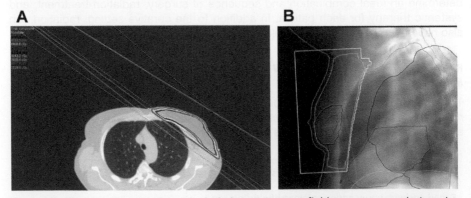

Fig. 1. (*A*). Planning CT axial view of whole breast tangent field arrangement designed to encompass the target volume while minimizing dose to the heart, lung, and contralateral breast. (*B*). Whole breast radiation tangent port corresponding to CT image (*A*). Field minimizes dose to the ipsilateral lung (*green*) and heart (*magenta*).

techniques include: photons, electrons, gamma rays (ie, iridium-192), and protons. Photon radiation is used for most external beam treatments and is the most common type of radiation. Iridium-192 is a radioactive isotope that is commonly used in brachytherapy. Proton therapy is not currently routinely used for breast cancer treatment, but there is an ongoing study for its potential expanded indications.[4]

External beam radiation is the most common type of treatment, including 3-dimensional conformal radiation treatment (3DCRT) and intensity-modulated radiation treatment (IMRT). Brachytherapy is a technique that involves placing a radiation source inside or next to an area requiring treatment; it is typically subdivided into intracavitary and interstitial techniques. Intraoperative radiation treatment (IORT) can be performed with an intraoperative beam (electron or photon) or as high-dose rate brachytherapy. Different techniques can be utilized to deliver doses to different targets. For example, brachytherapy is very effective at delivering a higher dose to a smaller volume, hence it is a technique used in partial breast radiation. The radiation is confined to the lumpectomy cavity with a small margin. The dosimetry for a brachytherapy plan is shown in **Fig. 2**. Partial breast treatment is typically done over ≤1 week, which is why it is called accelerated partial breast irradiation (APBI).

RADIATION TREATMENT IN THE NONMETASTATIC SETTING
Breast Conservation-Invasive Cancer

For women who have breast-conserving surgery, adjuvant radiation is a well-established treatment for both invasive breast cancers and ductal carcinoma in situ (DCIS). For invasive breast cancer, a large meta-analysis of 17 trials published in 2011 by the Early Breast Cancer Trialists' Collaborative Group (EBCTCG) showed the benefit of adjuvant whole breast radiation treatment (WBRT).[5] Ten-year risk of locoregional recurrence (LRR) was decreased by approximately half from 35 to 19 percent. Fifteen-year risk of breast cancer death was reduced from 25 to 21 percent. **Fig. 3** illustrates these curves.[5]

More modern studies have evaluated the benefit in low-risk patients, which are more commonly seen as screening continues to improve early detection. Cancer and Leukemia Group B (CALGB) 9343 evaluated women ≥70 years of age with T1N0, estrogen-receptor positive invasive ductal carcinoma treated by lumpectomy to receive tamoxifen plus adjuvant radiation or tamoxifen alone. The adjuvant radiation

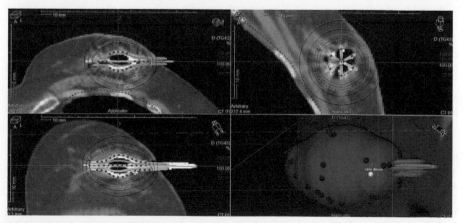

Fig. 2. APBI brachytherapy plan using SAVI multicatheter device. Rapid falloff of dose can be seen from 150% isodose line to 50% isodose line.

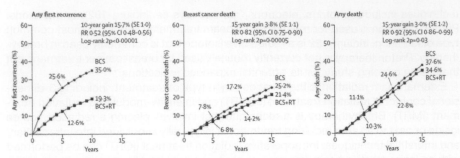

Fig. 3. This figure was published in Lancet, Vol. 378, Issue 9804; EBCTCG (Early Breast Cancer Trialists' Collaborative Group). "Effect of radiotherapy after breast-conserving surgery on 10-year recurrence and 15-year breast cancer death: meta-analysis of individual patient data for 10,801 women in 17 randomized trails" pp 1707-1716, Copyright Elsevier (2011), with permission.

had a statistically significant 10-year local recurrence reduction from 10 to 2 percent, but this did not impact breast cancer-specific survival or overall survival.[6] PRIME II evaluated women ≥65 years of age with invasive ductal carcinoma up to 3 cm in size treated by lumpectomy to receive adjuvant endocrine treatment plus whole breast radiation or adjuvant endocrine treatment only. This also showed that adjuvant radiation had a statistically significant 10-year local recurrence reduction from 9.8 to 0.9 percent, but no difference in overall and breast cancer-specific survival.[7] OncotypeDX may offer additional information on local recurrence risk in these low-risk patients, and the NRG Oncology study BR007 is further investigating this question.

WBRT with a hypofractionated regimen of 40–42.5 Gy in 15–16 fractions with or without a lumpectomy cavity boost of 10 Gy in 4–5 fractions has become the standard approach as studies have shown no significant differences in tumor control nor adverse effects when comparing the prior standard 5–6 week regimen to this shortened hypofractionated approach.[8-10] The 2018 American Society for Therapeutic Radiology and Oncology (ASTRO) Radiation Therapy for the Whole Breast Guidelines strongly recommended hypofractionated WBRT regardless of tumor grade, laterality, systemic therapy, and breast size. These guidelines also recommend a boost for all patients with higher risk of local recurrence, including patients ≤50 years of age with any grade disease, age 51–70 years of age with high-grade disease, or a positive margin.[11]

In regards to further hypofractionation, newer data also suggest the future potential of ultrashort whole breast radiation options from the FAST (28.5 Gy in 5 once-weekly fractions) and FAST-Forward (26 Gy in 5 fractions in 1 week) trials.[12-14] NRG/Radiation Therapy Oncology Group (RTOG) 1005 has been evaluating the option of 40 Gy in 15 fractions with a simultaneous integrated boost (SIB) of 48 Gy in 15 fractions to the lumpectomy cavity. This study was closed to accrual in 2014 and outcomes are still unpublished.[15]

APBI can be utilized to treat only the lumpectomy cavity with an appropriate margin, which is the area at highest risk of recurrence. This has been studied primarily using external beam radiation (typically 38.5 Gy in 10 fractions, twice daily) and brachytherapy (34 Gy in 10 fractions, twice daily) techniques. The National Surgical Adjuvant Breast and Bowel Project (NSABP) B-39/RTOG 0413 is a large phase 3 randomized trial of WBRT compared to APBI, which showed a 10-year cumulative incidence of ipsilateral breast tumor recurrence of 3.9 percent for WBRT versus 4.6 percent for APBI.[16] There was no difference in cosmesis. The ASTRO consensus statement on

APBI states that "suitable" candidates are $\geq$50 years of age, $\leq$2 cm invasive ductal carcinoma with at least 2 mm margins, no lymphvascular invasion, estrogen receptor positive, and gBRCA negative.[17] Additional partial breast fractionation schedules include a 5 fraction partial breast IMRT plan to 30 Gy delivered every other day, which was studied in the Florence trial (10-year ipsilateral breast tumor recurrence of 2.5% for WBRT and 3.7% for APBI).[18] In addition, 40 Gy in 15 fractions partial breast radiation was found to be noninferior to WBRT in the UK IMPORT LOW trial.[19]

Intraoperative radiation treatment is a unique option as it is delivered at the time of breast-conserving surgery. This can be delivered with low-energy photons or electrons using an intraoperative applicator. The TARGIT trial used a mobile machine delivering approximately 20 Gy to the surface using 50 kV photons. The intraoperative radiation could be supplemented by EBRT when postoperative pathology revealed higher risk factors. Compared to standard WBRT, the intraoperative approach showed no statistically significant difference for local recurrence-free survival, mastectomy-free survival, distant disease-free survival, overall survival, and breast cancer mortality at a median follow-up of 8.6 years.[20] TARGIT was associated with improved breast cosmesis. The ELIOT trial used intraoperative electron treatment to deliver a dose of 21 Gy and was compared to WBRT. At a median follow-up of 12.4 years, there was an increase in 15-year ipsilateral breast tumor recurrence of 12.6 percent compared to 2.4 percent.[21]

Key Points-Invasive Breast Cancer

- Adjuvant radiation with a boost is recommended for patients $\leq$50 years of age with any grade disease, age 51–70 years of age with high-grade disease, or a positive margin.
- Individualized shared decision-making with provider and patient is important to decide which individuals may elect the de-escalation of radiation (no radiation lumpectomy boost or completely omit adjuvant WBRT).
- There is increasing use of hypofractionation for patients that have adjuvant radiation.
- APBI is a well-studied adjuvant radiation treatment option for selected patients.
- Genomic assays may become increasingly important to select appropriate low-risk patients who can forego adjuvant radiation.

Breast Conservation-Ductal Carcinoma In Situ

For DCIS, there is also a large meta-analysis by the EBCTG published in 2010 showing the reduction of local recurrence with adjuvant WBRT after breast-conserving surgery. 10-year risk of any ipsilateral breast event (either recurrent DCIS or invasive cancer) was decreased by approximately half from 28.1 to 12.9 percent.[22] However, there was no significant impact on overall survival. NSABP B-17 and NSABP B-24 further evaluated adjuvant radiation with tamoxifen. These trials demonstrated that radiation had a relatively greater impact on preventing local recurrence than tamoxifen. A combined analysis of these trials showed a 15-year cumulative incidence of ipsilateral breast tumor recurrence of 19.4 percent for lumpectomy alone, 8.9 percent for lumpectomy with radiation, 10 percent for lumpectomy with radiation + placebo, and 8.5 percent for lumpectomy with radiation + tamoxifen.[23] These results can be seen in **Fig. 4**.[23]

More modern studies have further evaluated adjuvant radiation for low-risk DCIS. NRG/RTOG 9804 evaluated patients with mammographically detected DCIS, $\leq$2.5 cm, final margins $\geq$3 mm, and low or intermediate nuclear grade. Adjuvant radiation significantly reduced the 15-year cumulative incidence of ipsilateral breast

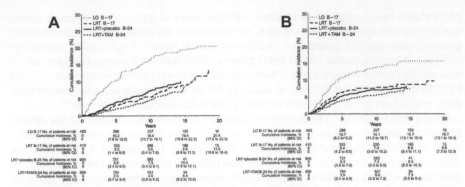

LO B-17 No. of patients at risk 403 ... 288 207 153 10
Cumulative Incidence, % 0 10.2 16.4 19.4 20.4
(95% CI) 0 (7.8 to 12.6) (13.7 to 19.1) (16.6 to 22.2) (17.6 to 23.3)

LRT B-17 No. of patients at risk 410 ... 535 256 196 13
Cumulative Incidence, % 0 3.2 5.5 8.9 13.5
(95% CI) 0 (1.4 to 5.0) (3.4 to 7.6) (6.5 to 11.3) (10.6 to 16.4)

LRT+placebo B-24 No. of patients at risk 900 731 563 41
Cumulative Incidence, % 0 3.9 7.3 10.0
(95% CI) 0 (2.4 to 5.5) (5.4 to 9.1) (7.8 to 12.1)

LRT+TAM B-24 No. of patients at risk 899 764 621 54
Cumulative Incidence, % 0 2.0 4.5 6.5
(95% CI) 0 (0.7 to 3.4) (3.0 to 6.3) (6.2 to 10.5)

LO B-17 No. of patients at risk 403 ... 288 207 153 10
Cumulative Incidence, % 0 10.7 14.1 15.7 15.7
(95% CI) 0 (8.3 to 13.2) (11.5 to 16.7) (13.1 to 18.4) (13.1 to 18.4)

LRT B-17 No. of patients at risk 410 ... 535 250 196 13
Cumulative Incidence, % 0 6.4 7.6 8.8 8.8
(95% CI) 0 (4.2 to 8.5) (5.6 to 10.2) (6.4 to 11.1) (7.3 to 12.3)

LRT+placebo B-24 No. of patients at risk 900 731 563 41
Cumulative Incidence, % 0 5.3 7.2 8.3
(95% CI) 0 (3.6 to 7.0) (5.3 to 9.0) (6.3 to 10.3)

LRT+TAM/B-24 No. of patients at risk 800 764 621 54
Cumulative Incidence, % 0 3.5 5.6 7.5
(95% CI) 0 (2.4 to 5.5) (3.9 to 7.3) (5.5 to 9.4)

Fig. 4. Effects of radiation and tarnoxifen on the cumulative incidence of breast cancer events. (*A*) Invasive ipsilateral breast tumor recurrences (I-ISTR), (*B*) ductual carcinoma in situ-ipsilateral breast tumor recurrences (DCIS-IBTR). (Wapnir IL, Dignam JJ, Fisher B, et al. Long-term Outcomes of Invasive Ipsilateral Breast Tumor Recurrences After Lumpectomy in NSABP B-17 and B-24 Randomized Clinical Trials for DCIS. J Natl Cancer Inst. 2011; 103(6):478-88 by permission of Oxford University Press.)

recurrence from 15.1 to 7.1 percent; invasive local recurrence was reduced from 9.5 to 5.4 percent.[24] There was no significant difference in overall survival. ECOG 5194 followed 2 cohorts of women with DCIS treated with lumpectomy alone. 12-year rates of ipsilateral breast events were 14.4 percent for cohort 1 (low- or intermediate-grade DCIS with tumors ≤2.5 cm, negative margins ≥3 mm) and 24.6 percent for cohort 2 (high-grade DCIS, tumor size ≤1 cm, negative margins ≥3 mm), respectively.[25] These studies show that there is still significant recurrence even in women with favorable pathology. Genomic assays such as DCIS Score and DCISion RT can provide additional guidance on recurrence risk.[26,27]

In regards to the specifics of radiation treatment of DCIS, the 2018 ASTRO Radiation Therapy for the Whole Breast Guidelines recommend hypofractionated WBRT as an alternative to conventional fractionation in patients with DCIS.[11] It also stated that a tumor bed boost may be used for patients with any of the following criteria: ≤50 years of age, high grade, or margins <2 mm. In addition, ASTRO would consider patients ≥50 years of age with screening-detected DCIS, low or intermediate grade, and with margins ≥3 mm as "suitable" candidates for APBI.[17]

Key Points-Ductal Carcinoma In Situ

- Adjuvant radiation with a boost is recommended for high-grade DCIS, premenopausal patients, patients <50 years of age, tumors >2.5 cm, or margins <2 mm.
- Individualized shared decision-making with provider and patient is important to decide which individuals may elect the de-escalation of radiation (no radiation lumpectomy boost or completely omit adjuvant WBRT).
- There is increasing use of hypofractionation for patients that have adjuvant radiation.
- Genomic assays may become increasingly important to select appropriate low-risk patients who can forego adjuvant radiation.

Radiation for Locally Advanced Breast Cancer

Adjuvant radiation treatment of T2 lesions with high-risk features, T3/T4 lesions, and node-positive patients is typically more extensive than for early-stage breast cancers.

Historically, radiation for patients with locally advanced disease would comprehensively include the breast/chest wall and all regional nodes (dissected and undissected axilla, supraclavicular region, and internal mammary chain nodes).

A meta-analysis by the EBCTG of 22 trials published in 2014 showed an improvement in 10-year recurrence and 20-year breast cancer mortality in women with 4 or more positive nodes who received adjuvant radiation to the chest wall and regional lymphatics.[28] 10-year risk of local recurrence was decreased from 32.1 to 13.0 percent. The 20-year breast cancer mortality was decreased from 80 to 70.7 percent. These results can be seen in **Fig. 5**.[28]

Over time, there have been significant changes in systemic therapy, as well as diagnostic procedures. Multiple studies have continued to help refine the role of regional lymph node radiation treatment. National Cancer Institute of Canada (NCIC) MA.20 is a randomized trial that evaluated adding regional nodal radiation to whole breast radiation in patients with 1–3 positive axillary lymph nodes or negative nodes with high-risk features. High-risk features were defined as primary tumor measuring ≥5 cm or ≥2 cm with fewer than 10 axillary nodes removed with at least one additional

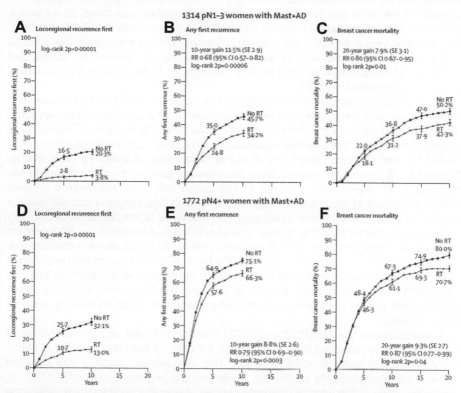

Fig. 5. Effect of radiotherapy (RT) after mastectomy and axillary dissection (Mast AD) on 10-year risks of locoregional and overall recurrence and on 20-year risk of breast cancer mortality in 1314 women with 1 to 3 pathologically positive nodes (pN1-3) and in 1772 women with 4 or more pathologically positive nodes (pN4+). (The Lancet, 2014, 383 (9935), p.2127-2135. EBCTCG (Early Breast Cancer Trialists' Collaborative Group), "Effect of radiotherapy after mastectomy and axillary surgery on 10-year recurrence and 20-year breast cancer mortality: meta-analysis of individual patient data for 8135 women in 22 randomised trials".)

high-risk feature (grade 3, estrogen-receptor negativity, or lymphvascular invasion). The regional nodal radiation significantly improved isolated local recurrence-free survival (95.2 versus 92.2 percent, p = 0.009), distant recurrence-free survival (86.3 versus 82.4 percent, p = 0.03) and overall disease-free survival (82 versus 77 percent, p = 0.01) at 10 years.[29]

EORTC 22922 is also a randomized trial that showed benefit to regional nodal radiation in patients with involved axillary nodes or central or medially located primary tumors. At a median follow-up of 15.7 years, regional nodal radiation was associated with a significant reduction in breast cancer mortality from 19.8 to 16.0 percent (p = 0.0055) and any breast cancer recurrence from 27.1 to 24.5 percent (p = 0.024).[30] At a median follow-up of 10.9 years, EORTC 22922 had shown a significant benefit with radiation to disease-free survival (72.1 versus 69.1%), distant disease-free survival (78 versus 75%), breast cancer mortality (12.5 versus 14.4%), and overall survival (82.3 versus 80.7%).

AMAROS evaluated the use of axillary radiation treatment in lieu of full axillary lymph node dissection (ALND) in patients with T1 or T2 disease with a positive sentinel lymph node dissection (SLND). This study included both breast conservation as well as patients with mastectomy (17%). The axillary radiation included all 3 levels of the axilla and the medial part of the supraclavicular fossa. At 10 years, AMAROS showed noninferior overall survival of 81.4 percent in the SLND with axillary radiation versus 84.6 percent in the ALND group, distant metastasis-free survival of 78.2 percent for SLND with axillary radiation versus 81.7 percent for ALND, and locoregional relapse-free survival of 83.0 percent for SLND with axillary radiation versus 81.2 percent for ALND.[31]

ACOSOG Z0011, similar to AMAROS, also included clinical T1 or T2 cancers with positive sentinel lymph nodes (1–2). All patients were treated with breast conservation. These patients were not treated with radiation specifically to the axilla.[32] However, it should be noted that there can be incidental dose to the low axilla with standard whole breast tangent fields, although this is highly dependent on patient's body shape. Moreover, 15 percent of patients were recorded as also receiving treatment in the supraclavicular region, and a review of 142 cases with sufficient records showed that 51.4 percent of those patients were treated with high tangents (cranial tangent border ≤2 cm from the humeral head) which would have a higher likelihood of covering more of the upper axilla.[33] The 10-year overall survival was noninferior at 86.3 percent in the SLND alone group versus 83.6 percent in the ALND group, as were disease-free survival (80.2% for SLND alone versus 78.2% for ALND) and locoregional recurrence (4.07% for SLND versus 3.59% for ALND). Given the decreased morbidity of lymphedema without the axillary dissection, these studies do not support the routine use of ALND in this patient population with limited axillary disease as defined by sentinel node excision.[32]

As stated above, the AMAROS and Z0011 trials did not treat comprehensive nodal volumes. A study published in 2022 evaluated the utility of including the internal mammary nodes with regional nodal radiation. This randomized, phase 3 trial included women with pathologically confirmed, node-positive breast cancer with ALND. As for the inclusion of the internal mammary nodes, there was no significant difference in 7-year disease-free survival rates if these nodes were included. However, a subgroup analysis of mediocentrally located tumors showed a 7-year disease-free survival rate improvement with internal mammary nodal radiation of 91.8 v. 81.6 percent and a breast cancer mortality reduction from 10.2 to 4.9 percent. There were no differences between the 2 groups in the incidence of adverse effects, including cardiac toxic effects and radiation pneumonitis.[34]

For node-positive patients who have had neoadjuvant chemotherapy, most patients receive postmastectomy radiation treatment, especially if there is any residual disease. There are 2 major ongoing trials that will help to define the role of adjuvant radiation treatment after the assessment of response to neoadjuvant chemotherapy. Alliance A011202 is a randomized phase 3 trial comparing axillary lymph node dissection to axillary radiation in patients with breast cancer (cT1-3 N1) who have positive sentinel lymph node disease after neoadjuvant chemotherapy. NSABP B-51/RTOG 1304 is a randomized phase 3 trial evaluating the role of postmastectomy chest wall/regional nodal radiation and postlumpectomy whole breast/regional nodal radiation in patients with documented positive axillary nodes before neoadjuvant chemotherapy who convert to pathologically negative axillary nodes after neoadjuvant chemotherapy.

As with early-stage invasive breast cancer and DCIS, there is also investigation into using a genomic-based assay to assess the risk of locoregional recurrence in patients with node-positive disease. The TAILOR RT trial (Canadian Cancer Trials Group MA 39) is currently accruing breast cancer patients with the following: ER positive, HER2 negative, 1–3 positive lymph nodes, and oncotype DX test recurrence scores <18. Patients are randomized to receive or omit adjuvant regional nodal radiation.

Key Points for Locally Advanced Breast Cancer

- Adjuvant radiation is recommended in patients with $\geq$4 axillary lymph nodes.
- Adjuvant radiation is recommended for patients with residual disease after neoadjuvant chemotherapy and/or patients with clinically node positive disease prior to neoadjuvant chemotherapy. There are 2 major ongoing trials that will help to clarify the role of adjuvant treatment in this setting.
- Individualized shared decision-making is important to decide which patients should have adjuvant radiation for patients with T2 tumors and 1–3 positive lymph nodes.
- Genomic assays may become increasingly important to select appropriate low-risk patients who can forego adjuvant radiation.

Radiation for Metastatic Breast Cancer

Although systemic therapy is the main treatment option for stage IV breast cancer, radiation can be an important local treatment for a specific site of cancer. This can include tumors compressing the spinal cord, tumors blocking an airway, painful chest wall lesions, bone metastases, and brain metastases. These courses of palliative radiation tend to be short in duration (1–10 fractions). Treatments can range from a very simple beam arrangement for bone metastasis to a complex stereotactic radiosurgery treatment of brain oligometastasis.

TOXICITIES/CONTRAINDICATIONS
Toxicities

Radiation toxicities will be less with lower doses and smaller treatment volumes. Therefore, these can vary based on techniques. Other treatments can also affect the extent of toxicities, including chemotherapy and extent of surgery. Overall, modern radiation treatment machines/techniques have contributed to a great reduction in the severity of toxicities compared to older studies. Skin reactions are still common, including erythema, hyperpigmentation, and peeling. Mild fatigue can also occur during the course of radiation treatment. Generally, these side effects resolve within 2–4 weeks after the completion of treatment.

Long-term complications are much less common and more difficult to calculate given the multifactorial nature of these side effects (such as age, genetic predisposition, medical comorbidities, other treatments, smoking history, and radiation techniques). Some representative estimates of these include cardiotoxicity (0.3% absolute increase in cardiac mortality in nonsmokers, 1.2% in smokers),[35] $\geq$ grade 2 pneumonitis (<2%),[29] secondary malignancy (generally low increased absolute risk of approximately 1:1000),[36] and lymphedema (increase after regional nodal radiation from 13% to 24% compared to ALND alone and from 2% to 6.1% after SLND).[37] In regards to the potential complications with breast reconstruction, there are many factors including radiation field size/dose of radiation, immediate versus delayed reconstruction, autologous versus implant-based reconstruction, and individual patient characteristics.[38]

Contraindications to Radiation Treatment

Relative contraindications to radiation treatment include active connective tissue disease involving the skin (ie, scleroderma) and prior radiation therapy at/near the chest wall or breast. Absolute contraindications include radiation treatment during pregnancy and being homozygous for ATM mutation.[39]

SUMMARY

Radiation is an important component of breast cancer treatment. The role of radiation will continue to be refined with advancing radiation technology as well as improvements in diagnostics, surgery, systemic therapies, and tumor biology assessment. Multidisciplinary management and addressing individual patient factors remain critical for excellent breast cancer patient care.

CLINICS CARE POINTS

- Radiation oncology should be included in decisions regarding adjuvant radiation for local control in breast conservation and locally advanced disease.

DISCLOSURE

The author has nothing to disclose.

REFERENCES

1. Grubbe EH. Priority in the therapeutic use of X-rays. Radiology 1933;21(2): 156–62.
2. Bergom C, Currey A, Desai N, et al. Deep inspiration breath hold: techniques and advantages for cardiac sparing during breast cancer irradiation. Front Oncol 2018;8:87.
3. Bergom C, Kelly T, Morrow N, et al. Prone whole-breast irradiation using three-dimensional conformal radiotherapy in women undergoing breast conservation for early disease yields high rates of excellent to good cosmetic outcomes in patients with large and/or pendulous breasts. Int J Radiat Oncol Biol Phys 2012;83:3.
4. Mutter RW, Choi JI, Jimenez RB, et al. Proton therapy for breast cancer: a consensus statement from the particle therapy cooperative group bresat cancer subdommittee. Int J Radiat Oncol Biol Phys 2021;111(2):337–59.

5. EBCTG. Effect of radiotherapy after breast-conserving surgery on 10-year recurrence and 15-year breast cancer death: meta-analysis of individual patient data for 10801 women in 17 randomised trials. Lancet 2011;378:1707–16.

6. Hughes KS, Schnaper LA, Bellon JR, et al. Lumpectomy plus tamoxifen with or without irradiation in women age 70 years or older with early breast cancer: long-term follow-up of CALGB 9343. J Clin Oncol 2013;31(19):2382–7.

7. Kunkler IH, Williams LJ, Jack W, et al. Prime 2 Randomised trial (postoperative radiotherapy in minimum-risk elderly): wide local excision and adjuvant hormonal therapy +/- whole breast irradiation in women =/> 65 years with early invasive breast cancer: 10 year results. Cancer Res 2021;81(4_Supplement):GS2-03.

8. Whelan TJ, Pignol JP, Levine MN, et al. Long-term results of hypofractionated radiation therapy for breast cancer. N Engl J Med 2010;362(6):513–20.

9. Haviland JS, Owen JR, Dewar JA, et al. The UK standardisation of breast radiotherapy (START) trials of radiotherapy hypofractionation for treatment of early breast cancer: 10-year follow-up results of two randomised controlled trials. Lancet Oncol 2013;14:1086–94.

10. Shah C, Al-Hilli Z, Vicini F. Advances in breast cancer radiotherapy: implications for current and future practice. JCO Oncol Pract 2021;17(12):697–706.

11. Smith BD, Bellon JR, Blitzblau R, et al. Radiation therapy for the whole breast: executive summary of an american society for radiation oncology (ASTRO) evidence-based guideline. Pracital Radiat Oncol 2018;8:145–52.

12. Brunt AM, Haviland JS, Wheatley D, et al. Hypofractionated breast radiotherapy for 1 week versus 3 weeks (FAST-Forward): 5-year efficacy and late normal tissue effects results from a multicentre, non-inferiority, randomised, phase 3 trial. Lancet 2020;395(10237):1613–26.

13. Brunt AM, Haviland JS, Syndenham M, et al. Ten-year results of FAST: a randomized controlled trial of 5-fraction whole-breast radiotherapy for early breast cancer. J Clin Oncol 2020;38(28):3261–72.

14. Krug D, Baumann R, Combs SE, et al. Moderate hypofractionation remains the standard of care for whole-breast radiotherapy in breast cancer: considerations regarding FAST and FAST-forward. Strahlenther Onkol 2021;197:269–80.

15. ClinicalTrials.gov 2022;. https://clinicaltrials.gov/ct2/show/results/NCT01349322.

16. Vicini FA, Cecchini RS, White JR, et al. Long-term Primary results of accelerated partial breast irradiation after breast-conserving surgery for early-stage breast cancer: a radndomised, phase 3, equivalence trial. Lancet 2019;394(10215):2155–64.

17. Correa C, Harris EE, Leonardi MC, et al. Accelerated partial breast irradiation: executive summary for the update of an ASTRO evidence-based consensus statement. Pract Radiat Oncol 2017;7:73–9.

18. Meattini I, Marrazzo L, Calogero S, et al. Accelerated partial-breast irradiation compared with whole-breast irradiation for early breast cancer: long-term results of the randomized phase III APBI-IMRT-florence trial. J Clin Oncol 2020;38(35):4175–83.

19. Coles CE, Griffin CL, Kirby AM, et al. Partial-breast radiotherapy after breast conservation surgery for patients with early breast cancer (UK IMPORT LOW trial): 5-year Results from a multicentre, randomised, controlled, phase 3, non-inferiority trial. Lancet 2017;390:1048–60.

20. Vaidya JS, Bulsara M, Baum M, et al. Long term survival and local control outocomes from a single dose targeted intraoperative radiotherapy durin gLumpectomy (TARGIT_IORT) for early breast cancer: TARGIT-A randomised clinical trial. BMJ 2020;370:m2836. https://doi.org/10.1136/bmj.m2836.

21. Orecchia R, Veronesi U, Maisonneuve P, et al. Intraoperative irradiation for early breast cancer (ELIOT): long-term recurrence and survival outcomes from a single-centre, randomised, phase 3 equivalence trial. Lancet Oncol 2021;22: 597–608.

22. EBCTG. Overview of the randomized trials of radiotherapy in ductal carcinoma in situ of the breast. J Natl Cancer Inst Monographs 2010;41:162–77.

23. Wapnir IL, Dignam JJ, Fisher B, et al. Long-term outcomes of invasive ipsilateral breast tumor recurrences after lumpectomy in NSABP B-17 and B-24 randomized clinical trials for DCIS. J Natl Cancer Inst 2011;103(6):478–88.

24. McCormick B, Winter KA, Woodward W, et al. Randomized phase III trial evaluating radiation following surgical excision for good-risk ductal carcinoma in situ: long-term report from NRG oncology/RTOG 0984. J Clin Oncol 2021; 39(32):3574–82.

25. Solin LJ, Gray R, Hughes LL, et al. Surgical excision without radiation for ductal carcinoma in situ of the breast: 12-year results from the ECOG-ACRIN E5194 study. J Clin Oncol 2015;33(33):2938–44.

26. Solin LJ, Gray R, Baehner FL, et al. A multigene expression assay to predict local recurrence risk for ductal carcinoma in situ of the breast. J Natl Cancer Inst 2013; 105(10):701–10.

27. Weinmann S, Leo MC, Francisco M, et al. Validation of a ductal carcinoma in situ biomarker profile for risk of recurrence after breast-conserving surgery with and without radiotherapy. Clin Cancer Res 2020;26(15):4054–63.

28. EBCTG. Effect of radiotherapy after mastectomy and axillary surgery on 10-year recurrence and 20-year breast cancer mortality: meta-analysis of individual patient data for 8135 women in 22 randomized trials. Lancet 2014;383:2127–35.

29. Whelan TJ, Olivotto IA, Parulekar WR, et al. Regional nodal irradiation in early-stage breast cancer. N Engl J Med 2015;373(4):307–16.

30. Poortmans PM, Weltens C, Fortpied C, et al. Internal mammary and medial supraclavicular lymph node chain irradiation in stage I-III breast cancer (EORTC22922/ 10925): 15-year results of a randomised, phase 3 trial. Lancet Oncol 2020;21(12): 1602–10.

31. Rutgers E, Donker M, Poncet C, et al. Radiotherapy or surgery of the axilla after a positive sentinel node in breast cancer patients: 10 year follow up results of the EORTC AMAROS trial (EORTC 10981/22023). Cancer Res 2019;79(4). GS4–01.

32. Giuliano AE, Ballman KV, McCall L, et al. Effect of axillary dissection vs no axillary dissection on 10-year overall survival among women with invasive breast cancer and sentinel node metastasis the ACOSOG Z0011 (Alliance) randomized clinical trial. JAMA 2017;318(10):918–26.

33. Jagsi R, Chadha M, Moni J, et al. Radiation field design in the ACOSOG Z0011 (Alliance) trial. J Clin Oncol 2014;32(32):3600–6.

34. Kim YB, Byun HK, Kim DY, et al. Effect of elective internal mammary node irradiation on disease-free survival in women with node-positive breast cancer. JAMA Oncol 2022;8(1):96–105.

35. Taylor C, Correa C, Duane FK, et al. Estimating the risks of breast cancer radiotherapy: evidence from modern radiation doses to the lungs and heart and from previous randomized trials. J Clin Oncol 2017;35(15):1641–9.

36. Clarke M, Collins R, Darby S, et al. Effects of radiotherapy and of differences in the extent of surgery for early breast cancer on local recurrence and 15-year survival: an overview of the randomised trials. Lancet 2005;366:2087–106.

37. Warren LE, Miller CL, Horick N, et al. The impact of radiation therapy on the risk of lymphedema after treatment for breast cancer: a prospective cohort study. Int J Radiat Oncol Biol Phys 2014;88(3):565–71.
38. Ho A, Hu Z, Mehrara B, et al. Radiotherapy in the setting of breast reconstruction: types, techniques, and timing. Lancet Oncol 2017;18:e742–53.
39. Jordan RM, Oxenberg J. Breast cancer conservation therapy. [Updated 2021 Sep 22]. In: StatPearls [Internet]. Treasure Island (FL). StatPearls Publishing; 2022. Available at: https://www.ncbi.nlm.nih.gov/books/NBK547708.

Preoperative Systemic Therapy for Breast Cancer

Abhigna Kodali, MD[a],*, Vijayakrishna K. Gadi, MD, PhD[b]

KEYWORDS

- Preoperative therapy • Neoadjuvant therapy • TNBC • HER2 positive breast cancer
- Hormone receptor–positive breast cancer

INTRODUCTION

Conventionally, systemic chemotherapy has been used in the adjuvant setting following breast and regional lymph node surgery in a significant percentage of breast cancer patients with operable disease. The use of preoperative or neoadjuvant systemic therapy for management of advanced, nonmetastatic breast cancer was previously restricted to clinical indications primarily focused on "debulking" in the breast or regional lymph nodes. For instance, typical candidates for neoadjuvant chemotherapy included only patients with inoperable or locally advanced breast cancer including inflammatory breast cancer, patients with N2 and N3 regional lymph node disease, and patients with T4 tumors. Another indication was to use systemic preoperative therapy in patients for whom a delay in surgery is preferable (i.e., during pregnancy, management of medical comorbidity). However, indications for preoperative therapy in early-stage breast cancer have evolved to include a wider spectrum of patients.[1] It is now routinely offered to patients with operable disease not only to down-stage disease to spare them the morbidity of more extensive breast and/or lymph node surgery, but also to use the response in the breast and nodes as an indicator for prognosis and to better individualize adjuvant therapy. Here, the authors review these updates and offer some guidelines for specific clinical scenarios (**Fig. 1** and **Table 1**).

One accepted goal of neoadjuvant systemic therapy is to debulk an invasive breast cancer to increase the proportion of patients eligible for breast conservation surgery. Neoadjuvant trials from cancer cooperative groups and/or industry that incorporate patients from multiple sites and/or countries such as CALGB (Cancer and Leukemia Group B) 40601, CALGB 40603, and BrighTNess showed that the conversion rate from breast conservation surgery (BCS) ineligible to BCS eligible in specific phenotypes of breast cancer ranged from 43% to 53% in prespecified secondary analyses.[2–4] Similarly, neoadjuvant chemotherapy has also been shown to downstage

a Division of Hematology and Oncology, Maimonides Cancer Center, 6300 Eight Avenue, Brooklyn, NY 11220, USA; b Division of Hematology and Oncology, University of Illinois Chicago and Translational Oncology Program, University of Illinois Cancer Center, 818 South Wolcott Avenue, 410 SRH, Chicago, IL 60612, USA
* Corresponding author.
E-mail address: akodali@maimonidesmed.org

Surg Clin N Am 103 (2023) 201–217
https://doi.org/10.1016/j.suc.2022.08.017
0039-6109/23/© 2022 Elsevier Inc. All rights reserved.

surgical.theclinics.com

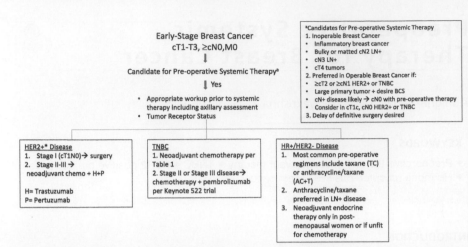

Fig. 1. Suggested guidelines for preoperative systemic therapy in breast cancer subtypes.
[a]HER2+ = IHC 3+ staining or ISH amplified.

axillary disease and allow for minimization of surgery in the axilla. Several large prospective trials such as ACOSOG (American College of Surgeons Oncology Group) Z1071, SENTINA (Sentinel Neoadjuvant), and SN FNAC (Sentinel Node Biopsy Following Neoadjuvant Chemotherapy) demonstrated that after preoperative chemotherapy, pathologic complete response (pCR) in the breast and lymph nodes determined on a sentinel lymph node surgery ranged from 19% to 41%, thereby avoiding axillary dissection in those patients with acceptable false-negative rates.[5–7] Therefore, neoadjuvant chemotherapy is now a strategy for deescalation of surgery in both the breast and axilla.

Pathologic responses following the addition of biological therapies to chemotherapy have been shown to provide prognostic information particularly in patients diagnosed with triple-negative breast cancer (TNBC) and human epidermal growth factor receptor 2 (HER2) overexpressing/gene-amplified (HER2+) tumors.[8,9] One noteworthy concept under development is the standardized measurement of residual cancer burden (RCB) with scores ranging from 0 (equivalent to pCR) to III ranked from none to progressively higher residual disease following neoadjuvant therapy.[10] The depth of response to combination preoperative therapy (pCR/RCB-0 vs residual disease) has become useful for guiding subsequent selection of adjuvant therapy.[11] In summary, neoadjuvant therapy has evolved from a less frequently used approach to debulk a large breast cancer to a more commonplace approach for certain operable, breast cancer subtypes.

TRIPLE-NEGATIVE BREAST CANCER

Approximately 15% to 20% of all breast cancers fall into the category of TNBC indicated by the absence of ER/PR expression and low/absent HER2 staining or absence of HER2 gene amplification. Fundamentally, the TNBC classifier is a confusing term because it categorizes disease based on what is missing and not necessarily on what is actionable. Fortunately, with the advent of expression and tumor genomic profiling, this heterogenous group can be further subclassified into a handful of distinct biologies.[12] Most of the TNBC tumors (60%–80%) are of the basal type. The basal type includes hallmark features of membrane expression of basement membrane

Table 1
Sample of preferred neoadjuvant/adjuvant regimens in triple-negative breast cancer

Trial	Treatment Regimen	Results
CALGB 9741	Dose-dense AC x 4 cycles → dose-dense paclitaxel q2 wk x 4 cycles	Dose-dense regimen led to improved DFS (RR = 0.74; P = .010) and OS (RR = 0.69; P = .013).
Sparano et al	Dose-dense AC x 4 cycles → weekly paclitaxel x 12 wks	5-y DFS 81.5% (odds ratio, 1.27; P = 0.006) 5-y OS 89.7% (odds ratio, 1.32; P = 0.01)
US Oncology Research Trial 9735	Docetaxel/cyclophosphamide (TC) x 4 cycles	At 7 y follow-up, 6% DFS and 5% OS improvement with TC regimen compared with AC regimen
Keynote 522[a]	Preoperative pembrolizumab/carboplatin/paclitaxel → pembrolizumab/cyclophosphamide/doxorubicin → adjuvant pembrolizumab	pCR 64.8% (95% CI, 59.9–69.5) EFS at 36 mo: 84.5% (95% CI, 81.7–86.9)
CREATE-X Trial[b]	Adjuvant capecitabine x 6–8 cycles	5-y DFS 69.8% (HR 0.58; 95% CI, 0.39–0.87) OS rate 78.8% (death HR 0.52; 95% CI, 0.30–0.90)
OlympiA Trial[c]	Adjuvant olaparib x 1 y	3-y invasive DFS 85.9% (HR 0.58; 95% CI, 0.41–0.82)

Abbreviation: RR, risk ratio.
[a] Indicated in the high-risk patients with TNBC (stage II–III).
[b] If residual disease after preoperative therapy with taxane, alkylator, anthracycline-based regimen in patients with TNBC.
[c] Consider In germline BRCA 1/2 mutations and: • TNBC: if residual disease after preoperative therapy or if ≥ pT2 or ≥ pN1 after adjuvant chemotherapy. • HR+, HER2−: residual disease and clinical, pathologic, ER status, tumor grade score ≥3 or if ≥ 4 LN + after adjuvant chemotherapy (both category 2A NCCN recommendations)[26]

protein markers (cytokeratin [CK] 5 and CK6) and absence of hormone receptors. Basal breast cancers also harbor evidence of DNA repair defects in homologous recombination with strong overlap with germline loss of BRCA1 and related genes. These tumors are chemotherapy sensitive, particularly to anthracyclines, taxanes, and platinum agents and targeted drugs such as poly(ADP-ribose) polymerase (PARP) inhibitors.[13–15] Approximately half of basal TNBC are infiltrated with effector immune cells and when treated with the addition of checkpoint inhibitors to standard chemotherapy, have improved clinical responses. Another large proportion (approximately 10%) of TNBC is notable for the presence of androgen receptor with an underlying luminal biology not dissimilar to the aggressive luminal B category of ER+ breast cancers. These tumors, although responsive to chemotherapy, are notable for responsiveness to antiandrogen treatments and diminished responses to targeted agents that might work in basal TNBC.[13,14] The remainder of TNBC categories (eg, normal-type, claudin-low, luminal A/B, driver mutation driven [epidermal growth factor receptor (EGFR)/HER2 mutated]) are numerically smaller subgroups for which precise approaches are in development.[13–15] These molecular classifying principals have been applied in clinical studies to identify patients for whom specific therapies when optimally delivered might increase clearance of in-breast/in-node disease.

Table 2
Sample of preferred neoadjuvant/adjuvant regimens in HER2+ breast cancer

Trial	Treatment Regimen	Results
TRYPHAENA	Docetaxel/carboplatin/trastuzumab ± pertuzumab x 6 cycles → trastuzumab ± pertuzumab (complete 1 y)	pCR (ypT0/is ypN0) with pertuzumab regimen: 66% (95% CI 51%-77%)
BCIRG-006	Docetaxel/carboplatin/trastuzumab x 6 cycles → trastuzumab (complete 1 y)	5-y DFS 81% (HR: 0.75; P = .04) 5-year OS 91% (HR: 0.77, P = .04)
BERENICE	Doxorubicin/cyclophosphamide x 4 cycles → paclitaxel + trastuzumab ± pertuzumab x 12 wk → trastuzumab ± pertuzumab (complete 1 y)	pCR 61.8% (95% CI 54.7% to 68.6%)
APT Trial[a]	Paclitaxel and trastuzumab weekly x 12 wk → trastuzumab (complete 1 y)	7-y invasive DFS 93% (95% CI 90.4–96.2) 7-y OS 95% (95% CI 92.4–97.7)
KATHERINE[b]	Adjuvant TDM-1 in residual disease	3-y invasive DFS 88.3% (HR: 0.50, 95% CI 0.39–0.64)
ExteNET[c]	Adjuvant neratinib x 1 y	When started within 1 y of post-trastuzumab therapy: Absolute 5-y invasive DFS benefit 5.1% (HR 0.58; 95% CI 0.41–0.82) Absolute 8-y OS benefit 2.1% (HR 0.79; 95% CI 0.55–1.13)

[a] Consider for clinical, low-risk Stage I (cT1N0M0) HER2+ tumors.
[b] Indicated in adjuvant setting if residual disease after preoperative therapy.
[c] Consider adjuvant neratinib following adjuvant trastuzumab-containing therapy in HR+, HER2+ disease with high risk of recurrence (ie, residual disease after neoadjuvant therapy).

Neoadjuvant Treatments

Traditionally, the regimens for neoadjuvant chemotherapy in TNBC have been the same regimens used in the adjuvant setting. The Early Breast Cancer Trialists' Collaborative Group's 15-year meta-analysis comparing different chemotherapy regimens among 100,000 women in 123 randomized trials demonstrated a one-third reduction in the 10-year breast cancer mortality with chemotherapy regimens consisting of anthracyclines, cyclophosphamide, and taxane compared with no chemotherapy.[16] However, because of the hematologic and cardiac side effects of anthracycline regimens, deescalation regimens were subsequently evaluated. The ABC trials evaluated the efficacy of a taxane-based regimen (taxane-cyclophosphamide [TC]) versus several triple drug regimens composed of cyclophosphamide, doxorubicin, and a taxane (Tax-AC; where the taxane was docetaxel) in 3 sequentially conducted randomized phase III trials in women with HER2-negative disease (any ER status). The joint efficacy analysis from these studies identified an improved 4-year invasive disease-free survival (IDFS) with TaxAC compared with TC in patients with high-risk HER2 negative tumors (IDFS 90.7% for TaxAC vs 88.2% for TC, p = 0.04). Subsequent secondary analyses also suggested increased benefit in patients with hormone receptor–negative, HER2-negative tumors (i.e., TNBC) and those with highest category of positive lymph nodes, therefore establishing anthracycline, taxane, cyclophosphamide regimens as a standard.[17]

Evolving Role of Platinum Agents

Preclinical data suggest that TNBC may be more sensitive to interstrand cross-linking agents that lead to DNA damage such as platinum chemotherapies due to deficiencies in homologous recombination repair.[18] The addition of carboplatin to standard neoadjuvant regimens has been evaluated in several studies and shown to augment achievement of pCR but resulted in additional toxicity. Moreover, long-term benefits after treatment completion (overall survival [OS]) are unknown.

In CALGB 40603 study, the largest randomized trial evaluating carboplatin to date, the percentage of patients who achieved pCR in breast/axilla increased from 41% to 54% (odds ratio, 1.71; P = 0.0029) with addition of carboplatin.[3] However, on further follow-up analysis, carboplatin did not seem to improve event-free survival (EFS) despite higher pCR rates, calling into question the benefit of therapy escalation with platinum drugs.[19] In the GeparSixto study, 53.2% of patients with TNBC achieved pCR with carboplatin compared with 36.9% of patients without carboplatin (p = 0.005), which translated to a better disease-free survival (DFS) (hazard ratio [HR] 0.56, 95% confidence interval [CI], 0.34–0.93; p = 0.022).[20,21] A post-hoc analysis comparing pCR in patients with carboplatin and paclitaxel versus paclitaxel followed by doxorubicin and cyclophosphamide in the BrighTNess trial showed significantly improved results pCR rate of 58% versus 31%, p < 0.0001.[4] Long-term data from the BrighTNess trial recently demonstrated an improved EFS (4-year absolute EFS ~10% higher) in patients who received paclitaxel plus carboplatin, with or without veliparib, compared with those who received paclitaxel alone, consistent with carboplatin being responsible for the improvement in EFS. However, because none of these 3 studies (CALGB 40603, GeparSixto, BrighTNess) were powered for definitive assessment of DFS/EFS or OS endpoints, pooled analysis of long-term outcomes from these trials is planned.[4]

Neoadjuvant Immunotherapy in TNBC

Chemotherapy is believed to prime endogenous anticancer immunity following increased release of tumor-specific antigens for processing by antigen-presenting cells to effector cells.[22] However, in many TNBC's, active suppression of the immune response is maintained by expression of immune checkpoints by the tumor cells or inhibitory immune cells within the tumor microenvironment (TME). Key aspects of inhibition of immune responses in the TME include the interaction between checkpoint protein programmed cell death 1 (PD-1) and programmed cell death ligand 1 (PD-L1). Pembrolizumab is an anti-PD-1 monoclonal antibody that has been shown in several clinical studies to augment immune activity in patients with metastatic TNBC. Based on these observations, the phase 2, adaptive design I-SPY2 trial evaluated pembrolizumab in combination with neoadjuvant chemotherapy versus neoadjuvant chemotherapy alone. This trial demonstrated a higher percentage of patients attaining pCR with addition of pembrolizumab (60%) versus with chemotherapy alone (22%).[23] Subsequently, KEYNOTE-522, a phase 3 trial, evaluated the efficacy of neoadjuvant pembrolizumab plus platinum containing chemotherapy followed by adjuvant maintenance pembrolizumab in patients with early stage TNBC. Initial results showed that 64.8% of patients who perceived pembrolizumab plus neoadjuvant chemotherapy had a pCR versus 51.2% with chemotherapy alone, with a treatment difference of 13.6% (95% CI, 5.4–21.8; p < 0.001).[24] The EFS at 36 months was 84.5% (95% CI, 81.7 to 86.9) in the pembrolizumab–chemotherapy group, as compared with 76.8% (95% CI, 72.2 to 80.7) in the placebo–chemotherapy group (HR 0.63; 95% CI, 0.48 to 0.82; P < 0.001).[25] Based on these data, neoadjuvant pembrolizumab is now Food and

Drug Adminstration (FDA) approved in high-risk patients with early stage TNBC (high risk defined as > T1N0) regardless of tumor PD-L1 status. Indeed, guidelines such as those published by the National Comprehensive Cancer Network (NCCN) now reflect this lower tumor size for consideration of a preoperative approach specifically to tailor adjuvant therapies that have been associated with survival benefits. The EFS data continue to mature at the time of this article's preparation. Additional investigations to evaluate the subset of tumors in KEYNOTE-522 most likely to benefit are ongoing.

Tailoring Adjuvant Therapy After Neoadjuvant Chemotherapy in TNBC

Compared with patients with TNBC achieving pCR following neoadjuvant therapy, individuals with residual disease identified following surgery have poorer EFS outcomes. For these patients with residual disease, there have only been a few rigorously tested adjuvant therapy options to consider. The CREATE-X trial, conducted in Japan and South Korea, randomized HER2-negative patients with residual disease after neoadjuvant chemotherapy (containing anthracycline, taxane, or both) to receive 6 to 8 cycles of adjuvant oral capecitabine versus placebo. Patients in the TNBC subset drove most of the benefit in the trial population, with 5-year DFS of 69.8% in capecitabine group versus 56.1% in control group (HR 0.58; 95% CI, 0.39 to 0.87) and OS rate 78.8% versus 70.3% (death HR 0.52; 95% CI, 0.30–0.90).[27] The benefit of adjuvant capecitabine in TNBC has been reported in other studies,[28–30] and practice guidelines have indicated this option to be a standard treatment of patients who receive preoperative chemotherapy but still have residual disease. However, because data show improved EFS even in patients with residual disease following treatment with neoadjuvant pembrolizumab plus chemotherapy and later with adjuvant pembrolizumab, the benefit of capecitabine in residual disease following checkpoint inhibitor therapy is unclear.[25]

More recently, PARP inhibitors have been studied in early stage TNBC. Pathogenic BRCA1 or BRCA2 mutations occur in about 5% of patients with breast cancer. Patients with germline BRCA1 or BRCA2 mutations are deficient in proteins critical for homologous recombination DNA repair, and PARP inhibitors selectively kill tumor cells that have a deficiency in homologous recombination repair. The OlympiA trial evaluated the role of PARP inhibitor olaparib in high-risk patients with HER2-negative early breast cancer with germline BRCA1 or BRCA2 pathogenic or likely pathogenic variants who received local treatment and neoadjuvant or adjuvant chemotherapy. In this phase 3, double-blinded, randomized controlled trial evaluating 1 year of adjuvant olaparib, the 3-year invasive DFS was 85.9% in the olaparib group and 77.1% in the placebo group (difference, 8.8 percentage points; 95% CI, 4.5–13.0; HR for invasive disease or death, 0.58; 99.5% CI, 0.41–0.82; P < 0.001).[31] It is important to note that patients who received postneoadjuvant capecitabine were not permitted participation in the OlympiA trial, and therefore, the relative efficacy of olaparib compared with capecitabine (as studied in CREATE-X) is unknown. In addition, with results from KEYNOTE-522 establishing a role for neoadjuvant pembrolizumab followed by adjuvant maintenance pembrolizumab in high-risk early-stage TNBC, the optimal timing of adjuvant olaparib is unclear.

Key Points

- In operable TNBCs, neoadjuvant chemotherapy is the standard except in very low-stage tumors.
- Anthracycline-/taxane-based chemotherapy regimens lead to higher benefit compared with taxane-only regimens.

- Keynote 522 study demonstrated improved EFS with addition of neoadjuvant immune checkpoint inhibitors regardless of PD-L1 tumor status.
- Additional studies are needed to determine the role of capecitabine in residual disease.
- Adjuvant olaparib for high-risk, early-stage HER2 negative breast tumors in patients with germline BRCA1 or BRCA2 pathogenic or likely pathogenic variants is associated with significantly higher invasive DFS.

HUMAN EPIDERMAL GROWTH FACTOR RECEPTOR 2-POSITIVE BREAST CANCER

Human epidermal grown factor receptor 2 (HER2) is overexpressed in 15% to 20% of all breast cancers and is one of the most aggressive breast cancer phenotypes.[32] However, with the 2 prior decades of focused advancements in HER2-targeted therapies and treatment optimization, the prognosis has improved greatly.

As observed in TNBC, HER2+ breast cancer is associated with high-quality response rates to neoadjuvant chemotherapy and therefore allowing for surgical minimization. Moreover, the addition of HER2-directed therapies to chemotherapy has increased response rates substantially, with pCR approaching almost 50% to 75% depending on the specific therapies and degree of enrichment for specific molecular subtypes. Similar to TNBC, a strong association between pCR and long-term survival has been shown in HER2+ breast cancers, with significant improvement in relapse-free survival and OS when compared with women with residual disease.[2]

Neoadjuvant therapy now plays an integral role, as it optimizes treatment and allows for risk stratification in HER2+ breast cancers. It is therefore now the standard of care for HER2+ disease except in very small, clinically low-risk tumors (ie, **Table 2**, T1N0).[33]

Evolution of Treatment Regimens in Human Epidermal Growth Factor Receptor 2-Positive Breast Cancer

Anti-human epidermal growth factor receptor 2–directed therapies

There are 4 HER2-directed therapies that are now approved in the adjuvant setting, some of which are now also used in the neoadjuvant setting: (1) monoclonal antibodies trastuzumab and (2) pertuzumab; (3) an oral irreversible tyrosine kinase inhibitor that blocks signal transduction through the EGFR family including the HER2 kinase neratinib; and (4) an antibody-drug conjugate (ADC) of trastuzumab and emtansine (cytotoxic payload agent) trastuzumab emtansine (T-DM1).

In several adjuvant trials, the addition of HER2-targeted therapy to chemotherapy as opposed to placebo has been associated with higher response rates. A joint analysis of the NCCTG N9831 and NSABP B-31 trials found that addition of 1 year of trastuzumab to chemotherapy in patients with HER2+ operable breast cancer led to a 37% relative improvement in OS (HR, 0.63; 95% CI, 0.54 to 0.73; P < .001) and a 40% improvement in DFS (HR, 0.60; 95% CI, 0.53 to 0.68; P < .001).[34] Subsequently and as discussed further later, addition of dual anti-HER2 therapy with pertuzumab added to trastuzumab and chemotherapy showed a significantly improved invasive DFS (HR, 0.72; 95% CI, 0.59 to 0.87 at 6-year follow-up), specifically in patients with node-positive disease regardless of hormone receptor status.[35,36]

Because of the benefit in the adjuvant setting, trastuzumab has since been studied in the neoadjuvant setting combined with chemotherapy and demonstrated improved survival outcomes. The NOAH study evaluated open-label neoadjuvant trastuzumab combined with chemotherapy followed by adjuvant trastuzumab and demonstrated a significantly improved EFS in the trastuzumab group (71%, 95% CI 61–78) compared with control nontrastuzumab group (56%, 95% CI 46–65) with HR of 0.59 (95% CI 0.38–0.90; p = 0.013) and almost doubled the rates of pCR from 19% to 38%.[37]

Next, dual HER2-directed therapy was evaluated in the neoadjuvant setting. The open-label NeoSphere study randomized treatment-naïve HER2+ patients to 4 cycles of neoadjuvant docetaxel with either trastuzumab, pertuzumab, or both versus combination pertuzumab and trastuzumab without chemotherapy. There was a significantly improved pCR in pertuzumab and trastuzumab plus docetaxel group (45·8% [95% CI 36.1–55.7]) compared with trastuzumab plus docetaxel group (29·0% [20.6–38.5]; p = 0.0141).[38]

Other dual HER2 regimens such as trastuzumab and lapatinib with neoadjuvant chemotherapy have also been studied and have shown to increase the pCR rate. However, the role of lapatinib in this setting is unclear due to discordant results in regard to survival outcomes observed among these studies. A recent meta-analysis included 4 randomized trials (CALGB 40601, Cher-LOB, NSABP-B41, NeoALTTO) that included patients to receive neoadjuvant chemotherapy with trastuzumab, lapatinib, or their combination. Dual blockade with trastuzumab and lapatinib led to significantly improved OS (HR 0.65, 95% CI 0.43–0.98) when given with neoadjuvant chemotherapy, suggesting that there could be a role for lapatinib in the neoadjuvant setting.[39] However, further studies are needed to define the role of lapatinib in the current neoadjuvant treatment paradigm. Nonetheless, treatment with lapatinib in the adjuvant setting is FDA approved and appears on professional guidelines following the full year of HER2-directed monoclonal antibody treatment in the (neo)adjuvant setting in what is now termed "extended" adjuvant therapy based on the results of the EXTENET trial. In this trial, neratinib demonstrated a 2-year invasive DFS rate of 93.9% (95% CI 92.4–95.2) compared with 91.6% (95% CI 90.0–93.0) in placebo group.[40] Based on subset analyses, an enrichment of benefit in patients with hormone receptor–positive (HR+) and HER2+ disease who were also contemporaneously being treated with endocrine therapy was observed.

Finally, T-DM1 has also been studied but so far has not shown clear-cut advantage with improved survival over dual monoclonal antibody therapy when given in the neoadjuvant setting. The KRISTINE trial assessed the efficacy of T-DM1 plus pertuzumab compared with trastuzumab plus pertuzumab with traditional neoadjuvant chemotherapy. The results showed that patients who received neoadjuvant chemotherapy plus dual HER2-directed therapies had a numerically higher pCR rate (55%) versus 44% of patients who received T-DM1 plus pertuzumab.[41] T-DM1 plus pertuzumab was better tolerated than systemic chemotherapy containing regimens and there remains interest in understanding which type of tumor is best targeted. A small single-arm phase II trial demonstrated that heterogeneity of HER2 expression differentiates which tumors may fully respond to ADC such as T-DM1.[42] This concept of using nonsystemic chemotherapies regimens focused on ADC in combination with pertuzumab is being reevaluated in ongoing clinical studies with this refined understanding of the tumor composition.

Role of anthracyclines

Different chemotherapy backbones have also been studied in combination with dual HER2-directed therapy. More specifically, because of cardiac toxicities associated with both HER2-targeted therapies and commonly used anthracyclines in breast cancer treatment (epirubicin, adriamycin), investigation into the tolerability of all treatments combined is an important factor to consider. The BCIRG-006 study evaluated the efficacy and safety of trastuzumab with anthracycline and nonanthracycline regimens in the adjuvant setting. The 5-year DFS were 75% among chemotherapy-only group, 84% among anthracycline plus trastuzumab group, and 81% in nonanthracycline plus trastuzumab group. OS rates were 87%, 92%, and 91%, respectively, showing that there was no significant difference in efficacy in anthracycline versus nonanthracycline regimens. However, the rates of cardiac side effects were notably higher in anthracycline group compared with nonanthracycline group.[43]

In the neoadjuvant setting, the TRAIN-2 study investigated the benefit of anthracyclines compared with a carboplatin-taxane regimen when given with dual HER2 targets trastuzumab and pertuzumab. At 19-month follow-up, pCR was noted in 67% (95% CI, 60–73) in the anthracycline group and in 68% (95% CI, 61–74) in nonanthracycline group (p = 0.95). The study did note a higher number of grade 3 or more neutropenia in the anthracycline group versus nonanthracycline group (60% vs 54%), increase in secondary malignancies, and symptomatic left ventricular dysfunction.[44] A 3-year follow-up showed similar EFS (92.7% vs 93.6% in the nonanthracycline group). OS at 3 years was also similar in both groups (97.7% in the anthracycline group vs 98.2% nonanthracycline group).[45] Because a similar proportion of pCR in both groups was observed and similar long-term survival noted, this study indicated that a nonanthracycline containing regimen could represent a preferred approach.

Tailoring Adjuvant Therapy in Residual Disease After Neoadjuvant Chemotherapy in HER2 Positive Breast Cancer

Patients with HER2+ breast cancer who are identified with residual disease at surgery after neoadjuvant chemotherapy have a higher risk of disease recurrence and death compared with patients with pCR.[5] The KATHERINE trial evaluated patients with residual disease after neoadjuvant therapy (taxane with or without anthracycline and trastuzumab) to receive adjuvant T-DM1 or trastuzumab for 14 cycles. The DFS at 3 years was significantly higher in the T-DM1 group than trastuzumab group (HR 0.50, 95% CI, 0.39–0.64; p < 0.001). Because of the 50% lower risk of recurrent breast cancer or death with adjuvant T-DM1, it has now become the standard of care treatment in patients with residual disease.[46] Interestingly, the pattern of recurrences in KATHERINE was notable because nearly 50% of all recurrences were intracranial in both randomized groups and indicated that optimization with brain-penetrant HER2-targeting agents is desirable and is formally being evaluated in multiple studies at the time of this article's preparation (ie, Compass HER2 trials).

Key Points

- Neoadjuvant chemotherapy is standard in HER2+ disease except in very low-risk tumors
- Addition of neoadjuvant trastuzumab almost doubles pCR rates.
- Dual HER2-directed neoadjuvant therapy (trastuzumab and pertuzumab) improves outcomes in more advanced disease.
- Adjuvant T-DM1 decreases risk of breast cancer recurrence in patients with residual disease after neoadjuvant chemotherapy.
- Adjuvant neratinib in high-risk, HR+ and HER2+ tumors should be considered as an adjunct therapy for patients with residual disease after neoadjuvant therapy.

HORMONE RECEPTOR–POSITIVE, HUMAN EPIDERMAL GROWTH FACTOR RECEPTOR 2-NEGATIVE BREAST CANCER

Estrogen receptor positive (ER+) breast cancer is the most common subtype of breast cancer, making up approximately 75% of all cases. The mainstay treatment is endocrine therapy, which targets estrogen via different strategies. One mechanism is by inhibiting production of estrogen by blocking aromatase (aromatase inhibitors) or inhibiting ovarian estrogen production via gonadotropin releasing hormone agonists. A second mechanism is by targeting ER (tamoxifen, fulvestrant) and rendering it inactive.[47]

Both chemotherapy and endocrine therapy are most commonly used in the adjuvant setting. However, in select cases, they can be used in the neoadjuvant setting but unlike in TNBC and HER2+ breast cancer, HR+ breast tumors are less sensitive to chemotherapy in terms of achieving pCR.[48,49]

Neoadjuvant Chemotherapy in Hormone Receptor Positive, Human Epidermal Growth Factor Receptor 2– Breast Cancer

In HR+ breast cancers, indication of neoadjuvant chemotherapy is based on the tumor characteristics such as tumor grade and nodal status and is offered to render inoperable disease operable or reduce the extent of surgery to optimize local therapy. The most common neoadjuvant regimens in HR+ breast cancer include taxane-based regimen or anthracycline/taxane regimen. These 2 regimens were assessed in the aforementioned ABC trials, which demonstrated the noninferiority of taxane-based regimen compared with anthracycline/taxane regimen. However, in patients with HR+, node positive disease, the change in four-year invasive DFS was modest at 2.0% in 1-3 lymph node positive but approximately 6.0% in 4 or more lymph nodes, indicating a benefit with anthracycline/taxane regimen, especially in multi-node disease.[17] Genomic profiles such as Oncotype Dx Recurrence Score and MammaPrint have shown to predict benefit from adjuvant chemotherapy; however, because of limited data for application in the neoadjuvant setting, expert guidelines presently do not recommend using genomic profiles to determine use of neoadjuvant chemotherapy or endocrine therapy at this time.[33]

Neoadjuvant Endocrine Therapy in Hormone Receptor Positive, Human Epidermal Growth Factor Receptor 2– Breast Cancer

Neoadjuvant endocrine therapy can be used for disease control in patients who are not candidates for surgery or deemed unsuitable for chemotherapy. In postmenopausal women, aromatase inhibitors (AI) can also be used to increase locoregional treatment options.[50,51] When compared with neoadjuvant chemotherapy, in a meta-analysis of 20 randomized clinical trials, neoadjuvant AI had similar clinical response rate and BCS rate as neoadjuvant combination chemotherapy but with lower toxicity.[47] In addition, using neoadjuvant treatment response to later tailor adjuvant therapy in HR+, HER2– breast cancer remains under investigation. Although pCR rates are low following neoadjuvant endocrine therapy, one emergent strategy is using biomarkers such as Ki67 in residual tumor integrated into a post-treatment model referred to as preoperative endocrine prognostic index (PEPI) to determine prognosis and optimize adjuvant treatments.[52–54] In premenopausal women, neoadjuvant endocrine therapy is not routinely recommended and remains investigational.

Role of CDK4/6 Inhibitors and PI3K Inhibitors in the Early-Stage Hormone Receptor Positive, Human Epidermal Growth Factor Receptor 2– Breast Cancer

Although HR+ breast cancers are highly responsive to endocrine therapy, a major concern is innate or acquired resistance. One such mechanism that drives resistance is the regulation of cyclin D-CDK4/6-Rb axis. Inhibitors of this pathway (CDK4/6 inhibitors such as abemaciclib, ribociclib, palbociclib) arrest tumor growth and are approved and commonly used for early lines of treatment in the metastatic setting.[55] More recently, addition of abemaciclib to standard adjuvant endocrine therapy in HR+, HER2− early-stage breast cancer with high-risk features who are at increased risk for early recurrence was investigated in the phase III MonarchE trial. High-risk patients were defined as those with 4 or more pN-positive disease or 1 to 3 positive nodes with large tumor size, high grade, or Ki-67 greater than 20%. The study showed that adding abemaciclib to endocrine therapy significantly improved invasive DFS with a 25% risk reduction (P = .01; HR, 0.75; 95% CI, 0.60–0.93) and a 3.5% absolute improvement in 2-year IDFS rates (92.2% vs 88.7%) and is now FDA approved.[56]

In addition, CDK 4/6 inhibitors are now being evaluated as a way to improve the efficacy of neoadjuvant endocrine therapy or to overcome de novo resistance to neoadjuvant endocrine therapy. The neoMONARCH and PALLET trials evaluated abemaciclib and palbociclib with neoadjuvant endocrine therapy, respectively. Results from the neoMONARCH study showed that abemaciclib alone or in combination with neoadjuvant AI led to significant decrease in Ki67 expression compared with AI alone, and 46% of patients achieved a radiologic response at the end of treatment.[57] The PALLET trial showed that adding palbociclib to AI once again led to significant decrease in Ki67 expression but did not show an increase in clinical response.[58] The FELINE trial evaluated efficacy of neoadjuvant ribociclib and AI therapy by assessing changes in biomarkers (PEPI and Ki67). A PEPI score 0 after neoadjuvant endocrine therapy is associated with low risk of relapse even without adjuvant chemotherapy in ER+ breast cancer.[59] The results from FELINE trial showed that addition of ribociclib to neoadjuvant AI did not lead to more women with a PEPI score of 0.[60] Of note, these aforementioned trials were phase II studies. Presently, phase III trials to elucidate the role of CKD4/6 inhibitors in the neoadjuvant setting are ongoing.

Another mechanism of endocrine resistance is through increased PI3K/AKT/mTOR signaling, and in the metastatic setting, PI3K inhibitors such as alpelisib in combination with fulvestrant have been shown to have enhanced activity against PIK3CA-mutated tumors and is now approved for use in patients with advanced disease.[61] Neoadjuvant taselisib with letrozole versus letrozole alone was evaluated in a phase II, randomized, double blinded trial and showed that a higher proportion of patients achieved an objective response in taselisib group, indicating a potential role in the neoadjuvant setting in PIK3CA mutation harboring tumors.[62]

Key Points

- HR+ tumors are less sensitive to neoadjuvant chemotherapy when compared with TNBC or HER2+ tumors.
- Taxane or anthracycline/taxane regimens are used in the neoadjuvant setting.
  - There is a slightly increased benefit of neoadjuvant anthracycline/taxane regimen in node-positive patients.
- Neoadjuvant endocrine therapy can be used in postmenopausal women to increase locoregional treatment options but remains investigational in premenopausal women.
- Role of neoadjuvant CKD4/6 inhibitors and PI3K inhibitors is currently being investigated.

FUTURE DIRECTIONS

Patients who achieve a pCR after neoadjuvant chemotherapy have a significant survival advantage over those who did not.[9] However, the data are less clear on predicting metastatic recurrence in patients with residual disease. One area of emerging research is evaluating the role of biomarkers in monitoring response to neo-adjuvant chemotherapy and resistance to treatment.

One such biomarker is circulating tumor DNA (ctDNA), which is being evaluated in the neoadjuvant setting in breast cancer. A substudy of the NeoALTTO phase III trial evaluated whether ctDNA was associated with response to anti-HER2–targeted ther-apy and concluded that its detection before neoadjuvant anti-HER2 therapies was associated with decreased pCR rates.[63] Another substudy of the neoadjuvant I-SPY2 TRIAL retrospectively evaluated cell-free DNA (cfDNA) from high-risk patients with early breast cancer and showed that persistent detection was a significant pre-dictor of poor response and metastatic recurrence, whereas clearance was associ-ated with improved survival even in patients who did not achieve pCR.[64] Detection of minimal residual disease (MRD) by ctDNA is also being evaluated in the adjuvant setting, especially in HR+ breast cancer subtype where a large proportion of metasta-tic recurrences occur more than 5 years after initial diagnosis. In the CHiRP study that interrogated samples from high-risk HR+ breast cancer with no evidence of recur-rence 5 years after diagnosis, ctDNA identified MRD in all cases associated with distant recurrences.[65] Additional prospective studies are needed to establish the clin-ical utility of ctDNA and cfDNA assays and determine whether intervention after MRD detection improves patient outcomes.

The use of tumor expression profiles as a predictive biomarker of treatment response is another area of emerging research. The 70-gene MammaPrint prognostic score was further stratified into "high-" or "ultra-high"-risk groups in the I-SPY2 trial and was used as a biomarker to assess response of receptor subtypes and variety of therapeutic agents/combinations. Results showed that this further stratification of MammaPrint score predicted chemosensitivity and can guide treatment prioritization of targeted agents.[66] Similarly, in the NBSRT study, BluePrint, an 80-gene molecular classifier, reclassified 15% of ER+, HER2− tumors as basal-type (ER+/Basal) group and found pCR to neoadjuvant therapy was similar to TNBC/basal tumors and had a higher rate of pCR than ER+/luminal A and ER+/luminal B tumors; this highlights the role of tumor expression profiles in identifying tumors with higher chemosensitivity and their role in treatment planning.[67] Another predictive biomarker of interest is tumor-infiltrating lymphocytes percentage, which has been shown to predict response to neoadjuvant chemotherapy, particularly in TNBC and HER2-driven cancers.[68] Further research into these biomarkers can pave the way to a more tailored treatment approach to optimize toward a balance of effectiveness while minimizing harm from cytotoxic and other therapies.

CLINICS CARE POINTS

- Neoadjuvant chemotherapy is indicated in inoperable disease and is strongly preferred in certain operable settings.

- Benefits of neoadjuvant chemotherapy include increased rates of breast conservation surgery and surgical minimization in the axilla.

- Response to neoadjuvant chemotherapy (eg, pCR or RCB classification) provides prognostic information and guides subsequent adjuvant therapy.

- Incorporation of targeted and immunotherapy agents into neoadjuvant therapy is specific to tumor biology (ie, particularly in TNBC and HER2).

DISCLOSURE

A.K: nothing to disclose. V.K. Gadi: Founder (equity) in SEngine Precision Medicine, Novilla, and 3rdEyeBio; Scientific board member for Puma Biotechnology, New Equilibrium Biosciences, Phoenix Molecular Designs. Member of speakers' bureaus for Puma Biotechnology, Genentech/Roche, Hologics. Recipient of research support to his institution from Agendia and Tizona Therapeutics.

REFERENCES

1. Gralow JR, Burstein HJ, Wood W, et al. Preoperative therapy in invasive breast cancer: pathologic assessment and systemic therapy issues in operable disease. J Clin Oncol 2008;26(5):814–9.

2. Fernandez-Martinez A, Krop IE, Hillman DW, et al. Survival, pathologic response, and genomics in CALGB 40601 (Alliance), a neoadjuvant phase III trial of paclitaxel-trastuzumab with or without lapatinib in HER2-positive breast cancer. J Clin Oncol 2020;38(35):4184–93.

3. Sikov WM, Berry DA, Perou CM, et al. Impact of the addition of carboplatin and/or bevacizumab to neoadjuvant once-per-week paclitaxel followed by dose-dense doxorubicin and cyclophosphamide on pathologic complete response rates in stage II to III triple-negative breast cancer: CALGB 40603 (Alliance). J Clin Oncol 2015;33(1):13–21.

4. Geyer CE, Sikov WM, Huober J, et al. Long-term efficacy and safety of addition of carboplatin with or without veliparib to standard neoadjuvant chemotherapy in triple-negative breast cancer: 4-year follow-up data from BrighTNess, a randomized phase III trial. Ann Oncol 2022;33(4):384–94.

5. Boughey JC, Suman VJ, Mittendorf EA, et al. Sentinel lymph node surgery after neoadjuvant chemotherapy in patients with node-positive breast cancer: the ACOSOG Z1071 (Alliance) clinical trial. JAMA 2013;310:1455–61.

6. Kuehn T, Bauerfeind I, Fehm T, et al. Sentinel lymph node biopsy in patients with breast cancer before and after neoadjuvant chemotherapy (SENTINA): a prospective, multicentre cohort study. Lancet Oncol 2013;14:609–18.

7. Boileau JF, Poirier B, Basik M, et al. Sentinel node biopsy after neoadjuvant chemotherapy in biopsy-proven node-positive breast cancer: the SN FNAC study. J Clin Oncol 2015;33:258–64.

8. von Minckwitz G, Untch M, Blohmer JU, et al. Definition and impact of pathologic complete response on prognosis after neoadjuvant chemotherapy in various intrinsic breast cancer subtypes. J Clin Oncol 2012;30(15):1796–804.

9. Cortazar P, Zhang L, Untch M, et al. Pathological complete response and long-term clinical benefit in breast cancer: the CTNeoBC pooled analysis. Lancet 2014;384(9938):164–72. https://doi.org/10.1016/S0140-6736(13)62422-8. Epub 2014 Feb 14. Erratum in: Lancet. 2019 Mar 9;393(10175):986.

10. Symmans WF, Peintinger F, Hatzis C, et al. Measurement of residual breast cancer burden to predict survival after neoadjuvant chemotherapy. J Clin Oncol 2007;25(28):4414–22.

11. Symmans WF, Wei C, Gould R, et al. Long-term prognostic risk after neoadjuvant chemotherapy associated with residual cancer burden and breast cancer subtype. J Clin Oncol 2017;35(10):1049–60.

12. Gadi VK, Davidson NE. Practical Approach to Triple-Negative Breast Cancer. J Oncol Pract 2017;13(5):293–300.

13. Lehmann BD, Bauer JA, Chen X, et al. Identification of human triple-negative breast cancer subtypes and preclinical models for selection of targeted therapies. J Clin Invest 2011;121(7):2750–67.

14. Burstein MD, Tsimelzon A, Poage GM, et al. Comprehensive genomic analysis identifies novel subtypes and targets of triple-negative breast cancer. Clin Cancer Res 2015;21(7):1688–98.

15. Cheang MC, Martin M, Nielsen TO, et al. Defining breast cancer intrinsic subtypes by quantitative receptor expression. Oncologist 2015;20(5):474–82.

16. Early Breast Cancer Trialists' Collaborative Group (EBCTCG), Peto R, Davies C, Godwin J, et al. Comparisons between different polychemotherapy regimens for early breast cancer: meta-analyses of long-term outcome among 100,000 women in 123 randomised trials. Lancet 2012;379(9814):432–44.

17. Blum JL, Flynn PJ, Yothers G, et al. Anthracyclines in early breast cancer: the ABC Trials-USOR 06-090, NSABP B-46-I/USOR 07132, and NSABP B-49 (NRG Oncology). J Clin Oncol 2017;35(23):2647–55.

18. Hurley J, Reis IM, Rodgers SE, et al. The use of neoadjuvant platinum-based chemotherapy in locally advanced breast cancer that is triple negative: retrospective analysis of 144 patients. Breast Cancer Res Treat 2013;138:783–94.

19. Shepherd JH, Ballman K, Polley MC, et al. CALGB 40603 (Alliance): Long-Term Outcomes and Genomic Correlates of Response and Survival After Neoadjuvant Chemotherapy With or Without Carboplatin and Bevacizumab in Triple-Negative Breast Cancer. J Clin Oncol 2022;40(12):1323–34.

20. von Minckwitz G, Schneeweiss A, Loibl S, et al. Neoadjuvant carboplatin in patients with triple-negative and HER2-positive early breast cancer (GeparSixto; GBG 66): a randomised phase 2 trial. Lancet Oncol 2014;15(7):747–56.

21. Loibl S, Weber KE, Timms KM, et al. Survival analysis of carboplatin added to an anthracycline/taxane-based neoadjuvant chemotherapy and HRD score as predictor of response-final results from GeparSixto. Ann Oncol 2018;29(12):2341–7.

22. Farkona S, Diamandis EP, Blasutig IM. Cancer immunotherapy: the beginning of the end of cancer? BMC Med 2016;14:73.

23. Nanda R, Liu MC, Yau C, et al. Effect of pembrolizumab plus neoadjuvant chemotherapy on pathologic complete response in women with early-stage breast cancer: an analysis of the ongoing phase 2 adaptively randomized I-SPY2 trial. JAMA Oncol 2020;6(5):676–84.

24. Schmid P, Cortes J, Pusztai L, et al. KEYNOTE-522 Investigators. Pembrolizumab for Early Triple-Negative Breast Cancer. N Engl J Med 2020;382(9):810–21.

25. Schmid P, Cortes J, Dent R, et al. KEYNOTE-522 investigators. Event-free Survival with Pembrolizumab in Early Triple-Negative Breast Cancer. N Engl J Med 2022;386(6):556–67.

26. National Comprehensive Cancer Network (NCCN). NCCN Clinical practice guidelines in oncology. Breast cancer version 4.2022. https://www.nccn.org/professionals/physician_gls/pdf/breast.pdf. Accessed August 15, 2022.

27. Masuda N, Lee SJ, Ohtani S, et al. Adjuvant Capecitabine for Breast Cancer after Preoperative Chemotherapy. N Engl J Med 2017;376(22):2147–59.

28. Joensuu H, Kellokumpu-Lehtinen PL, Huovinen R, et al. Adjuvant capecitabine, docetaxel, cyclophosphamide, and epirubicin for early breast cancer: final analysis of the randomized FinXX trial. J Clin Oncol 2012;30(1):11–8.

29. O'Shaughnessy J, Koeppen H, Xiao Y, et al. Patients with Slowly Proliferative Early Breast Cancer Have Low Five-Year Recurrence Rates in a Phase III Adjuvant Trial of Capecitabine. Clin Cancer Res 2015;21(19):4305–11.

30. Natori A, Ethier JL, Amir E, et al. Capecitabine in early breast cancer: a meta-analysis of randomised controlled trials. Eur J Cancer 2017;77:40–7.
31. Tutt ANJ, Garber JE, Kaufman B, et al. OlympiA Clinical Trial Steering Committee and Investigators. Adjuvant Olaparib for Patients with BRCA1- or BRCA2-Mutated Breast Cancer. N Engl J Med 2021;384(25):2394–405.
32. Slamon DJ, Godolphin W, Jones LA, et al. Studies of the HER-2/neu proto-oncogene in human breast and ovarian cancer. Science 1989;244:707–12.
33. Korde LA, Somerfield MR, Carey LA, et al. Neoadjuvant chemotherapy, endocrine therapy, and targeted therapy for breast cancer: ASCO guideline. J Clin Oncol 2021;39(13):1485–505.
34. Perez EA, Romond EH, Suman VJ, et al. Trastuzumab plus adjuvant chemotherapy for human epidermal growth factor receptor 2-positive breast cancer: planned joint analysis of overall survival from NSABP B-31 and NCCTG N9831. J Clin Oncol 2014;32(33):3744–52.
35. von Minckwitz G, Procter M, de Azambuja E, et al. APHINITY Steering Committee and Investigators. Adjuvant Pertuzumab and Trastuzumab in Early HER2-Positive Breast Cancer. N Engl J Med 2017;377(2):122–31.
36. Piccart M, Procter M, Fumagalli D, et al. APHINITY Steering Committee and Investigators. Adjuvant Pertuzumab and Trastuzumab in Early HER2-Positive Breast Cancer in the APHINITY Trial: 6 Years' Follow-Up. J Clin Oncol 2021; 39(13):1448–57.
37. Gianni L, Eiermann W, Semiglazov V, et al. Neoadjuvant chemotherapy with trastuzumab followed by adjuvant trastuzumab versus neoadjuvant chemotherapy alone, in patients with HER2-positive locally advanced breast cancer (the NOAH trial): a randomised controlled superiority trial with a parallel HER2-negative cohort. Lancet 2010;375(9712):377–84.
38. Gianni L, Pienkowski T, Im YH, et al. Efficacy and safety of neoadjuvant pertuzumab and trastuzumab in women with locally advanced, inflammatory, or early HER2-positive breast cancer (NeoSphere): a randomised multicentre, open-label, phase 2 trial. Lancet Oncol 2012;13(1):25–32.
39. Guarneri V, Griguolo G, Miglietta F, et al. Survival after neoadjuvant therapy with trastuzumab-lapatinib and chemotherapy in patients with HER2-positive early breast cancer: a meta-analysis of randomized trials. ESMO Open 2022;7(2): 100433.
40. Chan A, Delaloge S, Holmes FA, et al, ExteNET Study Group. Neratinib after trastuzumab-based adjuvant therapy in patients with HER2-positive breast cancer (ExteNET): a multicentre, randomised, double-blind, placebo-controlled, phase 3 trial. Lancet Oncol 2016;17(3):367–77.
41. Hurvitz SA, Martin M, Symmans WF, et al. Neoadjuvant trastuzumab, pertuzumab, and chemotherapy versus trastuzumab emtansine plus pertuzumab in patients with HER2-positive breast cancer (KRISTINE): a randomised, open-label, multicentre, phase 3 trial. Lancet Oncol 2018;19(1):115–26.
42. Metzger Filho O, Viale G, Trippa L, et al: HER2 heterogeneity as a predictor of response to neoadjuvant T-DM1 plus pertuzumab: Results from a prospective clinical trial. 2019 ASCO Annual Meeting. Abstract 502. Presented June 3, 2019.
43. Slamon D, Eiermann W, Robert N, et al, Breast Cancer International Research Group. Adjuvant trastuzumab in HER2-positive breast cancer. N Engl J Med 2011;365(14):1273–83.
44. van Ramshorst MS, van der Voort A, van Werkhoven ED, et al. Dutch Breast Cancer Research Group (BOOG). Neoadjuvant chemotherapy with or without anthracyclines in the presence of dual HER2 blockade for HER2-positive breast cancer

(TRAIN-2): a multicentre, open-label, randomised, phase 3 trial. Lancet Oncol 2018;19(12):1630–40.

45. van der Voort A, van Ramshorst MS, van Werkhoven ED, et al. Three-year follow-up of neoadjuvant chemotherapy with or without anthracyclines in the presence of dual ERBB2 blockade in patients with ERBB2-positive breast cancer: a secondary analysis of the TRAIN-2 randomized, phase 3 trial. JAMA Oncol 2021; 7(7):978–84.

46. von Minckwitz G, Huang CS, Mano MS, et al. KATHERINE Investigators. Trastuzumab Emtansine for Residual Invasive HER2-Positive Breast Cancer. N Engl J Med 2019;380(7):617–28.

47. Spring LM, Gupta A, Reynolds KL, et al. Neoadjuvant endocrine therapy for estrogen receptor-positive breast cancer: a systematic review and meta-analysis. JAMA Oncol 2016;2(11):1477–86.

48. Colleoni M, Viale G, Zahrieh D, et al. Chemotherapy is more effective in patients with breast cancer not expressing steroid hormone receptors: a study of preoperative treatment. Clin Cancer Res 2004;10(19):6622–8.

49. Colleoni M, Viale G, Zahrieh D, et al. Expression of ER, PgR, HER1, HER2, and response: a study of preoperative chemotherapy. Ann Oncol 2008;19(3):465–72.

50. Cataliotti L, Buzdar AU, Noguchi S, et al. Comparison of anastrozole versus tamoxifen as preoperative therapy in postmenopausal women with hormone receptor-positive breast cancer: the Pre-Operative "Arimidex" Compared to Tamoxifen (PROACT) trial. Cancer 2006;106(10):2095–103.

51. Smith IE, Dowsett M, Ebbs SR, et al, IMPACT Trialists Group. Neoadjuvant treatment of postmenopausal breast cancer with anastrozole, tamoxifen, or both in combination: the Immediate Preoperative Anastrozole, Tamoxifen, or Combined with Tamoxifen (IMPACT) multicenter double-blind randomized trial. J Clin Oncol 2005;23(22):5108–16.

52. Chia YH, Ellis MJ, Ma CX. Neoadjuvant endocrine therapy in primary breast cancer: indications and use as a research tool. Br J Cancer 2010;103(6):759–64.

53. Suman VJ, Ellis MJ, Ma CX. The ALTERNATE trial: assessing a biomarker driven strategy for the treatment of post-menopausal women with ER+/Her2- invasive breast cancer. Chin Clin Oncol 2015;4(3):34.

54. Ellis MJ, Suman VJ, Hoog J, et al. Ki67 proliferation index as a tool for chemotherapy decisions during and after neoadjuvant aromatase inhibitor treatment of breast cancer: results from the american college of surgeons oncology group Z1031 trial (Alliance). J Clin Oncol 2017;35(10):1061–9.

55. Hosford SR, Miller TW. Clinical potential of novel therapeutic targets in breast cancer: CDK4/6, Src, JAK/STAT, PARP, HDAC, and PI3K/AKT/mTOR pathways. Pharmgenomics Pers Med 2014;7:203–15.

56. Johnston SRD, Harbeck N, Hegg R, Toi M, Martin M, Shao ZM, Zhang QY, Martinez Rodriguez JL, Campone M, Hamilton E, Sohn J, Guarneri V, Okada M, Boyle F, Neven P, Cortés J, Huober J, Wardley A, Tolaney SM, Cicin I, Smith IC, Frenzel M, Headley D, Wei R, San Antonio B, Hulstijn M, Cox J, O'Shaughnessy J, Rastogi P, monarchE Committee Members, Investigators. Abemaciclib Combined With Endocrine Therapy for the Adjuvant Treatment of HR+, HER2-, Node-Positive, High-Risk, Early Breast Cancer (monarchE). J Clin Oncol 2020;38(34):3987–98.

57. Hurvitz SA, Martin M, Press MF, et al. Potent Cell-Cycle Inhibition and Upregulation of Immune Response with Abemaciclib and Anastrozole in neoMONARCH, Phase II Neoadjuvant Study in HR+/HER2- Breast Cancer. Clin Cancer Res 2020;26(3):566–80.

58. Johnston S, Puhalla S, Wheatley D, et al. Randomized Phase II Study Evaluating Palbociclib in Addition to Letrozole as Neoadjuvant Therapy in Estrogen Receptor-Positive Early Breast Cancer: PALLET Trial. J Clin Oncol 2019;37(3): 178–89.

59. Ellis MJ, Tao Y, Luo J, et al. Outcome prediction for estrogen receptor-positive breast cancer based on postneoadjuvant endocrine therapy tumor characteristics. J Natl Cancer Inst 2008;100(19):1380–8.

60. Khan QJ, O'Dea A, Bardia A, et al. Letrozole + ribociclib versus letrozole + placebo as neoadjuvant therapy for ER+ breast cancer (FELINE trial). J Clin Oncol 2020;38(15_suppl):505.

61. André F, Ciruelos E, Rubovszky G, et al. SOLAR-1 Study Group. Alpelisib for PIK3CA-Mutated, Hormone Receptor-Positive Advanced Breast Cancer. N Engl J Med 2019;380(20):1929–40.

62. Saura C, Hlauschek D, Oliveira M, et al. Neoadjuvant letrozole plus taselisib versus letrozole plus placebo in postmenopausal women with oestrogen receptor-positive, HER2-negative, early-stage breast cancer (LORELEI): a multicentre, randomised, double-blind, placebo-controlled, phase 2 trial. Lancet Oncol 2019;20(9):1226–38.

63. Rothé F, Silva MJ, Venet D, et al. Circulating Tumor DNA in HER2-Amplified Breast Cancer: a translational research substudy of the NeoALTTO Phase III Trial. Clin Cancer Res 2019;25(12):3581–8.

64. Magbanua MJM, Swigart LB, Wu HT, et al. Circulating tumor DNA in neoadjuvant-treated breast cancer reflects response and survival. Ann Oncol 2021;32(2): 229–39.

65. Lipsyc-Sharf M, De Bruin E, Santos K, et al. Circulating tumor DNA (ctDNA) and late recurrence in high-risk, hormone receptor–positive, HER2-negative breast cancer (CHiRP). J Clin Oncol 2022;40(suppl 16):abstr 103.

66. Wolf DM, Yau C, Brown-Swigart L, Hirst G, Buxton M, Paoloni M, I-SPY2 TRIAL Investigators, Olopade O, DeMichele A, Symmans F, Rugo H, Berry D, Esserman L, van t Veer L. Gene and pathway differences between MammaPrint High1/ High2 risk classes: results from the I-SPY 2 TRIAL in breast cancer [Abstract]. In: AACR 107th Annual Meeting 2016 April 16-20, Abstract nr 859.

67. Whitworth PW, Beitsch PD, Pellicane JV, et al, NBRST Investigators Group. Distinct Neoadjuvant Chemotherapy Response and 5-Year Outcome in Patients With Estrogen Receptor-Positive, Human Epidermal Growth Factor Receptor 2-Negative Breast Tumors That Reclassify as Basal-Type by the 80-Gene Signature. JCO Precis Oncol 2022;6:e2100463.

68. Denkert C, von Minckwitz G, Darb-Esfahani S, et al. Tumour-infiltrating lymphocytes and prognosis in different subtypes of breast cancer: a pooled analysis of 3771 patients treated with neoadjuvant therapy. Lancet Oncol 2018;19(1): 40–50.

Moving?

Make sure your subscription moves with you!

To notify us of your new address, find your **Clinics Account Number** (located on your mailing label above your name), and contact customer service at:

Email: journalscustomerservice-usa@elsevier.com

800-654-2452 (subscribers in the U.S. & Canada)
314-447-8871 (subscribers outside of the U.S. & Canada)

Fax number: 314-447-8029

Elsevier Health Sciences Division
Subscription Customer Service
3251 Riverport Lane
Maryland Heights, MO 63043

*To ensure uninterrupted delivery of your subscription, please notify us at least 4 weeks in advance of move.

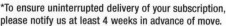

Printed and bound by CPI Group (UK) Ltd, Croydon, CR0 4YY

03/10/2024

01040471-0002